Radiology of the Foot

Radiology of the Foot

STEPHEN D. WEISSMAN, D.P.M.

*Associate Professor of Podiatric Medicine
and Orthopaedics
Pennsylvania College of Podiatric Medicine
Philadelphia, Pennsylvania*

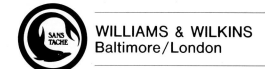

WILLIAMS & WILKINS
Baltimore/London

Copyright ©, 1983
Williams & Wilkins
428 East Preston Street
Baltimore, MD 21202, U.S.A.

Made in the United States of America

Library of Congress Cataloging in Publication Data

Weissman, Stephen D.
  Radiology of the foot.
  Includes index.
  1. Foot—Radiography. 2. Foot—Diseases—Diagnosis. I. Title. [DNLM: 1. Foot—
Radiography. 2. Foot diseases—Diagnosis. WE 880 R129]
RC951.W45 1983   617'.585'07572   82-23806
ISBN 0-683-08927-7

Composed and printed at the
Waverly Press, Inc.
Mt. Royal and Guilford Aves.
Baltimore, MD 21202, U.S.A.

To Lee and Frank

Preface

After seven years of teaching podiatric radiology, one fact became very obvious: there was a desperate need for *a single textbook that includes all of the material covered in current podiatric radiology courses.*

I have found myself referring students to portions of many different texts, none of which were intended to be used specifically for the lower extremity.

At our College, in the past few years, we have spent a great deal of time making videotapes and other teaching aides, each of which made a small contribution and none of which accomplished anything major.

It is with this background that I undertook to compile this textbook. It is written with the podiatry student in mind, but certainly not to the exclusion of the practitioners of radiology of the foot. My intent was to cover the clinical subject as completely as possible without making the cost of the book prohibitive.

Radiology is a subject that lends itself well to photographs. Therefore, I have included over 500 photographs, most of which are of the foot and ankle. We have included some of the newer x-ray techniques such as bone scans, CAT scans, and ultrasonography, and their uses as applied to the lower extremity.

Since practitioners must be able to recognize and distinguish between the normal and abnormal, Chapters 3 ("Normal Foot And Ankle") and 5 ("Radiology of the Foot in Pediatrics") begin with a thorough coverage of the normal radiograph.

Once the practitioner recognizes that an abnormality is present, he must determine with which category of problem he is dealing: mechanical, local, neoplastic, or systemic. The chapters are thus arranged to facilitate this process.

Contributors

Stephen D. Weissman, D.P.M.
Associate Professor of Podiatric Medicine
  and Orthopaedics
Pennsylvania College of Podiatric Medicine
Philadelphia, Pennsylvania

Irving H. Block, D.P.M.
Miami Beach, Florida

Vincent J. Hetherington, D.P.M., M.S.
Assistant Professor of Podiatric Medicine and Sur-
  gery
University of Osteopathic Medicine and Health
  Sciences
Des Moines, Iowa

Richard M. Jay, D.P.M.
Assistant Professor of Podiatric Orthopaedics
Pennsylvania College of Podiatric Medicine
Philadelphia, Pennsylvania

Robert Van Derslice, M.D.
Assistant Professor of Radiology
Medical College of Pennsylvania
Philadelphia, Pennsylvania

Louis P. Zulli, D.P.M.
Professor of Podiatric Medicine
Pennsylvania College of Podiatric Medicine
Philadelphia, Pennsylvania

Contents

Preface vii

Contributors ix

CHAPTER 1   Historical Overview and Public Health Concerns   1
IRVING H. BLOCK, D.P.M.

CHAPTER 2   X-ray Techniques   13

CHAPTER 3   Normal Foot and Ankle   38

CHAPTER 4   Biomechanically Acquired Foot Types   50

CHAPTER 5   Radiology of the Foot in Pediatrics   77
RICHARD JAY, D.P.M.

CHAPTER 6   Metatarsal and Digital Deformities   102

CHAPTER 7   Physiologically and Pathologically Induced X-ray Changes   132

CHAPTER 8   Osteochondritis   165

CHAPTER 9   Infections of Bone and Neurotrophic Foot   179

CHAPTER 10   Joint Disease and Arthritis   202

CHAPTER 11   Trauma   231

CHAPTER 12   Tumors of the Foot   278
LOUIS P. ZULLI, D.P.M.

CHAPTER 13   Systemically Induced Changes in Skeletal Structure   320
ROBERT VAN DERSLICE, M.D.

CHAPTER 14   Special Studies: Bone Scans and Computerized Axial Tomography   442
VINCENT J. HETHERINGTON, D.P.M., M.S.

Index   457

CHAPTER 1

Historical Overview and Public Health Concerns

IRVING H. BLOCK, D.P.M.

Wilhelm leaned forward. Carefully, deliberately, he placed one of his hands over a bit of luminescent cardboard which was lying in front of him. With the other hand he adjusted the angle of the Crooke's tube that was being stimulated from the sparks of the induction coil. The tube's rays, passing through his living hand, projected a silhouette of his bones upon the cardboard.[1]

Wilhelm Konrad Roentgen, a 50-year-old scientist who had never received a high school diploma, was for the very first time seeing through man's living flesh! The date was November 8, 1895, and for the next 7 weeks Roentgen "investigated the properties of these unknown rays so thoroughly that almost nothing new has been discovered and not one of Roentgen's observations have ever been proven wrong in the nearly eighty-six years since." Although Roentgen continued to be interested in the field for many years, he wrote and published only three papers on x-ray before concentrating his work in other areas of physics.

Ultimately, all of Wilhelm Roentgen's work earned for him a great deal of acclaim, including the first Nobel Prize in Physics (1901). His ingressive work in the field of x-ray, however, also gave to the peoples of the world a double-edged sword.

During the following decades man has become painfully aware of the dangers of x-ray.[1] The fluoroscopy box, a common object in the American shoe store during the first 30 years of the twentieth century, was used as an aide in the fitting of shoes. Adults and children alike would mount a platform and peer through a goggle-like device at the skeletal outline of their own feet as they lay in shoes which were being considered for purchase. The longer the foot remained inserted

in the machine, the greater was the emission of radiation. By the late 1930s, however, cumulative research findings began to point to the dangers inherent in this device that the public had unwittingly been abusing. After much debate and lobbying, several state health departments began removing the units from general use.

During this time, dentists whose fingers were frequently exposed to the primary beam of their machines as they held film in place and physicians who were setting fractures under the fluoroscope were learning first-hand of the tissue-destroying properties of the rays.[1]

As the health care professions became more aware of both the positive and negative potential of the x-ray, a great deal of effort was put forth to further the acquisition of knowledge about the subject. Indeed, "there has been more investigation into the mechanisms, nature and prevention of radiation injury than has been the case with most toxic agents.[1] A continuing dialogue among practitioners using medical diagnostic and therapeutic protective devices and systems has developed at the various levels in government, industry, and the professions. Podiatry has supported every aspect of this public health concern.

About a decade after the end of World War II, a small number of interested podiatrists organized themselves into a group which has come to be known as the American College of Podiatric Radiologists. It is a recognized speciality group within the American Podiatry Association whose members write textbooks on the subject of foot roentgenology, develop specialized devices to improve safety and functioning of x-ray machines, publish the *Journal of Podiatric Roentgenology*, and also produce audiovisual exhibits, regular roentgenology symposia, and maintain an up-to-date library. This is the largest library of its kind in the profession.

The American College of Podiatric Radiologists has observed that the goal of podiatric medicine in the field of radiology is "to encourage and develop interest (within the podiatry profession) in radiology, radiologic interpretation, diagnosis and research ... the preparation, study, and interpretation of radiographs for diagnostic purposes ... to improve the practice, elevate the standards and advance scientific proficiency in the field of radiology and thereby serve the cause of public health ..." through the promotion of radiation safety.[2]

In 1948, the Public Health Service received a budget of $17,000 as an appropriation in the area of radiological health. In 1958, a full division of Radiological Health was established within the Department of Health, Education and Welfare. After that time, the Surgeon General of the United States created the National Advisory Committee on Radiation to help control radiation hazards. In 1961, the outlays for this group surpassed $6,500,000 and within a few years approached $50,000,000.

Why had radiological health been receiving so much worldwide attention during the latter half of the twentieth century? The devastation of Nagasaki and Hiroshima that left an indelible mark on humanity and the peacetime progress of nuclear engineering with its potential dangers are but two reasons. As nuclear developments became more competitive with standard methods of energy production, a whole set of controls were promulgated.

In this chapter, we deal chiefly with low-level ionizing radiation produced by x-ray machines. The medical x-ray unit contributes the greatest amount of man-made radiation to the population of the United States. It is therefore important to find methods of reducing such exposure without sacrificing the great benefits of x-ray diagnosis or therapy. This aspect of public health requires continuing attention and quality control.

To this end, the National Council of Radiation Protection has identified areas of radiation concern and produced many documents relating to radiation standards for the public. The American Podiatry Association has collaborators on this council.

Since undergraduate schools of podiatric medicine teach radiology and the basic protection and safety methods, the American Podiatry Association has resolved that graduate level training should provide in-depth investigation of these matters on a continuing education basis. Several important seminars in various sections of the country have underscored the podiatrist's concern in this matter.

The need to achieve significant reduction in somatic and genetic changes for both present and future generations makes the concerns dealt with in this chapter a necessity for the health and welfare of the public. Therefore, in order to enable the student of podiatric medicine to better handle the multifaceted responsibilities concomitant with the use of x-ray, this chapter will investigate in-depth the following aspects of the effects of radiation on living tissue: types of energy transfer; types of ionizing radiation; radiation safety and exposure control; mutations; radiation sickness; and laws and documents.

RADIATION SAFETY AND THE EFFECTS OF RADIATION ON LIVING TISSUE

Mutation—sudden, permanent variation with offspring differing from parents in a marked characteristic as differentiated from gradual variation through many generations; a change in a gene potentially capable of being transmitted to offspring. Induced mutation—resulting from experiment or accident with x-ray, radioactive substances, etc.; not occurring in nature as an evolutionary change.[3]

Traditionally, health care professionals have striven to understand the biological effects produced by x-ray, not because of the esoteric nature of the study, but because of the potential harm inherent within the use of ionizing radiation. Thus, the scientific community has developed highly regulated restrictions concerning the use of x-ray, the performance of regulated machinery and devices, and the protection of individuals from unnecessary exposure.

At the outset of an investigation into these biological effects, it is of the utmost importance that two basic concepts be accepted and understood. First, radiation damage may be cumulative. Whereas much of the tissue damage which occurs in the human body can be repaired over a period of time by newly produced cells, some portion may not be repaired. Consequently, repeated doses of radiation will cause the damage to increase arithmetically according to the amount of radiation received. "The total amount of damage accumulated [will then be] greater than that from any individual dose."[4]

Hand-in-hand with this concept of the cumulative nature of radiation damage goes the dictum that radiation, regardless of quantity, may produce some degree of injury. Since the risk of injury is reduced in direct proportion to the reduction of the radiation dose, the responsibility of the podiatric radiologist becomes obvious. It is reassuring to know that in many instances of low-level diagnostic x-ray procedure, with proper safeguards, "the risk of harm can be so low as to be difficult to measure."[4]

Based on the above concept, researchers have promulgated a theory which maintains that *any* dose of radiation, no matter how small, can be considered harmful. Focusing on what is referred to as a non-threshold dose-response relationship, this theory advances the posture that there is no point on a continuum recording positive radiation emission which can be representative of a "safe," injury-free dose.

As a result of this, the podiatric radiologist must be aware of three factors that apply to the manner in which x-ray can affect human tissue. The first factor, dose rate, is the measurement by which one determines the amount of radiation which is being delivered within a given unit of time. This factor is of minimal concern to the podiatrist in diagnostic x-rays because it applies primarily to x-ray therapy.

The second factor concerns the amount of the body which is exposed to x-ray. Because the quantity of potential cell damage is in direct proportion to the area of the body which is exposed (keeping in mind the non-threshold dose-response relationship), the podiatric radiologist has as one of his/her greatest responsibilities the *effective shielding of non-essential tissue* from the x-ray beam. It is this very shielding which enables the benefits of diagnostic and therapeutic x-ray to outweigh its potential harm. Depending upon the part of the body being x-rayed and the angle of the tube head, partial-body or gonadal shielding may be appropriate.

Effective shielding of tissue outside the perimeter of the zone to be radiated would become an extremely difficult process were it not for the fact that the podiatric radiologist must take extreme care to decrease exposure to the area of concern by achieving good *collimation* of the x-ray beam prior to x-radiation. Obviously, any beam which overlaps the film is both wasted and hazardous to radio-sensitive organs (such as the reproductive organs) which need not be exposed during diagnostic examination by a podiatrist. Various techniques have been employed to achieve this end, among them the use of the Block washer,[5] a flat,

Table 1.1
Relative Sensitivity of Various Cells to Radiation[a]

Highest sensitivity
Immature blood cells
Immature sperm and egg cells
Intermediate sensitivity
Epithelial cells
Lowest sensitivity
Muscle cells
Nerve cells

[a] Based upon this general rule, the various types of cells in the body can be ranked according to how sensitive they are to radiation damage. Of highest sensitivity are immature white blood cells, particularly the lymphocytes, immature red blood cells, and immature sperm and egg cells. Of intermediate sensitivity are epithelial cells, particularly those which form the lining of the gastrointestinal tract. At the bottom of our sensitivity list, that is, among the most resistant cells in the body, are muscle and nerve cells. Note that the exception to this is the developing nervous system of the embryo or fetus, which is more radiosensitive than in the adult.

leaded disc with a small hole in the center, which is inserted behind a fixed cone of the x-ray unit.

The third factor of which the radiographer must be aware is the varying degrees of sensitivity of different cells in the body (Table 1.1). As a rule, it has been noted that those cells which are young, rapidly dividing, and not highly specialized in their function will be the most radiosensitive. Conversely, the least radiosensitive cells will be those which are highly specialized and do not reproduce themselves. Table 1.1 not only affords a visualization of the relative degrees of sensitivity of various cells, but will also reinforce an awareness of the need to carefully shield organs of the body from the x-ray beam.

As one progresses through current x-ray literature, one will often notice that the words *rad*, *roentgen*, and *rem* are used as roughly equivalent terms when soft tissue absorption is being discussed. In actuality, the biologically *absorbed* dose is a "rem" while the amount of x- (or gamma) ray *emitted* into the air is labeled a "roentgen" (abbreviated R).

Since the podiatrist is often involved in diagnostic rather then therapeutic radiology, it is extremely important that he/she be aware of the real and present danger which exists when small amounts of radiation are absorbed by the body over a long period of time. This is a situation which can occur for the individual living in an industrially and scientifically advanced society when cumulative doses of diagnostic radiation build up in the body. It is with this above-mentioned possible long-term effect, rather than the long-term effect produced by large amounts of radiation over a short period—or short-term effect produced by large amounts of radiation (usually over 100 rads) over a short period—that the practitioner must be concerned.

Although the podiatrist usually does not become involved in the administration of large amounts of x-ray, it is necessary at this point to give a brief overview of the effects of whole-body doses of radiation that occur through nuclear accident or malfunction of the x-ray unit. These effects, known as the acute radiation syndrome, may begin within hours—or as long as several weeks—after exposure. The individual may experience any or all of the following: nausea, vomiting, severe diarrhea, fluid loss, severe infection, widespread hemorrhage, and loss of hair. The resistance and general condition of the individual receiving the radiation—and, of course, the type of radiation and the amount received—will determine if there is gradual recovery from the acute radiation syndrome or eventual death.

Current research shows a relationship between the processes by which cancer cells multiply, genetic mutations occur, and the aging process proceeds. Although the precise mechanisms employed by these interrelated functions have not yet been fully investigated or understood, certain common grounds for their development have been observed.

One such observation concerns the formation of "free radicals," "short-lived but potent damaging agents"[6] that are formed when water molecules (which exist in abundance in living cells) receive radiation. Evidence indicates that the formation of these free radicals, which are a "byproduct of certain normal biochemical reactions in living cells," is accelerated by irradiation. Hence the link between the aging of cell tissue and carcinogenic growth which may be stimulated by x-radiation.[6]

LONG-TERM RADIATION EFFECTS

Investigation into the biological effects of x-ray may, at this point, focus on the two categories into which long-term radiation effects fall: *genetic* and *somatic.* The first category of change, genetic, does *not* manifest itself in life-threatening situations which are observable to the present generation. When sperm or egg cells (or their precursors) are radiated, the genetic material carried inside the cell can be altered. Although the possibility of such a genetic change or mutation increases as

the level of absorbed radiation increases, it is important to remember that genetic change occurs as a non-threshold dose-response situation. Therefore, any genetic damage which exists— regardless of how low its level—can be incorporated into a fertilized egg which will reproduce itself and its mutant billions of times as the life process progresses. This "damaged genetic information" will eventually become part of the egg or sperm cells of the next generation and will be passed on indefinitely since there can be no spontaneous recovery from genetic damage.[6]

Genetic mutation or damage may have a number of different results, all of which are harmful to the host organism. In extreme cases, the mutation may actually cause the death of the organism before birth. In other non-lethal situations, the mutation may produce physical defects which are observable. It is the last situation, however, which causes the greatest concern in the area of public health. It involves those mutations which are so subtle as to be difficult to observe but which "result in an increased susceptibility to certain chronic diseases or biochemical abnormalities." The long-range implications of these somewhat harmful and very common mutations cause the greatest concern".[6]

As was mentioned earlier in this chapter, individuals living in industrially and scientifically advanced societies are constantly being exposed to ever-increasing quantities and types of agents (radiation among them) within their environment that can cause low-level genetic mutations which will then threaten the overall level of health of future generations. The challenge and responsibility that this situation poses to health care professionals who work with x-ray is, therefore, enormous. To reiterate points made earlier, the primary x-ray beam must be effectively collimated, scatter radiation must be *greatly reduced or eliminated*, and scrupulous use of shielding must be employed.

The second category of change, referred to as "somatic" change, occurs when cells other than sperm or egg are exposed to radiation. Any damage that is done in somatic cells will exist only *within* the cells of the individual who has been radiated. It is important to note that somatic changes cannot be passed down to future generations.

Currently, the somatic effects which manifest themselves in living tissue have been divided into four areas: those which increase the incidence of cancer; those which have an effect on the developing embryo or fetus *during* pregnancy (as opposed to the genetic mutations discussed previously); those tending to induce cataract formation in the eye; and, finally, those which are considered to be life-span shortening.

Controlled experiments have induced the growth of many kinds of tumors in laboratory animals, as well as in human beings. Since cells in different areas of the body exhibit varying degrees of sensitivity to radiation, and since the amount of exposure can be controlled by adjusting the dose rate, scientists have been able to "implicate ionizing radiation as a causative agent in leukemia, as well as cancers of the skin, bone, lung, thyroid, and breast."[6]

Because there is a lengthy latency period (perhaps 20 years or more) before the carcinogenic effects of radiation become manifest, a great deal of damage had unknowingly been done during that period when radiology was in its infancy. Among those groups who have suffered these ill effects are those who—as infants during the 1940s and 1950s—received x-radiation for a variety of benign conditions such as enlarged thymus glands, adenoids, or sinuses, and even acne.

According to studies done on the above cases, therapy doses were generally in the *hundreds* of rads. Why, then, need there be concern over modern-day diagnostic doses that are in the millirad (thousandth-rad) range? Concern must exist because the non-threshold dose-response relationship points to the danger of possible somatic change to the unborn fetus. Studies have confirmed an increased risk of carcinogenic development (including leukemia) "in children whose mothers received diagnostic x-rays to the abdominal or pelvic areas during pregnancy."[6]

But even a small risk in the increase of cancer gives these studies special importance for those ... who work in the medical x-ray field, because it underscores the importance of protecting pregnant women against needless x-ray exposure.[6]

Fortunately, for those who work in the area of podiatry, a carefully controlled diagnostic extremity examination should produce no *scatter* radiation and should not expose the embryo or fetus to the primary x-ray beam.

The third area of possible somatic change resulting from ionizing radiation is cataract formation. Normally, when body cells die, they are sloughed off and carried away. This is not true of cells on the lens of the eye that are destroyed by direct radiation. These cells will remain and, if they accumulate in sufficient number, will pro-

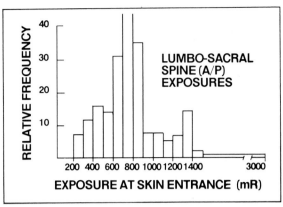

Figure 1.1. An ongoing study by the FDA's Bureau of Radiological Health and a number of state radiation control agencies gives some interesting answers to this question. The study is called NEXT, or Nationwide Evaluation of X-ray Trends, and it involves continuing surveys of x-ray facilities across the United States. It shows a very wide variation in radiation exposure produced in different medical offices and hospitals performing the same procedure on a standard-size patient. This illustration shows the tremendous variation in exposure for lumbosacral spine examinations. Notice that the patient's skin exposure per film might be anywhere from 200 to 3000 milliroentgens, depending on where the examination was performed.[6]

duce vision-blocking opacities. Fortunately, it takes a relatively high dose of direct radiation to the eye to cause this problem.

The final area of somatic change is life span shortening. Statistical evidence points to the fact that "irradiated animals tend to succumb sooner than non-irradiated ones to the same diseases and conditions from which they normally die."[6]* This very real hazard is controlled, however, by stringent government regulations and careful implementation of the safeguards which were discussed earlier in this chapter.

Figure 1.1 depicts a very interesting survey of a study called NEXT which will probably provide the basis for much future discussion in the field of radiology.

RADIATION SAFETY AND EXPOSURE CONTROL

Ultimately, what motivates the health care professional to better safeguard public health is a combination of effective prior scientific input and individual moral values.[7]

---

* "No life-span shortening has been observed in medical x-ray personnel working at today's levels of permissible occupational exposure."[6]

Table 1.2
Radiant Energy Spectrum Diagram with Approximate Wavelengths[a]

Forms	Ångström Units	Type of X-ray Radiation	Approximate kV at X-ray Tube
Cosmic rays	0.00001		
	0.001		
	0.01	Supervoltage therapy	1,000
	0.03		
	0.14	Deep therapy	200
	0.3	Superficial therapy	65–100
Gamma and x-rays	0.6		
	0.8	Contact therapy	50
	1.6	Grenz ray therapy	10
	2.06		
	15.0		
Ultraviolet	3,900		
	7,600		
Visible light	40,000		
Infrared Radio rays	3 meters		

[a] Note: X-rays for medical radiography have a useful wavelength of approximately 0.1 to 0.5 (1/10 to ½) Ångström units.

The podiatrist radiographer must be motivated to take only those x-rays that are necesary to make an effective diagnosis; and to combine good technique and sound judgment when doing so in order to reduce unnecessary exposure. Of course, graduate level continuing education courses and seminars—as well as continuous professional reading—will improve diagnostic acumen. But first it is necessary to be able to structure a sound x-ray environment in the podiatric workplace.

In order to do so, one must make use of a basic knowledge of physics. This includes an understanding of the types of energy transfer, the types of ionizing radiation, the proper exposure for diagnostic podiatric radiology, the geometry of image formation, and the factors effecting the image itself.

X-rays resemble visible light rays; however, unlike light waves, their wave lengths are very short: about 1/10,000 the wave length of visible light. X-rays, therefore, have the characteristic of being able to penetrate materials which would reflect light. The spectrum of radiant energy (Table 1.2) shows the position of x-rays as compared to cosmic rays, infrared rays, and radio waves. These wavelengths are measured in Ångström units when one Å (Ångström unit) is defined as 10^{-8} cm or 1/100,000,000 cm. Medical radiography is approximately 0.50 Ångström units.[8]

Radiolucency refers to matter which is penetrated by x-rays with relative ease; whereas radiopacity describes matter which absorbs x-ray in great measure. It was the discovery of these related facts which gave birth to the science of radiography.[8] It is the difference in opacity of gasses, fatty tissue, muscle, cartilage, connective tissue, bone, and heavy metals when reproduced on photosensitive film which makes possible the x-ray image range in the study of differentiating anatomy.

The production of x-rays depends upon the presence of highly energetic electrons that strike a target with great velocity. It is evident that in this process most of the electron energy is converted to heat, while only a small percentage (less than 1%) is converted to x-ray. After the x-rays are emitted from the x-ray tube's portal opening, they are directed toward the receptor or x-ray film. When the x-rays are emitted through the opening, window, or port, they are known as the primary beam. The central ray is at the geometric center of this primary beam. Productive, or hard, x-rays have a shorter wavelength and are therefore more penetrating; whereas non-productive, or soft, rays that have a longer wavelength do not penetrate deeper areas of bone. They only add to unnecessary radiation absorption at skin level.

It is important to become familiar with the following terms: matter, atom, and ionization. *Matter* is anything which occupies space and has mass. All matter is made up of a combination of atoms (two or more of which form a molecule). An *atom* is the smallest particle of any chemical element which cannot be further subdivided into smaller units by chemical or other means without losing its fundamental identifying characteristic. Protons, neutrons, and electrons are grouped together to form these units or atoms. All atoms are electrically neutral. *Ionization* refers to the adding or subtracting of orbital electrons. Ionization is an important principle in the production and control of x-rays and in the vital area of radiation safety because x-rays knock electrons off atoms when matter is struck. The atom, when left with a net positive charge, is thus ionized.

All radiation possesses energy either inherently, as in the case of electromagnetic radiation, or as kinetic energy or motion, as in the case of the particulate radiations. Absorption of radiation is the process by which this energy is being transferred to the atoms of the medium through which the radiation is passing. To say that *radiation interracts with* matter is to say that it is either absorbed or scattered.[9]

Transfer of energy may occur through ionization or through excitation, which is the addition of energy to an atomic or molecular system.

Theoretically, there are twelve processes by which x-rays interact with matter. The three most important ones are the photoelectric effect, the Compton effect, and pair production (Table 1.3). The attenuation of x-rays is dependent upon the absorber material and the x-ray energy.[9]

The angle at which the x-rays are emitted from the focal spot on the tube has an effect on their intensity. This is known as the *heel effect.* Since the cathode side of the x-ray tube emits a more intense ray, a better balanced radiograph can be obtained when the cathode side is placed over the heaviest body part being rayed. (This effect has only minimal application to podiatric radiology.)

STRUCTURED X-RAY ENVIRONMENT IN THE PODIATRIC WORKPLACE

When implemented, the following methods and techniques will help reduce radiation exposure to both the patient and office personnel.[10]

Professional Judgment

Professional judgment exercised by the podiatrist is a very important aspect in the limiting of unnecessary radiation exposure. Careful consideration of the podiatric and general health needs of the individual patient should determine the extent of the radiographic examination. Such examination should never be an automatic or routine procedure.

Collimation

The adaptation of adequate collimation has been determined to be one of the most effective methods for the reduction of radiation. This method of beam restriction not only prevents unnecessary radiation from reaching areas above the foot or leg, but also reduces backscatter radiation which contributes to the patient dose and results in a fogged film.

The collimators that have been used to restrict the beam in stationary cones work quite well in dental-converted x-ray units and low amperage general-purpose machines. The beam limitation can be adjusted by changing the diameter of the

**Table 1.3
Characteristics of the Three Most Important X-ray Interactions with Matter**

Process	Type of Transfer	X-ray Energy Level	Atomic Number Absorber Material[a]
Photoelectric effect	Complete	Low	High
Compton effect	Partial	Intermediate	Low
Pair production	Complete[b]	High	High

[a] The attenuation of x-rays is dependent upon the absorber.
[b] With production of annihilation photons.

aperature of the cone. It is possible to purchase a collimator that has adjustable plates which will change the circular or rectangular aperature beam size. The more modern variable collimating units will allow the aperature to respond automatically to the size of the film being exposed after the area of interest is set on the control. This unit is usually available with an indicator that will show by a light beam reflected on the part (foot or leg) exactly where the primary beam will be entering the object that is superimposed on the film. Such an indicator is required in most states.

Filtration

By placing an aluminum filter in the beam, most of the long (soft) radiation which is of the low energy range and has no useful effect for diagnostic radiology is not allowed to pass through the skin. However, the shorter wavelengths which are of higher energy range are allowed to pass through the filter in order to reach the patient and the film. Thus, the radiation dose of the patient is lowered and film fog is reduced. Most states require filtration of 1.5 mm for equipment operating below 70 kVp and 2.5 mm of aluminum filtration for equipment operating at or above 70 kVp.

Kilovoltage

Since the photon's ability to penetrate is increased with higher kilovoltage (thus allowing a greater number of x-rays to reach the film), one can expect a decrease in the exposure time. This will reduce the absorbed dosage to the patient and body part being radiographed. Also, a difference in contrast of the radiograph will be obtained. This may be a desired technique when visualizing soft tissue in which a reduction of kVp is predetermined.

Film Speed

High speed or fast film (a combination of various screen films and intensifying cassettes) will account for tremendous reduction in patient exposure. The reduced exposure time also eliminates the need for frequent retakes caused by patient movement. This is particularly helpful when children are being radiographed.

Exposure Time

Reduced exposure time will definitely enable the radiographer to deliver less radiation to the film. Mechanical timers—found on most older units—can be set at a fair range of time increments, usually to within one-eighth of a second. Electronic timers can further reduce exposure to 1/25 of a second when necessary. It should be noted that mechanical or spring-wound timers usually lack the ability to reproduce the time increments with any reliability.

Milliamperage

The quantity of radiation is proportional to the milliamperage. Reduction of mA will reduce the amount of radiation reaching the film. It will also reduce the heat generated in the tube element so that one may expect longer tube life.

Darkroom Processing Technique

Good quality diagnostic radiographs depend upon the techniques employed in the darkroom. Adequate film development will not only make a quality film available, but will allow for the reduction of radiation exposure to all concerned.

The best method of film development is the use of automatic processors. The essentials of time and temperature are constantly maintained. When manual methods are employed, the film manufacturer's time/temperature chart should be followed using a thermometer and a timer. These methods are far superior to sight development. The tendency to overexpose when taking the x-ray and to underdevelop as a means of compensation only causes needless exposure to the patient.

The darkroom must be so constructed that there is no leakage of outside light. The use of proper safety lights will then prevent unnecessary fogging of the film. The Wratten 6B filter with a 7½ watt bulb will usually work well with screen film. There are also other good safety lights available. It is important that there are no areas around the mechanism that emit unfiltered light. The distance of the safety light from the film is impor-

tant; if fogging occurs, a greater distance or a smaller bulb may be indicated.

Screens

An intensifying screen consists of a thin layer of calcium tungstate crystals which emit a bluish light when exposed to radiation. The faster the screen, the more solidly packed are the layers of crystals. In order to prevent a loss of diagnostic detail in the finished radiograph, a medium-par screen may be the choice for podiatric use since it offers little or no loss in readability.

Reduction of Radiation Exposure to Personnel

Judicious implementation of those factors which create a structured office environment will reduce radiation exposure to office personnel. Protective barriers should be made of materials appropriate for the stoppage of x-rays, and unit controls should be placed outside the radiographic room whenever possible. If the latter cannot be done, the operator should be at least 6 feet from the tube and primary beam. The use of leaded aprons and film holders (such as Monee) are essential when leg and knee exposures are taken. An Ortho-X-Poser will reduce scatter to both patient and personnel. Also, a variety of personnel monitoring devices and services are available in most communities which will estimate and identify exposure received by both the operator and the other office personnel.

Direction of Beam

The beam should never be directed to any area where other office personnel would receive exposure. Structural barriers should be evaluated for x-ray protection effectiveness if the primary beam is in any way pointed in the direction of an occupied room. No one but the radiographer and patient should be in or close to the x-ray room.

X-raying Children

Small children should be held by a parent, not by office personnel. Adequate shielding, aprons, and lead-lined gloves should be used, particularly if an adult is in the direct path of the primary beam. Fast film and intensifying cassettes must also be employed.

Radiographic Techniques

The following guidelines will not only increase the quality of the finished radiograph, but will ultimately reduce unnecessary radiation in the workplace by reducing the number of retakes.

SCATTER RADIATION

This radiation decreases contrast by adding exposure to the film. Gradations on the film are lost and the soft tissue is less apt to be recognized when infection, infusion, and other details are present. Proper collimation will decrease photon output for scatter or bounce-off.

OBJECT-FILM DISTANCE

The greater the distance from the object to the film, the greater the magnification and distortion (Fig. 1.2).[11]

FILM POSITION

The film should be parallel to the long axis of the object being radiographed in both the horizontal and vertical plane. This will limit the distortion that might otherwise occur (Fig. 1.3).[11]

TARGET-FILM DISTANCE

As one increases the target-to-film distance, the x-ray beam becomes less divergent, resulting in a sharper image and less distortion. In podiatry, the best distance should range from 24–30 inches.

The following three physical factors can be adjusted by the radiographer to suit the specific need and technique being employed during exposure.

1. *Distance:* The target-to-film distance is a factor which can be altered to fit the technique. The intensity of radiation is inversely proportional to the square of the distance. This is known as the "inverse square" law. As one doubles the distance from the source to the object, the intensity is reduced to one-fourth. Similarly, the intensity is increased four times when the distance from the source to the object is halved (Fig. 1.4).[11]

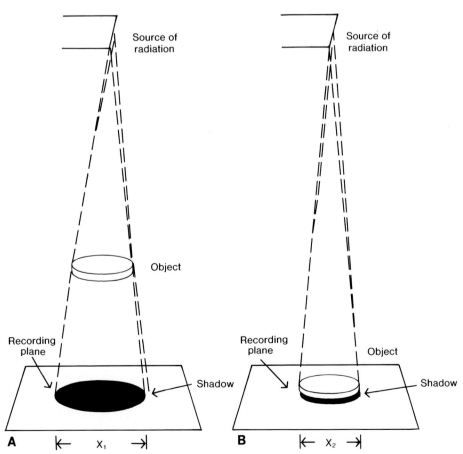

Magnification resulting from increased object film distance

Figure 1.2. Diagrams showing geometrical effects on image sharpness. *A,* improvement in sharpness produced by a small focal spot. *B,* superior result of a small focal spot and minimal distance between the object and recording plane. Notice also the enlargement (X_1) caused by the distance of the object from recording plane as compared to the more accurate size (X_2) produced when the object is close to the plane. (From *X-Rays In Dentistry*, Radiography Markets Division, Eastman Kodak Company, with permission.)

Distortion of image as a result of
improper film position

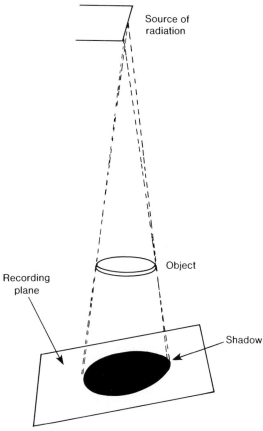

Figure 1.3. Distortion results when the object and the recording plane are not parallel. (From *X-Rays In Dentistry*, Radiography Markets Division, Eastman Kodak Company, with permission.)

2. *Milliamperage times Time*: The quantity of radiation is directly proportional to the milliamperage and the time. Therefore, the milliamperage times time (seconds) is proportional to the quantity of radiation. It is then possible to vary the milliamperage and time with each other and still maintain the original mas of quantity; for example, 15 mA × 1 second = 15 mas; 30 ma × 0.5 seconds = 15 mas.

3. *Kilovoltage*: The penetrating ability of x-rays is increased when the kVp is increased, thus enabling more x-rays to reach the film. Overall intensity is also increased. This in turn decreases the reader's ability to visualize contrast. When contrast is to be increased, the kVp will have to be reduced so that a wider variation of material absorption will take place.

In summary, there are a number of things the podiatrist can do to limit unnecessary radiation exposure to himself, his office personnel, and his patients:

1. Use professional judgment
2. Collimate the x-ray beam
3. Provide adequate filtration
4. Utilize the correct kilovoltage
5. Utilize lead aprons
6. Use high speed film
7. Use high speed screens
8. Utilize adequate time/temperature method of development
9. Use fresh processing solutions
10. Maintain adequate darkroom
11. Maintain adequate operator position
12. Evaluate direction of beam
13. Use film holders
14. Use personnel monitoring devices[11]

LAWS AND RADIATION CONTROL

"At present, radiation health and safety is a particularly complex and varied field, including a large number of ... departments, commissions, and agencies. The public rightfully expects an orchestrated ... approach to ... [radiation] hazards."[12]

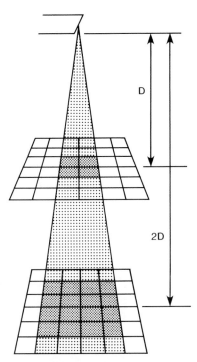

Radiation intensity decreases as
the distance increases

Figure 1.4. Diagram showing how the intensity of an x-ray beam is altered by changing the focus-film distance (the "inverse square" law). (From *X-Rays In Dentistry*, Radiography Markets Division, Eastman Kodak Company, with permission.)

For the past several decades, there has been little argument against the need for judicious regulation of both ionizing radiation equipment and the actions of those that use it. About the year 1958, radiological health activities escalated with the creation of the United States Public Health Service. At about the same time, there was established within the Office of the Surgeon General the National Advisory Committee on Radiation a group of consultants dealing with questions of policy related to the *control of radiation hazards.*

The foundation for all of these modern developments had actually been laid in the late 1920s by the National Committee on Radiation Protection which was established for the purpose of making recommendations concerning safe operating practices in the field of radiology. One of the first recommendations by this committee has become known as the maximum permissible dose (MPD) or weekly dose, that amount which individuals working with ionizing radiation may be expected to receive without developing serious biological damage. It is interesting to note that this value has been reduced repeatedly over the years to its present recommended level of less than 0.1 roentgen per week.[12]

The setting of any standard without a threshold makes it impossible to decide "how safe is safe enough." Radiobiological research, therefore, puts its highest priority on the interrelationship between dose, dose rate, and latency period. There is increased probability that, with sufficient dose reduction, the latent period will exceed the lifespan. This is known as the "practical threshold," a term first proposed by Evans as a result of his studies of osteogenic sarcoma among radiation workers.

When dealing with and attempting to understand *any* method of ascertaining standards, one should be aware that such determinations are judgments which must be based on opinions of knowledgeable people in the field. It is these very opinions, directed through appropriate regulatory agencies, which ultimately formulate government policy.

During the past decade, many laws and rules have been passed on both federal and state levels. The Federal Performance Standards Act (Public Law No. 90-602), for example, was the first major act that applied to diagnostic x-ray equipment manufactured after August 1, 1974. It set a requirement that the beam diameter not be more than one inch beyond the border of the x-ray plate, at a minimum target-to-skin distance. Manufacturers were prevented from replacing x-ray

unit parts under certain conditions. Finally, the use of collimators with exact specifications and light-identifying devices were included in the standards for newer units. This did a great deal to eliminate unnecessary and unproductive ionizing radiation that was not directed to the area of concern.

The following guide should serve as an overview which will enable students and practicing podiatrists to better understand the regulatory aspects of the podiatric use of x-rays. It consists of an update of *Model Legislation* (reprinted February, 1972) for users of ionizing radiation in the healing arts; a synopsis of the Radiation Control for Health and Safety Act (Public Law No. 90-602); the standards and some of the major features that affect the podiatrist. (Specific regulations of state jurisdictions may be obtained from the various State Bureau of Radiological Health Agencies.)

Federal Register's Proposed Rules and Performance Standards Highlights

The following list contains some areas of interest to podiatry:

August 15, 1972, Vol. 37, No. 158; diagnostic x-ray systems; performance standards; regulations from the administration and enforcement of the recommended control for the Health and Safety Act of 1968.

October 15, 1973, Vol. 38, No. 198; policy and interpretation of Radiation Control Act of 1968 with definition of terminology.

November 4, 1975, Vol. 40, No. 213; requires manufacturers to provide information on the characteristics of films on screen combination devices.

July 15, 1975, Vol. 40, No. 136; suggested state regulations for control of radiation including the impact of this conference of Radiation Control Program Directors in preparation for model state regulations, registration of radiation machines, and safety requirements.

December 15, 1975, Vol. 40, No. 24; deals with criteria for medical radiation exposure for women of childbearing age.

March 12, 1976, Vol. 47, No. 50; who provides and orders diagnostic x-ray in federal health facilities?

May 7, 1976, Vol. 41, No. 90; quality assurance: responsibilities of *providers* of X-rays are addressed.

August 1976, HEW Publication (FDA) 76-8054, U.S. DHEW, subpart c, radiation protection requiring use of *gonad shielding.*

February 25, 1977, Vol. 42, No. 38; Deals with

certification of components, field size (SID).

November 8, 1977, Vol. 42, No. 215; final order on positive beam limitation; only impact for podiatry is in large facilities using higher mA and kVp units.

May 9, 1978, Vol. 43, No. 90; diagnostic x-ray systems and their components, podiatric implications, automatic x-ray field overriding, size of image receptor with 3% of SID (source-to-image) receptor, beam-limiting device ..." image receptor means any device, such as a fluorescent screen or *radiographic film,* which transforms incident x-ray photons either into a visible image or into another form...."

July 14, 1978, Vol. 43, No. 136; diagnostic x-ray systems and components. Highlights leakage factors, housing, combination of beam-limiting devices, spot filming, special cassette holders, and step-down collimation for fluoroscopy.

REFERENCES

1. BLOCK, I. H.: Podiatric involvement in radiologic health care. J.A.P.A., **67:** 7, 1977.

2. *Constitution of the ACPR,* 1974 revised edition, p. 8.

3. *Taber's Cyclopedic Medical Dictionary,* 12th Ed, p 74, FA Davis, Philadelphia, 1973.

4. Radiation Protection During X-Ray Examinations, Part 4: Biological Effects of X-rays. U.S. Department of Health, Education, and Welfare Bureau of Radiological Health, Rockville, Maryland. March, 1976.

5. BLOCK, I. H.: Collimation improvement: A means of adapting fixed cone devices for podiatric radiology. J.A.P.A., **67:** 409, 1977.

6. *State of Florida Basic X-Ray Operator Study Guide,* revised, 1980, p. 43.

7. BLOCK, I. H.: Lecture given at American Public Health Association Seminar. Detroit, 1980.

8. MESCHAN, I.: *Normal Radiographic Anatomy,* 2nd Ed, 1959, p. 3.

9. *Radiological Health Training Resource Material for Podiatrists.* Office of Training, Bureau of Radiological Health and Florida State Division of Health, December, 1967, pp. 1–22.

10. American Podiatry Association: Podiatric x-ray protection for diagnostic applications: A report prepared by the Ad Hoc Committee on Podiatric X-ray Protection. J.A.P.A. **60:** 432, 1970.

11. SILHA, R. E.: *X-rays in Dentistry,* Radiography Markets Division, Eastman Kodak, 1977.

12. MORGAN, R.: Radiation control in public health. Public Health Reports, **76:** July, 1961.

CHAPTER 2

X-ray Techniques

This chapter will cover the basic techniques utilized in Podiatric Radiology. While it in no way attempts to cover every view that is possible of the foot and ankle, it does cover the most frequently used projections, along with a discussion of x-ray film, its composition, intensifying screens, their uses, and definitions needed to understand the characteristics, and how to make a decision about these characteristics, when developing an office technique.

X-RAY FILM

X-Ray film consists of a transparent cellulose acetate or plastic base coated on each side with a photo-sensitive emulsion consisting primarily of one of the silver halides. While most films are coated on both sides, some films are only coated on one side. Changes in the layer of emulsion, which are caused by either light or x-ray emissions, will produce a visible pattern after proper chemical processing occurs. The emulsion layer consists of gelatin in which is suspended a large number of crystals of silver bromide and small amounts of the other silver halides. The crystals are distributed uniformly throughout the gelatin layer. The emulsion is designed to be most efficiently sensitized in particularly specific wavelengths so that it will be affected either by the x-ray beam directly or by certain specific intensifying screens. The size and number of crystals distributed in the emulsion determine the photographic properties of the emulsion. Variation of these parameters can be used to produce different characteristics and properties in the films. A small amount of blue dye is usually added to the base to help view the finished radiograph.

The film base, which serves to support the emulsion layers, must be constructed so as not to contract or expand in size during the chemical processing. If this occurs, distortion of the image

can occur. Usually, a final layer is coated on top of the clear gelatin to serve as a protective layer for the finished processed radiograph. This eliminates the need for extreme care in handling of the films.

Film may be classified either as screen or non-screen film, depending upon whether it is designed for use with a fluorescent screen or not.

SCREENS

When roentgen rays strike certain crystalline materials a phosphorescence occurs. The spectrum of light that is produced in this phosphorescence will vary with the crystalline substance. This fluorescence can vary from largely ultraviolet to largely visible light. The ultraviolet and the bluish light have proven to be the most advantageous with respect to x-ray screen emissions. This is primarily because of the ease in sensitizing x-ray film to emissions in these general spectra. Less than 5% of the density on a screen film radiograph is caused by the direct action of the x-rays. More than 95% of the film density is due to the light given off by the intensifying screens.

Intensifying screens consist mostly of a thin coating of the fluorescent crystals on a cardboard surface. The compound that is most commonly used today is the crystalline form of calcium tungstate. It is finely powdered and mixed with a binder and then coated in a thin, smooth layer onto the cardboard or plastic surface, which is used for support. Calcium tungstate crystals fluoresce primarily in the violet and near-violet regions of the spectrum. The base is usually colored white to reflect the emitted light optimally.

Intensifying screens are categorized with respect to brightness, speed and detail. Speed and detail seem to be the inverse of each other, thus requiring a compromise in selecting which qualities are most important. There are four classes of screens today, slow, medium, fast, and high speed. Medium speed seems to give a good balance between speed and detail, slow speed is used where sharpness and definition are of the most importance, and faster screens are used where shortness of exposure is the prime concern. It must be remembered that the size and number of calcium tungstate crystals in a screen are what determines its speed, sharpness, and definition.

The introduction of rare earth intensifying screens has made a large number of new film screen combinations available today in radiology. This of course means that there is an even wider range of system speeds available. With the various combinations available today of conventional and rare earth film/screen combinations, it is no longer necessary to expect a single film screen combination to meet all imaging needs. A number of fluorescent materials are used today for different screens, and are usually either blue-emitting or green-emitting (rare earth). The non-rare earth materials are calcium tungstate (most common), barium lead sulfate, barium strontium sulfate, zinc sulfide, and barium fluoral chloride. Rare earth screens are made up of lanthanum oty bromide, gadolinium compounds, or yttrium compounds. These screens are called rare earth because the elements responsible for x-ray absorption fall in the rare earth series in the periodic table. In general, they convert x-ray energy to light with more efficiency than the calcium tungstate screens. While absorption of an x-ray photon by calcium tungstate results in the emission of about 1000 light photons, rare earth phosphors produce up to 4000 light photons per x-ray photon. This would, of course, reduce the number of x-ray photons required for image formation.[1–8]

For years, non-screen film has been widely used in podiatric radiology as a standard. In 1980, with soaring silver prices, many of the film manufacturers discontinued their production of non-screen film because it is the richest in silver content. This left most podiatrists with a problem of which film screen combination to use. There are many factors about which the podiatrist must be cognizant in analyzing the myriad of films and film screen combinations. Non-screen film has become the benchmark to which we compare other films and film screen combinations.

Arithmetic Speed

The Cronex 4/PAR combination is the standard medium speed system used by the film manufacturer in industry for comparison. They arbi-

trarily assigned this combination a speed of 100 and compare all other films to it. This rates the film-screen combination, not just the film. We do not want to use a much faster system because many of the office x-ray machines have mechanical timers which are not capable of exposures shorter than $\frac{1}{4}$ second.

Resolution

Resolution is defined as the number of line pairs per millimeter that can be perceived on a film. Non-screen film has the highest resolution at 20+ LP/mm. It must be remembered, however, that the human eye without the aid of magnification can only see from 4–7 line pairs/mm at the top range. This is measured by Funk or Buckley-Mears grids. The lower the resolution, the fuzzier the image. Resolution is the property of rendering visible separate parts of the object.[12]

Average Gradient

Gradient is a measure of contrast. The lower the number the more gray we have. Non-screen film has a gradient of 1.90. If you increase the gradient you loose soft tissue definition.

Relative Noise or Graininess

This is affected by many factors: from screen type to speed to development technique. If a screen has poor phosphor distribution, it will lead to a grainy film. Similarly, a very high-speed exposure will lead to decreased graininess because fewer photons of x-radiation are used in making the exposure. Noise in a radiographic image is the fine mottle with fluctuation in film density from one area to another.[11]

Processing must be optimal to reduce grain size. High temperatures or excessive time in the developer can likewise blow up the size of the grains. Non-screen film has a relative noise level of very low.

Table 2.1 presents a few of the more commonly used film-screen combinations and compares them to non-screen film.

Contrast

Contrast is the visible difference between adjacent densities. It results from two independent but interacting causes: film contrast and subject contrast. The film contrast is unique to the type of film being used and the subject contrast is due to the general anatomical characteristics of the subject, including the type of tissue being x-rayed and

Table 2.1
Podiatry Imaging System Comparisons

Imaging System	Arithmetic Speed	Resolution (LP/mm)	Average Gradient	Relative Noise
Non-screen film (Monopak)	14	20+	1.90	Very low
Screen film (No Screen)	2	20+	1.60	Very very low
Mammography film/screen	7	17	1.70	Very very low
Extremity I/A	15	12	1.70	Very very low
Extremity I/B	30	12	2.00	Very low
Extremity II/C Very low	15	16	1.90	Very low
Cronex 4/Par	100	9	2.85	Moderate
Cronex 4/Hi Plus	200	7	2.85	Moderate-low
Cronex 4/QII	400	7	2.85	High
Cronex 4/QIII	700	6	2.85	High

the thickness and relative amounts of x-rays passing through the tissues to strike the film. Contrast may be quantified by the number of differences in density.

Contrast is further increased by using low kilovoltage with non-screen film, and by using non-screen film instead of screen film. It is decreased by using a high kilovoltage when non-screen film is used, or using screen film without a screen.[7,9,10]

Radiographic contrast can be controlled by the relationship between the kilovoltage and milleamperage seconds. A low kV and a high MAS will give a high contrast film. A high kV with a low MAS will give a low contrast film. The optimum contrast is that which makes visible as many variations in tissue density as possible. It must be realized that radiographic density will deteriorate as the amount of fog increases. Fog is any density which occurs on a processed film without a deliberate exposure. It usually appears as an extra density superimposed upon the desired density. It interferes with the interpretation of detail on the radiograph.

Density

Density is the amount of film blackening. "Density may be evaluated photo-metrically, and calculated as a function of the ratio between the amount of light incident to a film and the amount of light transmitted through a film. It can be measured with a densitometer."[7] If none of the light is transmitted through the film, there will be complete blackness or a density of 3.0. If 100% of

light is transmitted through the film, there is no density. 50% transmission of light would give a density of 0.3. The ideal radiographic density usually is no less than 0.25.[7] The density obviously is dependent upon the amount of silver that is left on the film following processing. It can thereby be controlled by controlling the amount of x-radiation that strikes the film.

Definition

Definition is the degree of distinctness or sharpness of the radiographic details on the x-ray film. It is dependent upon the optimum image sharpness.

Gradient

Gradient is the rate of change of density across an x-ray film. It is really a measure of contrast. The detail on the film depends upon a proper balance between contrast and density. Latitude permits the recording of variations of tissue density, while contrast permits these to be discernible to the viewer.

Filters

A filter is anything placed in the primary x-ray beam for the purpose of altering the quality of the x-radiation.[7] A filter is usually made of a sheet of aluminum and is placed between the x-ray source and the patient to cut out the soft radiation and leave the hard radiation which will not generally be absorbed by the body tissues.

Distortion

Distortion is defined as a perversion of shape in a radiographic image.[13] Distortion can be prevented by proper alignment of the x-ray tube with the object plane and the film plane. The plane of major interest should be parallel to the plane of the film in order to prevent distortion.

Lead Apron

It is of paramount importance to remember that total radiographic exposure given to a patient must be kept to a minimum. The simplest and most straightforward means of accomplishing this is through lead shielding. All patients should be afforded the use of either a lead apron or at the minimum a gonad shield. Pregnant women, in general, should not be x-rayed unless it is an emergency and those in their first trimester of pregnancy particularly should be kept clear of any x-ray exposure. Lead shielding should not be considered a chore, but should become a part of the routine in taking x-rays (Figure 2.37).

The object of a radiographic examination is to produce sufficient information to aid in arriving at a diagnosis of the patient's condition while minimizing the x-ray exposure to the patient. We must use views that can be duplicated at any time by any practitioner. Proper exposure should be performed so that the information on the radiographic film is optimal, and sufficient views should be taken to give all of the information that is required.

PROCESSING OF X-RAY FILMS

Developer

The developing solution consists of:
1. Hydroquinone
2. Metol, Elon or Phenidone—reducing agents (developing agents)
3. Sodium sulphite—preservative
4. Sodium carbonate—accelerator (activator, alkali)
5. Potassium bromide—fog preventor (restrainer)
6. Water

The reducing agent converts the grains of silver that have been activated by x-ray exposure to metallic silver, leaving minute particles of silver present in the emulsion. The sodium carbonate or activator (Alkali) acts by swelling the gelatin so that the reducing agents can work. Potassium bromide is a restrainer and aids in controlling the activity of the reducing agents, hence, preventing fog. Sodium sulphite is a preservative. It acts by preventing rapid oxidation of the developer. As the developer ages it will tend to become darker in color, indicating that oxidation has occurred. This lessens the effectiveness of the solution.[19–21]

Fixer

X-ray fixer has sodium thiosulphate as the main active ingredient. This fixer agent dissolves the silver salts that have not been acted upon by the developer in the unexposed and undeveloped areas. Potassium alum is usually present to act as a hardening agent. It restrains the swelling of the gelatin and hardens the emulsion by shrinking and tanning the gelatin. Sodium sulphite is present as a preservative. It prevents oxidation and discoloration of the fixer.[2,12–14]

Acid Neutralizer

An acid neutralizing solution composed of mild acetic acid is frequently used to neutralize the alkaline developer carried from the developing solution. This bath is set between the developer and the fixer. Use of an acid neutralizer will usually prolong the life of the fixer solution.

Projection

Projection is the manner in which the roentgen beam strikes the part to be x-rayed and exposes the film, according to Gamble and Yale.[9] When the x-ray beam reaches its roentgenographic objective, its course is described in anatomic terms with the surface of entry named first and exit last. A projection is named for the anatomical surface which the x-ray beams enters. For example, in a weightbearing position with the medial surface of the foot against the vertical x-ray film, the x-ray beam aimed at 90° at the cuboid, this is considered to be a lateral projection because the x-ray beam enters the lateral side of the foot.[9,15]

View

A view is the image formed on a radiograph or film. A view is named according to the anatomical part closest to the x-ray film or the area from which the x-ray beam exits, the opposite of a projection. In a position in which the film is vertical, the patient weightbearing with the medial surface of the foot next to the x-ray film, and the x-ray head at 90° with the central beam aimed at the cuboid bone, this view would be named the medial view because the medial surface of the foot is closest to the x-ray film, and it is the medial surface of the foot from which the x-ray beam exists. In podiatric medicine, most films are named for the projection.

Central Ray

Central ray designates the most direct radiation from the focal spot of the anode.

Collimation

The collimator is a device on an x-ray machine which delimits x-ray radiation to the area under examination. Collimators are required by federal law on all podiatric x-ray machines. This serves two purposes. It decreases the amount of radiation to the patient, and cuts out the scatter radiation on the film, which can give it a foggy appearance.

The diameter of the beam of radiation is reduced to the desired area (usually the size of the part being examined) by the use of shutters or diaphrams that are constructed of lead or another metal that has a high radiation absorption power. These lead shutters block out and absorb the radiation that would hit the undesirable areas of the film and subject. They are placed immediately under the radiation window of the x-ray tube head, and should be as close as possible to the tube target to perform properly. The collimator will usually have a light illuminating device in it for accurate centering and aiming of the x-ray beam.[12,16]

Focal Spot and Distance Factors

The manner in which an object placed in the path of an x-ray beam is projected depends on a number of factors. These include focal spot size (the size of the x-ray tube target) and distance of the object from the focal spot and from the film. If the focal spot is pinpoint in size, then the borders of the images will be sharper than if the focal spot is larger. The object to film distance should be as short as possible to give a sharp accurate reproduction of the object. If the object to film distance is increased, a magnification of the size of the object with a concomitant distortion will occur. The object to focal spot distance is usually dictated by the size of the focal spot. Furthermore, if the object is not centrally placed with respect to the central ray, this will cause an obliquing effect or a distortion of the x-ray image.[17]

Orthoposer

The orthoposer or ortho-X-poser is constructed and used to facilitate taking weightbearing x-ray views. It usually consists of a lead-lined box in which there is constructed a lead-lined well. The well is of the appropriate dimensions to accept and hold an x-ray film in either a cardboard or hard cassette in the vertical or upright position. There frequently is a spring-loaded tension knob which aids in maintaining the film in a perfectly vertical position (Fig. 2.1).

STANDARD X-RAY PROJECTIONS OF THE FOOT AND RADIOGRAPHIC FINDINGS ON THESE PROJECTIONS

Dorsoplantar Projection

In podiatric use, the dorsoplantar projection is

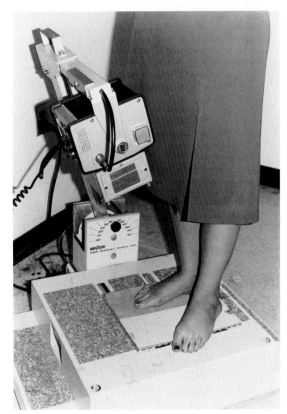

Figure 2.1. Weightbearing dorsoplantar projection. Note orthoposer.

usually taken with the patient weightbearing. It can be taken with both feet standing on one film at the same time, or each foot can be taken individually, if using the angle and base of gait techniques. The head is angled at 15° from the vertical. When x-raying one foot, the central ray is aimed directly at the lateral portion of the navicular. When x-raying both feet at the same time, it is aimed between the naviculars. It must be realized, however, that when taking both feet simultaneously, we are slightly obliquing each foot. On this projection, we are able to examine the transverse plane relationships of the entire midfoot area as well as the metatarsals and entire forefoot area. The anterior portion of the greater tarsus is also visible. We have an accurate representation of Lis Franc's joint, all the metatarsophalangeal joints and interphalangeal joints. We have a good approximation of the shape of the navicular and cuboid, the medial cuneiform, and to a lesser degree the middle and lateral cuneiforms. We can also observe the distal portion of the talus and calcaneus (Figures 2.1 to 2.3).

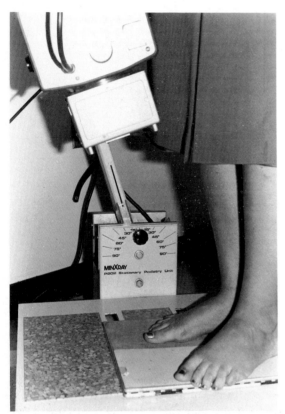

Figure 2.2.   Dorsoplantar projection.

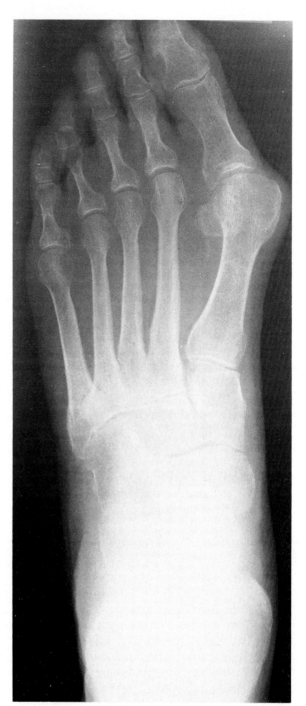

Figure 2.3.   Dorsoplantar projection.

Weightbearing Lateral Projection

This projection is taken with the head angled at 90° from the vertical with the foot placed with its medial side against the vertically placed x-ray film. The central ray is aimed at the cuboid. This projection affords us an accurate representation of the talus and calcaneus. Most of the cuboid is observable, and to a lesser extent we can examine the navicular and the medial cuneiform on this projection. The first and fifth metatarsals are clearly observable. The second through fourth metatarsals are overlapping each other as are the second through fifth digits. The first digit can be examined relatively well in this view. Variations of this view would be with the great toe extended to examine the phalanges of this digit or laterals can be taken using small dental films between the digits to examine any individual digit (Figures 2.4 and 2.5).

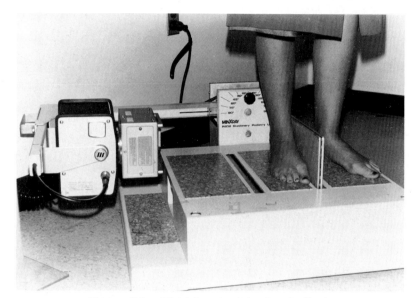

Figure 2.4. Weightbearing lateral projections.

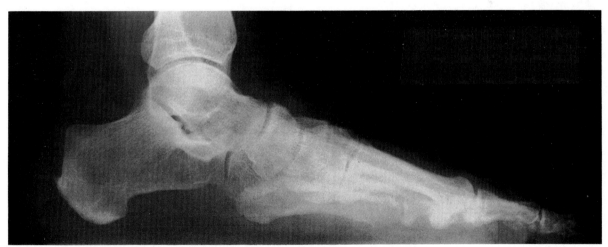

Figure 2.5. Weightbearing lateral projections.

Non-weightbearing Medial Projection
(Non-weightbearing Lateral View)

The patient must be sitting with the film flat on the orthoposer. The lateral side of both feet are placed on the film, with the plantar aspect of both feet either touching or not touching, but facing each other. The knees will be in an abducted position. The x-ray head is aimed at 0° with the central beam between the naviculars. This projection is useful in examining the talus, calcaneus, and various lesser tarsal bones. Although it does not give a functional appraisal of their positioning, it is useful in examining their shape and looking for the effects of trauma (Figures 2.6 to 2.8).

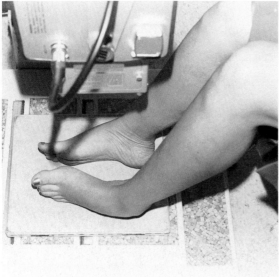

Figure 2.6. Non-weightbearing medial projection.

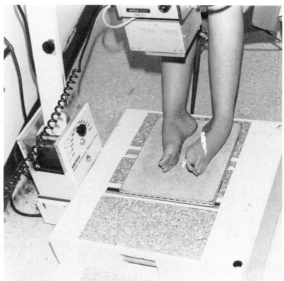

Figure 2.7. Non-weightbearing medial projection.

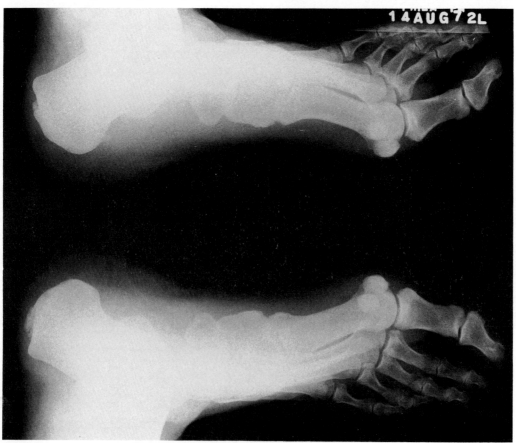

Figure 2.8. Non-weightbearing medial projection.

Medial Oblique Projection

The film is placed flat on the orthoposer. The medial aspect of the foot is placed along the border of the film closest to the x-ray head. The contralateral foot must be placed behind and out of the way. The x-ray head angle is 45° from the vertical and the central ray is aimed at the navicular. This projection is of limited value in examining the foot. It is most useful following trauma to the medial side of the foot or when examining for abnormalities in shape of the medial tarsal bones (Figures 2.9 to 2.11).

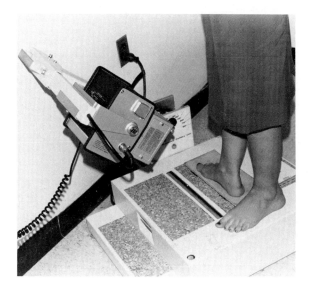

Figure 2.9. Medial oblique projection (weightbearing).

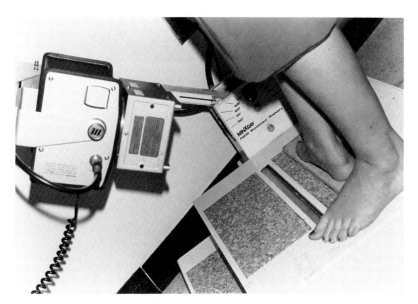

Figure 2.10. Medial oblique projection (weightbearing).

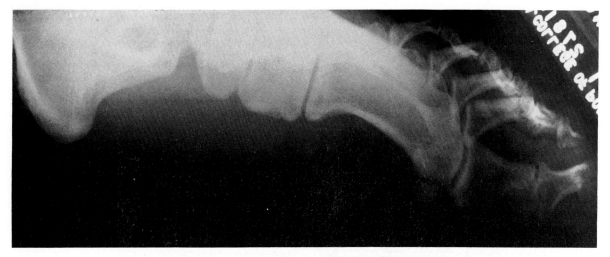

Figure 2.11.   Medial oblique projection (weightbearing).

Lateral Oblique Projection

The film is placed flat on the orthoposer with the lateral border of the foot along the border of the film closest to the x-ray head. The head angle is set at 45° from the vertical and the central ray is aimed at the cuboid bone. This is perhaps the most popular oblique in podiatric usage. It gives a slightly distorted and slightly magnified representation of most of the bones of the foot. It is most useful following trauma and occasionally when examining for abnormalities in shape of any of the bones of the foot. When the fifth digit exhibits a varus contracture, the lateral oblique projection gives the most accurate picture of the shape of the proximal phalanx of the fifth digit (Figures 2.12 and 2.13).

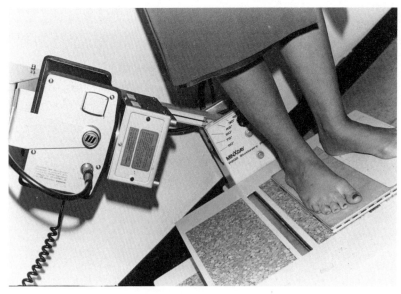

Figure 2.12.   Lateral oblique projection (weightbearing).

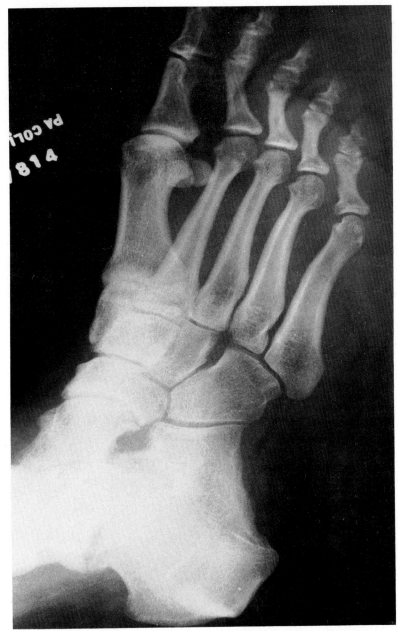

Figure 2.13. Lateral oblique projection (weightbearing).

Axial Sesamoidal Projection

For this projection, a block of foam rubber or an axial positioning device is usually used to aid in the positioning the patient. The film must be vertical with the patient facing the film. The digits and heels must be elevated. The head angle is set at 90° to the vertical and is aimed at the plantar aspect of the sesamoids. This view is useful in observing the sesamoids and their relationship with the first metatarsal head plantarally. It is also of questionable value in examining the plantar aspect of the metatarsal heads, and the relative declination heights (Figures 2.14 to 2.16).

Axial Calcaneal Projection

The film is placed flat on the orthoposer and the patient stands with his heel toward the x-ray machine. The head is angled 45° from the vertical and is aimed at the posterior surface of the calcaneus. This projection is useful when examining the calcaneus for fractures or possible abnormalities in shape (Figures 2.17 and 2.18).

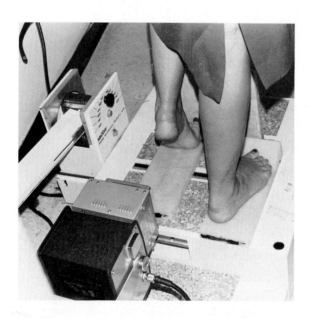

Figure 2.14. Axial sesamoidal projection.

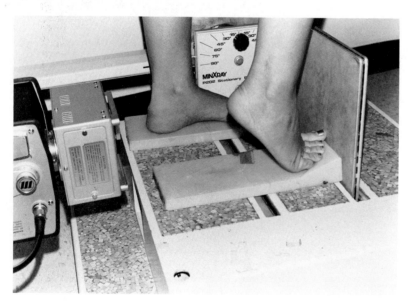

Figure 2.15. Axial sesamoidal projection.

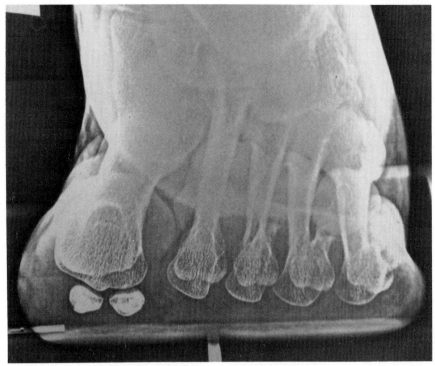

Figure 2.16. Axial sesamoidal projection.

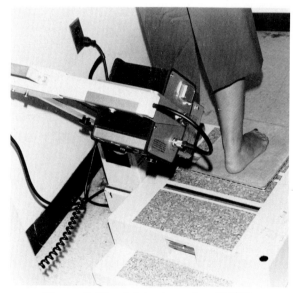

Figure 2.17. Axial calcaneal projection.

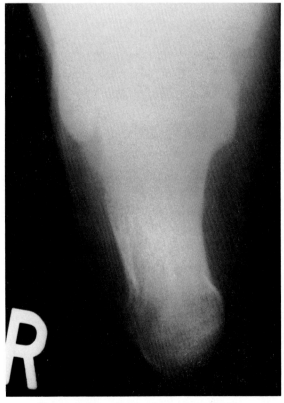

Figure 2.18. Axial calcaneal projection.

Ski-Jump or Harris and Beath Projections

These are special projections developed for use in examining the subtalar joints and sustentaculum tali. The film is flat on the orthoexposer with the patient standing on the film, heels toward the x-ray machine. This projection must be taken with the head set at three different angles; the first is taken at a 35° angle, next at a 40°, and lastly at a 45° angle. Because of the number of exposures to the patient, this projection is used only when absolutely necessary to determine if a fracture of the sustentaculum tali has occurred or if there is a talocalcaneal coalition in the area of the posterior or middle subtalar joints (Figure 2.19 and 2.20).[18]

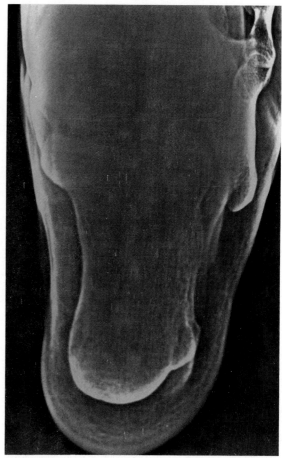

Figure 2.20.   Harris and Beath or ski-jump projection.

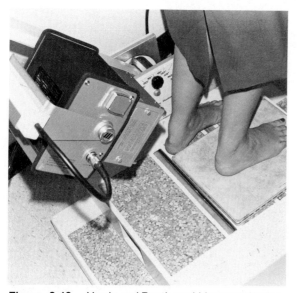

Figure 2.19.   Harris and Beath or ski-jump projection.

STANDARD X-RAY PROJECTIONS OF THE ANKLE AND RADIOGRAPHIC FINDINGS ON THESE PROJECTIONS

Mortise Projection

The film is placed in the upright position, with the patient standing heels toward the x-ray film and touching the film. The entire limb is internally rotated 15°. The x-ray head is set at 90° from the vertical and is aimed at the center of the ankle joint anteriorly. This projection gives a picture of the entire ankle joint and can be used to examine the joint space, as well as looking for the effects of trauma (Figures 2.21 to 2.23).

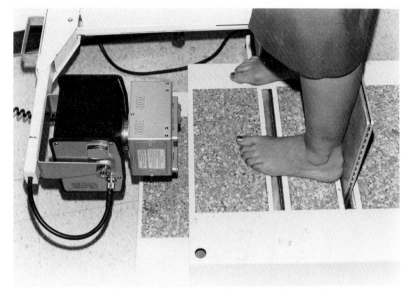

Figure 2.21. The mortise projection of the ankle.

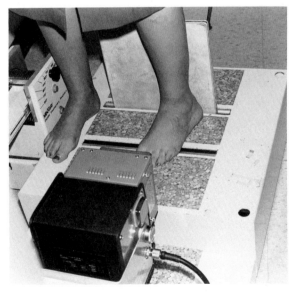

Figure 2.22. The mortise projection of the ankle.

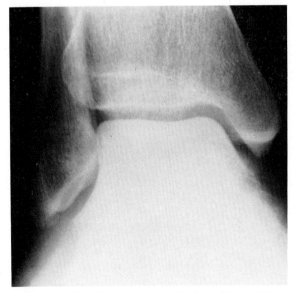

Figure 2.23. The mortise projection of the ankle.

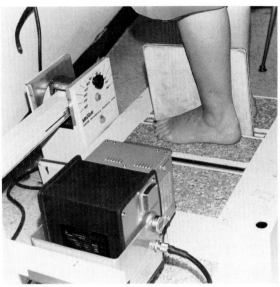

Figure 2.24. The lateral ankle projection.

Lateral Ankle Projection

This projection is taken using the same procedure as the lateral weightbearing projection of the foot, the only difference being that the film is placed with its long dimension vertically to include the lower leg. It shows the sagittal plane relationship of the ankle joint and lower leg (Figures 2.24 and 2.25).

Obliques of the Ankle

Obliques of the ankle are usually taken at 30° of internal rotation and possibly at 60° of external rotation of the limb. The x-ray head is aimed similarly to the mortise view of the ankle. These projections are usually taken following trauma to the ankle (Figures 2.26 to 2.29).

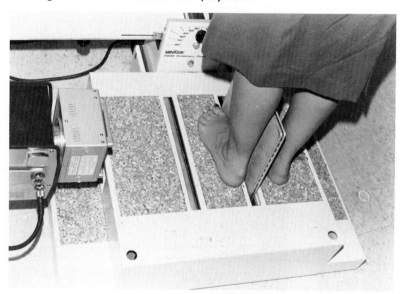

Figure 2.25. The lateral ankle projection.

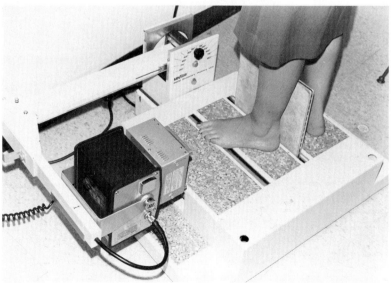

Figure 2.26. Lateral oblique projection of the ankle.

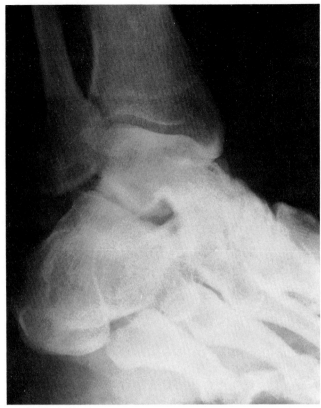

Figure 2.27. Lateral oblique projection of the ankle.

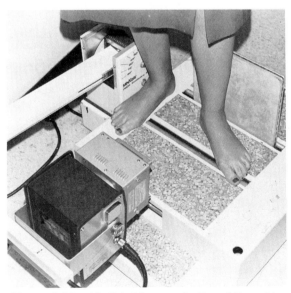

Figure 2.28. Medial oblique projection of the ankle.

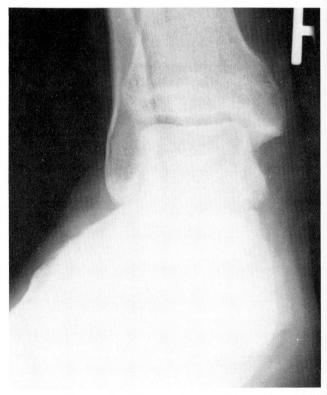

Figure 2.29. Medial oblique projection of the ankle.

The Stress Inversion Projection of the Ankle

Stress inversion projections are usually taken following inversion sprains of the ankle in which the practitioner suspects damage to the lateral ligaments of the ankle. Thefilm is placed upright in the orthoposer and the patient stands in the position similar to a mortise view of the ankle. The x-ray head is set at 90° and aimed at the center of the ankle joint. Uusally the ankle will be edematous and quite tender from the trauma so the injured area must be anesthetized. The technician must wear a lead apron and lead gloves and must forcibly invert the ankle joint to its limit and hold the patient in this position for the taking of the view. Bilateral views must be taken and should be taken in plantarflexion and at a right angle. (Figures 2.30, and 2.31).

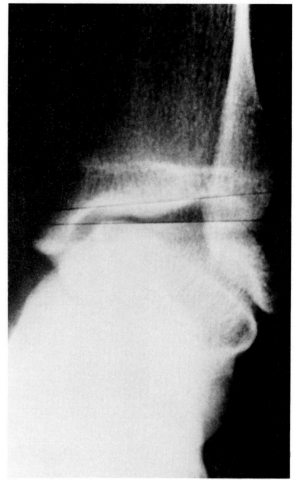

Figure 2.31.   Stress inversion projection of the ankle.

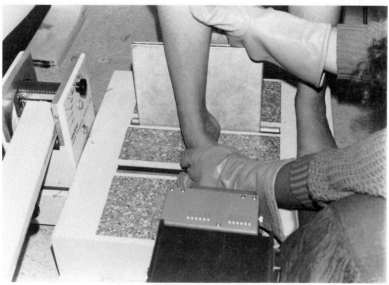

Figure 2.30.   Stress inversion projection of the ankle.

Anterior Drawer View

This view is taken following trauma to the ankle joint when a disruption of the soft tissues supporting the ankle joint are suspected. The view is set up similar to a lateral view of the ankle. However, the technician must be draped in lead and one hand must support the leg while the other hand forcibly pulls the foot anteriorly. Bilateral views should again be taken for comparison (Figure 2.32).

Stress Dorsiflexion Views

These views are set up similar to the lateral weightbearing projection of the foot with the difference being that the patient bends his knees forward as in a ski-jump position until he obtains a maximal dorsiflexion of the foot upon the leg. This view is useful in documenting an anterior ankle impingement as in an ankle equinus (Figure 2.33 and 2.34).

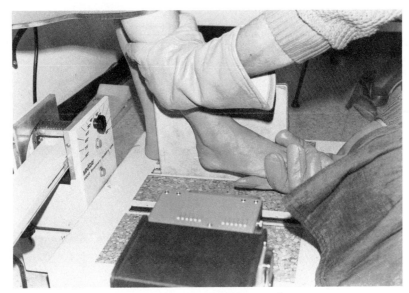

Figure 2.32. Anterior drawer view.

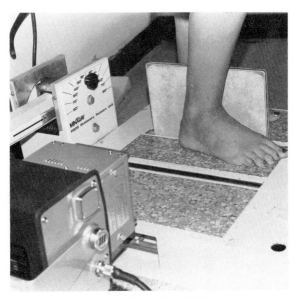

Figure 2.33. Stress dorsiflexion views.

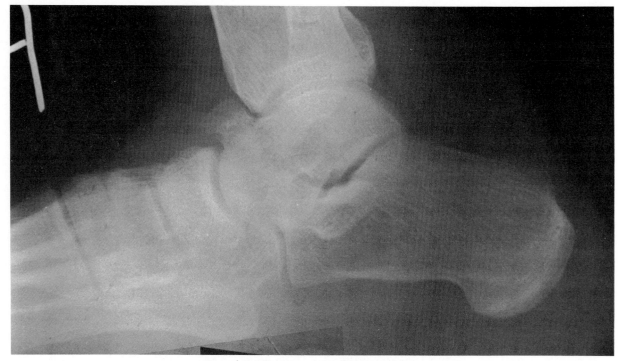

Figure 2.34. Stress dorsiflexion views.

ANGLE AND BASE OF GAIT X-RAYS

When x-rays are to be used for mechanoradiographical analysis, they must be taken in the proper angle and base of gait. Use of the angle and base of gait attempts to position the osseous segments of the foot in their representative functional position, as compared to non-functioning position, as in static stance. We must find a position that best represents the foot in function to get a better understanding of the positioning of the osseous segments during function. Since in gait, the foot is usually angulated in an abductory direction from the direction of movement, and the feet are a certain distance apart, this position must be duplicated to attempt to capture the most accurate position of function. The angle of gait is defined as the angle between a line bisecting each foot in the progression of gait. The base of gait is defined as the distance between the medial aspect of both heels in gait. To determine this position, observe the patient during gait. It is most helpful if the patient is walking on a floor that has markings to help to reproduce the appropriate angle and base. Once the actual angle and base figures have been determined, they should be used in positioning the foot for the dorsoplantar and lateral weightbearing films.

The foot being x-rayed is placed on the film with the contralateral side of the film covered by a lead plate. The contralateral foot is then positioned at the calculated angle to the first foot, and with the heels apart, corresponding to the base of gait. The patient's body is placed in the direction of progression. He is then repositioned accordingly for the opposite foot, the process repeated for the lateral projections.

Radiographs taken in the proper angle and base of gait afford us distinct advantages over those not taken in the angle and base of gait. The same angle and base of gait can always be reproduced for future radiographs. This gives a more accurate means of comparison to determine if therapy, whether surgical or mechanical, has indeed caused any change in the bony architecture. If one is inclined to measure angles, he can determine numerically whether a change has in fact occurred; for example, has the IM angle really changed as a result of a surgical procedure? When using random positioning techniques, we cannot rely on the fact that the position has been accurately duplicated from film to film.

MAGNIFICATION TECHNIQUE FOR PODIATRIC X-RAYS

From time to time, it becomes desirable to have an x-ray that is magnified, such as during surgical procedures, as pre- or postoperative films, or possibly in diagnostic films to examine an exostosis or in examining the digits. This can easily be accomplished on the original x-rays. If the distance between the object and the film is increased, magnification will occur naturally. It must be remembered that a certain amount of distortion can also occur during this magnification process, and the resolution and definition are affected adversely by the magnification. Accordingly, if magnification films are to be taken, you must use the film-screen combination that affords the smallest grain size with the greatest resolution. Generally, a magnification of 2–3 times is more than enough, and this can be accomplished by increasing the foot to film distance to approximately one-quarter of the film to tube distance (Figures 2.35 and 2.36).

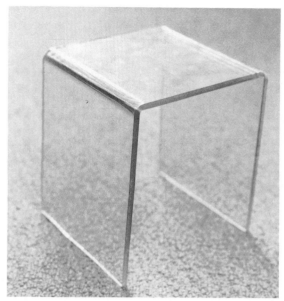

Figure 2.35. A magniposer is easily made of ¼-inch plexiglass.

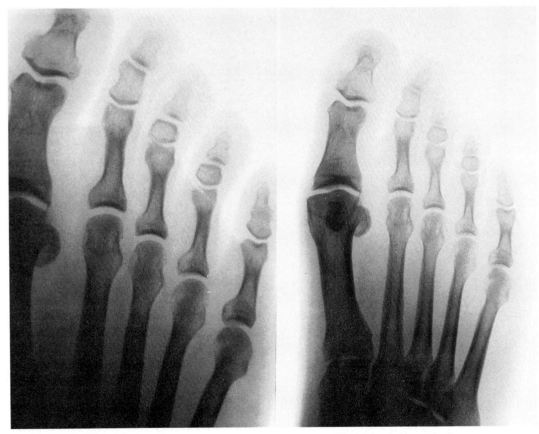

Figure 2.36. The projection on the left is magnified 2–3 times with very little loss of definition and clarity on a polaroid 8 × 10 positive film.

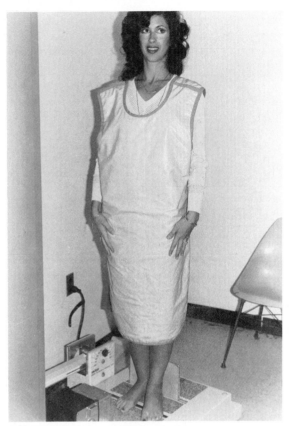

Figure 2.37. Lead shielding must be provided to all patients prior to x-ray exposure.

VIEW IMPROVISATION

It must be realized that x-ray projections can be improvised at any time to suit the needs of the viewer. There are times when the pathology to be examined is not shown on the standard DP lateral or oblique projections. In these instances, it is proper to determine the proper axial or oblique view to best show the pathology being examined and use it. In the examination of certain pathologies, many practitioners will develop a certain technique that differs slightly from the normal techniques. For example, to best show the medial exostosis of the first metatarsal head (a bunion deformity), both pre- and postoperatively, many practitioners will angulate the x-ray head 5° to 10° medially when taking a dorsoplantar film.

Similarly, when examining a fifth toe that exhibits a varus contracture, it must be realized that in order to get a good view of the head of the proximal phalanx, a lateral oblique projection at approximately 30° will best show the exact contour of the phalanx.

XERORADIOGRAPHY

Xeroradiography, which was developed in the 1950s, is a process in which an image is produced on a selenium-coated plate. The selenium plate is run through a special conditioning machine that applies an evenly distributed positive charge across the entire surface of the plate. It then loads the plate into a cassette. The cassette is exposed to x-ray in the usual manner and is then processed. When x-ray hits the selenium plate and interacts with it, it discharges portions of the original positive surface charge and creates charge carrier pairs in the selenium. The xeroradiographic cassette is then loaded into a processor, which automatically develops the electrostatic charge pattern on the selenium plate and transfers the developed image to paper for viewing and storage. The electrostatic image on the plate is made visible by applying a powderized blue toner to the surface of the plate. The toner is charged by particle to particle contact, and is attracted to the plate surface by the charge pattern. A sheet of specially sensitized paper is then placed in direct contact with the plate, and the toner in a certain pattern is transferred to the paper and fused with the paper, creating the image of the xeroradiograph.

Edge enhancement is a phenomenon of xeroradiography which improves the image detail over conventional film imaging. It tends to emphasize the characteristics of borders between tissues. This characteristic makes detailed information more easily seen. Xeroradiographs are particularly helpful in diagnosing neuromas, soft tissue masses, trauma to bones, joint effusions, soft tissue injuries, and in locating foreign bodies. Xeroradiography is even sensitive enough to visualize nonmetallic foreign bodies. Xeroradiography also has greater recording latitude than conventional radiography.[22-29]

POLAROID 8 × 10 RADIOGRAPHIC SYSTEM FOR PODIATRY

The Polaroid Instant 8 × 10 radiographic system for podiatry is a portable, self-contained system which produces finished, high-diagnostic quality positive radiographs without the need for conventional wet processing or a dark room. The system contains:
- Polaroid Land radiographic 8 × 10 film;
- Polaroid 8 × 10 radiographic cassette;
- Polaroid radiographic film processor and loading tray.

The radiographic film consists of two components, the orthochromatic negative in a light-protected envelope, and the transparent (blue tinted) positive imaging sheet which contains the processing chemicals in a small pod.

The cassette contains a single rare earth green-emitting screen. The negative in its light protected envelope is placed in the cassette, the cassette is closed, and the envelope removed. A uniquely designed pressure plate which maximizes film/screen contact is pressed into place and the exposure is made in normal fashion.

Processing is easily accomplished in 60 seconds by placing the positive imaging sheet containing the pod of processing chemicals into the tray.

The exposed cassette is then slipped into the tray and processing is initiated by pressing the process button. The exposed negative and the positive transparent imaging sheet are automatically fed through the processor rollers which break the pod and spread the processing chemicals over the image area. Upon completion of processing, the film unit is removed and peeled apart. The resulting dry image may be viewed immediately, although care must be taken to not scratch the image. Usually within a day the image is print-coated for storage.

Technically speaking, the Polaroid TPX film system utilized a very thin, green-sensitive, silver halide emulsion which is coated to much lower weight than any of the conventional wet processed negative materials; the emulsion is cast on a thin black polyester base. The combination of single rare earth screen and thin emulsion on a non-reflecting base for practical purposes eliminates crossover and light scattering present in conventional wet processed materials. Unlike many other rare earth systems, the TPX transparency has extremely low noise, lower than the non-rare earth systems of equal speed. The low noise coupled with high contrast for bony structures allows for the visualization of small osseous changes not easily identifiable with other silver halide systems.

The densitometric qualities of the film have been optimized in a way which allows physicians to obtain high contrast bone detail at no sacrifice to soft tissue information.

The TPX System is speed rated at 200–250 relative to par speed systems and yields detail normally associated with conventional systems 3–4 times the exposure.

Exposure latitude is equivalent to wet process conventional materials. Exposing the TPX at a little higher kilovoltage provides excellent contrast, detail, and aids in reducing the patient motion artifact.

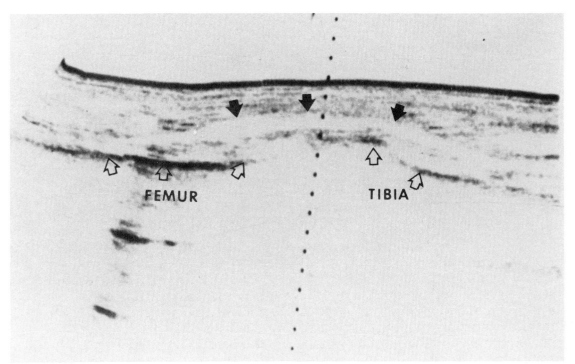

Figure 2.38. Ultrasonography is a relatively new technique in which high frequency sound waves are used to form images of portions of the body. Ultrasound of the popliteal region demonstrates the course of a normal popliteal artery (*solid arrows*).

The system has found application in magnification radiography, in-cast films, hospital and out-patient surgical suites, and normal first visit and follow-up radiographic procedures.[30]

ULTRASONOGRAPHY

Ultrasonography is a relatively new technique in medicine, and a very new technique in Podiatric Medicine. High-frequency sound waves are reflected differently depending upon the density of the reflecting tissues. They are received and used to form images of portions of the body. The technique is non-invasive and is harmless (Figures 2.38 to 2.41).

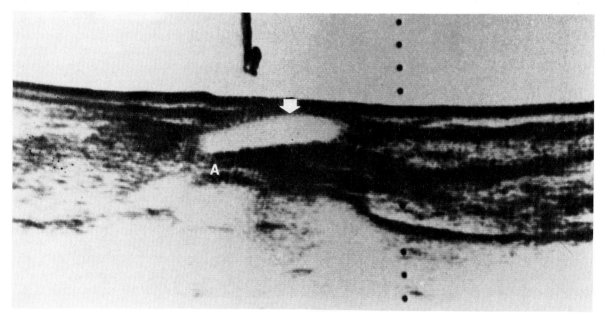

Figure 2.39. In this popliteal study, an elongated Baker's cyst (*arrow*) is identified posterior to the popliteal artery (*A*).

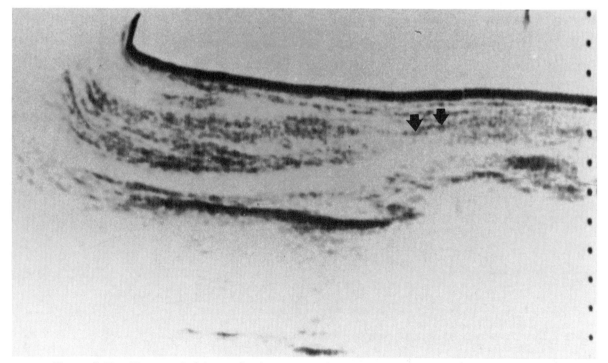

Figure 2.40. Ultrasound of the popliteal space reveals an aneurysm (*arrow*) of the popliteal artery.

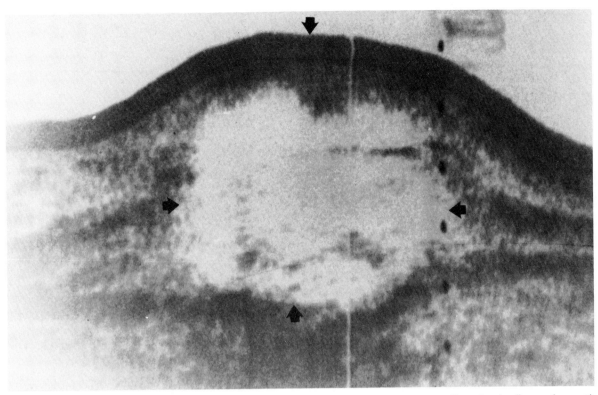

Figure 2.41. Ultrasound of the thigh reveals a well-circumscribed solid mass representing a benign lipoma (*arrows*).

REFERENCES

1. MEREDITH, W. J.: *Fundamental Physics of Radiation*, John Wright, Chicago, 1977.
2. CAHOON, J. B.: *Formulating X-Ray Techniques*, 7th Ed, Duke University, Durham, NC, 1970.
3. BRECHER, E. R.: *The Rays*, Williams & Wilkins, Baltimore, 1969.
4. CONLAM, M., CRAIG, M., ET AL.: *The Physical Basis of Medical Imaging*, Appleton-Century-Crofts, Englewood Cliffs, NJ, 1981.
5. CULLINAN, J. E., AND ANGELINE, M.: *X-Ray Technics*, JB Lippincott, Philadelphia, 1980.
6. JOHNS, H. E., AND CUNNINGHAM, J. R.: *The Physics of Radiology*, 3rd Ed, Charles C Thomas, Springfield, 1969.
7. FUCHS, A. W.: *Principles of Radiographic Exposure and Processing*, 2nd Ed, Charles C Thomas, Springfield, 1958.
8. EASTMAN, T. R.: *Dupont Imaging Management Magazine*, No. 3, 1981.
9. GAMBLE, F., AND YALE, I.: *Clinical Foot Roentgenology*, 2nd Ed, Krieger, Huntington, NY, 1975.
10. MILLER, F.: *College Physics*, 4th Ed, Harcourt Brace Javonovich, NY, 1977.
11. COULAM, C. M.: *The Physical Basis of Medical Imaging*, Appleton-Century-Crofts, Englewood Cliffs, NJ, 1981.
12. JACOBI, C. A., AND PARIS, D. Q.: *Text of Radiographic Techniques*, 4th Ed, CV Mosby, St. Louis, 1968.
13. BLOOM, W, HOLLENBACH, J., AND MORGAN, J.: *Medical Radiographic Technique*, Charles C Thomas, Springfield, 1965.
14. ROSS, J. A., AND GALLOWAY, R. W.: *A Handbook of Radiography*, JB Lippincott, Philadelphia, 1963.
15. CLARK, K. C.: *Positioning in Radiography*, 8th Ed, Intercontinental Medical Books, NY, 1967.
16. MERRILE, V.: *Atlas of Roentgenological Positioning and Standard Radiological Procedures*, 4th Ed, CV Mosby, St. Louis, 1975.
17. MESCHAN, I.: *Analysis of Roentgen Signs in General Radiology*, WB Saunders, Philadephia, 1973.
18. HARRIS, R. I., AND BEATH, I.: Hypermobile flatfoot with short tendoachilles. J. Bone Jt. Surg., *30A:* 116, 1948.
19. ROSS, J. A., AND GALLOWAY, R. W.: *A Handbook of Radiography*, JB Lippincott, Philadelphia, 1963.
20. BLOOM, W. L., JR., HOLLENBACK, J. L., AND MORGAN, J. A.: Medical Radiographic Technique, Charles C Thomas, Springfield, 1965.
21. CAHOON, J. B.: *Formulating X-Ray Technique*, 7th Ed, Duke University, Durham, NC, 1970.
22. PAGLIANO, J. D., AND WEXLER, C. E.: Xeroradiography for detection for neuromas in podiatry. J.A.P.A., **68:** 38, 1978.
23. WINIECKI, D. G., AND BIGGS, E. W.: Xeroradiography and its application in podiatry. J.A.P.A., **67:** 393, 1977.
24. WOLFE, J. N.: Xeroradiography of the bones, joints and soft tissues. Radiology, **93:** 583, 1969.
25. JING, B. S., VILLANUEVA, R., ET AL.: A new radiological technique in evaluation of prosthetic fitting. Radiology, **122:** 534, 1977.
26. NESSI, R., ET AL.: Xeroradiography of bone tumors. Skeletal Radiol., 2: 143, 1978.
27. GRIFFITHS, H. J., AND D'ORSI, C. J.: Use of xeroradiography in cruciate ligament injuries. Am. J. Roentgenol. Radium Ther. Nucl. Med. **121:** 94, 1974.
28. Xerox Corporation: What is edge enhancement and how does it affect the radiographic images? Technical Application Bulletin, #1, November, 1974.
29. Xerox Corporation: What are the most common xeroradiographic terms and what do they mean? Technical Application Bulletin, #3, November, 1975.
30. PEISACH, J.: Personal communication.

CHAPTER 3

Normal Foot and Ankle

THE NORMAL FOOT

The foot may be thought of as a bag of bones tied tightly together and functioning as a unit. The bones are expected to maintain their alignment without causing symptomatology to the patient. In a normal radiograph, the bones must have normal shape and normal alignment. The density of the soft tissues should be normal and there should be no fractures, tumors, or foreign bodies (Figs. 2.3 and 2.5).

BONES OF THE FOOT

The Talus

On the dorsoplantar projection, the talus appears as an irregularly shaped bone which articulates with the navicular. Only the distal portion of the bone, including the anatomical head and neck, can be seen, while its articulation with the calcaneus can be seen. Approximately 75% of its anterior surface articulates with the navicular, and the medial 25% usually is non-articular in the normal foot. In pronation, this articulation is greatly affected and usually results in less than 75% articulation with the navicular. In supination, the opposite occurs and the talus can articulate 100% with the navicular. In the normal foot, the long axis of the head and neck of the talus usually runs though the center of the first metatarsal head, while in pronation it falls medial to the first metatarsal head, and in supination it falls lateral to the first metatarsal head.

On the lateral projection, the talus is irregularly shaped, presenting with a head, neck, and body. On the normal lateral film, the long axis of the talus points approximately through the first metatarsal head. In pronation, the talus will plantarflex, so that the long axis falls plantar to the first metatarsal head, and conversely in supination, it will fall superior to the first metatarsal head. In

cases of long continuing microtrauma, as in some of the supinatory foot types or athletes, there is a filling in of the neck of the talus dorsally. The microtrauma is due to an impingement of the neck upon the distal anterior end of the tibia. On the lateral projection, the posterior and middle subtalar joint facets, as well as the articulation of the talus with the tibia, can be examined. The dome of the talus should be round and smooth.

The Navicular

On the dorsoplantar projection, the navicular is distal to the talus and in most cases is a rectangularly shaped bone. In cases of severe pronation, the navicular can become wedge-shaped with the apex being lateral. On the normal dorsoplantar film, the entire articulation of the navicular with the talus, as well as its articulation with the three cuneiforms, can be seen. Frequently, there will be an enlarged tuberosity of the navicular, which will cause a bulge on the medial side of the foot, just distal to the head of the talus. When this occurs, it distorts the amount of articulation with the head of the talus, making it appear greater than it really is.

On the lateral projection, the long axis of the navicular runs from dorsal to plantar. The bone should be rectangular. The articulation between the navicular and the first cuneiform is the only one present on the lateral, the second and third remaining unreadable. The talonavicular articulation should be smooth and curved, forming one-half the cyma line.

The Calcaneus or Os Calcis

On the dorsoplantar projection, only the distal end and a portion of the lateral border of the calcaneus is present. Occasionally, because of the saddle shape of the articulation between the calcaneus and cuboid, there appears to be two joint lines on the dorsoplantar view; one representing the dorsal aspect of the joint, and the second representing the plantar portion. The calcaneocuboid articulation is rarely incongruous. The lateral borders of the calcaneus and cuboid should lie roughly in a straight line. If angulation occurs between these two bones in a lateral direction, it is a sign of pronation, and is considered increased if it exceeds 5°.

In pronation, as the axis of the talus moves medially, the angulation between the talus and calcaneus increases, and a gap is observed between the distal portions of the talus and calcaneus called the talocalcaneal notch.

On the lateral projection, the entire bone is observable. The tuberosity of the calcaneus is located plantarly, and the medial tubercle forms a sclerotic line running through the tuberosity. The calcaneocuboid joint is completely observable on the lateral view and forms the plantar one-half of the cyma line. The posterior and middle subtalar joint facets are roughly parallel on the lateral projection. The posterosuperior angle of the calcaneus should be present. When this becomes enlarged and prominent, it is known as a Haglund's deformity. In the center of the body of the calcaneus, the trabeculations are sparse. This normal finding must be differentiated from a calcaneal cyst in which there are no trabeculations and the area may be circumscribed by a sclerotic ring. The sustentaculum tali is represented on the lateral view by a heavy white area rising up to the beak or distal superior portion of the calcaneus. The normal pitch or angulation of the calcaneus with the weightbearing plane is approximately 20°.

The Cuboid

The cuboid is an irregularly shaped bone, including both the dorsoplantar and lateral projections. On the dorsoplantar projection, the calcanecuboid joint and the articulation between the cuboid and the fourth and fifth metatarsals are seen. On the lateral projection, the articulation with the fifth metatarsal can be examined.

The Cuneiforms

The medial cuneiform has a rectangular dorsal surface. Its articulation with the navicular and with the first metatarsal are present on the dorsoplantar film. The distal articular surface should be flat and should form only a very mild angle with the long axis of the bone.

On the lateral film, the cuboid is a rectangular bone articulating with the navicular and the first metatarsal. Occasionally, the naviculocuneiform joint becomes deviated and appears to sag in a plantar direction. This is referred to as a naviculocuneiform fault.

The middle and lateral cuneiforms can be seen on the dorsoplantar view, but unclearly. Because they lie at an angle to the transverse plane, the joint space between the second and third cuneiforms and between the third cuneiform and cuboid are not seen. On the lateral projection they cannot be observed.

The First Metatarsal

The heaviest of the metatarsals, the first, shows the greatest girth and thickest cortex. The articulation between the first metatarsal and cuneiform and the lateral aspect of the base and its articulation with the second metatarsal can be seen. The first metatarsophalangeal joint is usually smooth, rounded, and congruous. The medial aspect of the head frequently is enlarged into a bunion deformity and can exhibit cystic degeneration, which occurs in the process of the formation of the bunion. The plantar aspect of the first metatarsal head articulates with the two sesamoids, and the length of the first metatarsal should be roughly the same length as the second metatarsal. A difference in length of plus or minus 2 mm is within the realm of normal. On the lateral projection, the first metatarsocuneiform joint, the first metatarsophalangeal joint, and the articulation of the first metatarsal head with the medial sesamoid can be seen. The smooth curve of the articular surface of the head is usually continued dorsally.

The Second through Fifth Metatarsals

The second through fifth metatarsals must be clearly examined on the dorsoplantar view. The second metatarsal should be approximately the length of the first metatarsal plus or minus 2 mm. The third metatarsal should be shorter than the second. The fourth should be shorter than the third and the fifth should be the shortest. The metatarsal heads should fall off from the second metatarsal head in a gentle curve. Metatarsophalangeal joints are usually clear and are rounded and congruous. The metatarsal bases two through five seem to overlap each other on the dorsoplantar projection making the tarsometatarsal joint fairly fuzzy. The tuberosity of the fifth metatarsal can be examined on the dorsoplantar film.

On the lateral projection there is a great deal of overlap between the second through fourth metatarsals. The fifth metatarsal usually can be made out fairly clearly. The phalanges of all the lesser toes cannot be clearly read on the lateral projection; however, on the dorsoplantar projection, they are usually very clearly visible.

THE ANKLE

The ankle is best examined on the mortise and lateral projections. On the mortise view, the entire ankle joint should be visible, including the dorsal, medial, and lateral aspects of the joint. The joint space should be even throughout, and there should not be sclerosis of the articulating surfaces. The contour of the dorsal aspect of the talus should be smooth with a small depression in the center, and there should be no erosions or areas of absent bone. The lower end of the tibia and fibular above the talus articulate with each other, and there should be a normal amount of space present at this articulation. This amount of joint space can increase in a diastasis of the ankle. The digital fossa at the tip of the fibular malleolus is observable, and the tips of both malleoli should be round and smooth in contour (Figs. 2.25).

On the lateral projection, the dome of the talus should be smooth and rounded, the fibular malleolus should be placed approximately in the center or slightly posterior to the center of the medial malleolus. If it is in a more posterior position, this usually indicates a tortional abnormality of the leg. The distal anterior aspect of the tibia and the neck of the talus should be examined for exostosis formation as would be found in an ankle or bony equinus (Fig. 2.5).

JOINTS

A congruous joint is a normal joint. As such, the two articular surfaces must be parallel and they must be wholly articular. A deviated joint is one in which the articular surfaces are still wholly articular, but are no longer parallel with each other. A subluxed joint is neither parallel nor wholly articular. A dislocated joint usually occurs following a trauma. Its radiographic evaluation shows that the articular surfaces are no longer parallel and are no longer articular. Frequently, they will overlap or be in a non-anatomical position (Figs. 6.8 to 6.10).

SUPERNUMERARY BONES

Supernumerary bones are the "extra" bones that are not normally present. They usually start from secondary centers of ossification that do not join or unite with the main centers of ossification. These bones are usually hereditary, and frequently are sesamoid bones, i.e., completely enclosed within a tendon. In the lower extremity, there are three constant sesamoid bones; the patella and the two sesamoids beneath the first metatarsal head.

OTHER SUPERNUMERARY BONES

Os Trigonum

If the lateral tubercle of the talus is separate from the body it is called as os trigonum. This is a very common finding and is usually asymptomatic. If the tubercle is enlarged, it is called a stiatas process, and it is best observed on the lateral projection of the foot and ankle (Fig. 3.1).

Os Tibiale Externum or Secondary Navicular

This forms from a secondary ossification center medial to the tuberosity of the navicular, and is a sesamoid bone within the tendon of the tibialis posterior. In some studies, it has been shown that the secondary navicular actually has a cartilage-linked joint for articulation with the navicular.[1] It is best observed on the dorsoplantar and the lateral oblique projections. Presence of a tibiale externum is frequently associated with a pronated foot and is referred to as a pre-hallux syndrome (Fig. 3.2).[2]

Os Supra Naviculare

This tiny ossicle is seen on the lateral projection over the dorsal aspect of the talonavicular joint. It must be distinguished from a fracture by observing bilateral x-rays. It is not a sesamoid bone (Figs. 3.3 and 3.4).

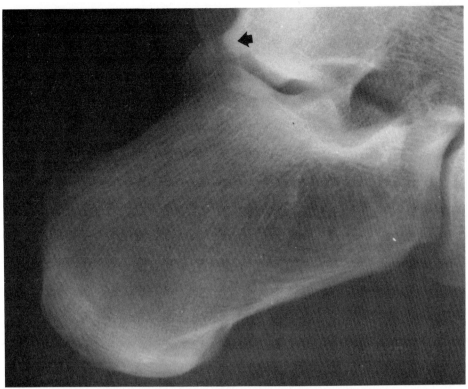

Figure 3.1. Os trigonum. A separate lateral tubercle of the talus.

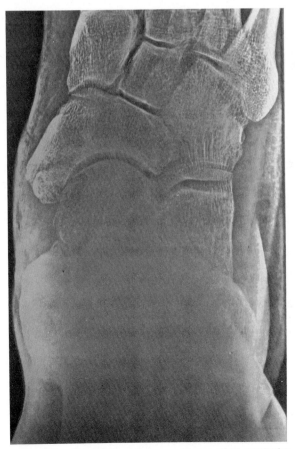

Figure 3.2. Os tibiale externum or secondary navicular.

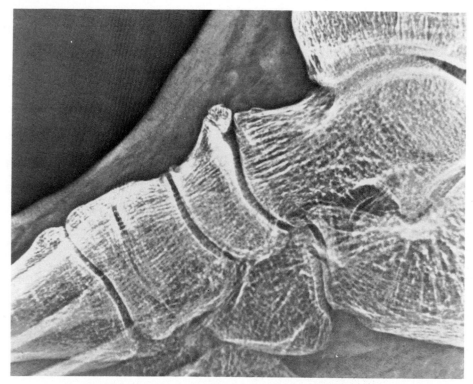

Figure 3.3.   Os supranaviculare or os supratalonaviculare.

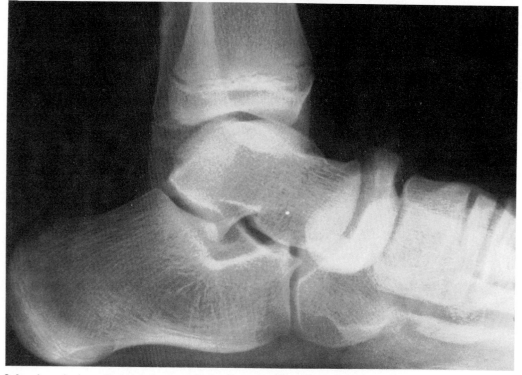

Figure 3.4.   A navicular with two primary centers of ossification must be distinguished from an os supranaviculare.

Os Interphalangeum of the Hallux

This is located below the interphalangeal joint of the hallux within the tendon of the flexor hallucis longus and is a sesamoid bone. Frequently, a nucleated clavus exists in the skin beneath this ossicle (Fig. 3.5).

Os Peroneum

The os peroneum is seen within the tendon of the peroneus longus and articulates with the plantar lateral aspect of the cuboid. While it is observable on both the DP and lateral projections, it is best viewed on the lateral oblique projection (Fig. 3.6).

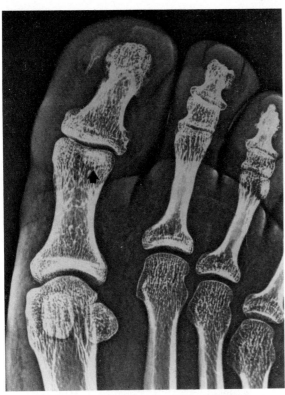

Figure 3.5.   Os interphalangeum of the hallux.

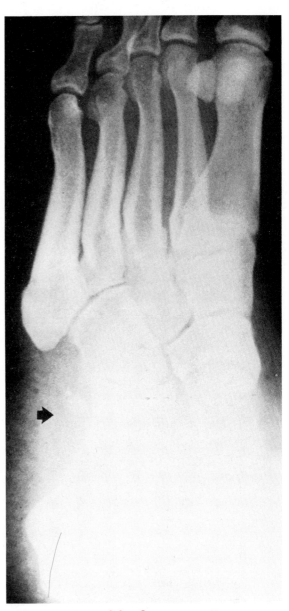

Figure 3.6.   Os peroneum.

Os Vesalianum

The os vesalianum represents a secondary ossification center of the base of the fifth metatarsal which has not fused with the shaft of the metatarsal. It is not commonly found, and must be distinguished from a fracture of the base of the fifth metatarsal via bilateral x-rays. It is not a sesamoid bone (Fig. 3.7).

Os Subtibiale

The os subtibiale is seen best on the mortise view of the ankle just below the tip of the tibia (Fig. 3.8).

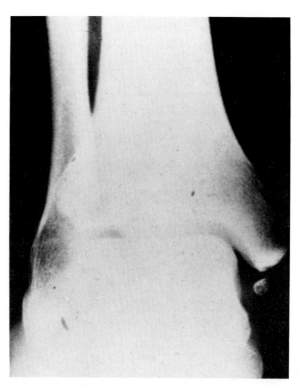

Figure 3.8.   Os subtibiale.

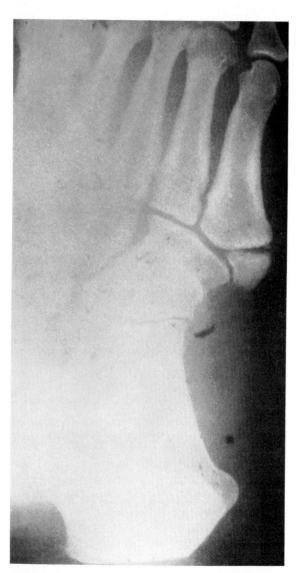

Figure 3.7.   Os vesaleanum must be distinguished from a fracture of the styloid of the fifth metatarsal.

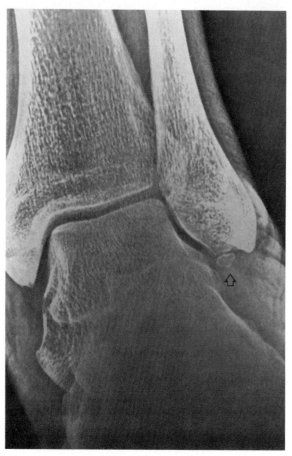

Figure 3.9.   Os subfibulare.

Os Subfibulare

This ossicle named for its location is best observed on the mortise view of the ankle just below the tip of the fibular malleolus. Os subfibulare and subtibiale must be distinguished from fractures of the malleoli (Fig. 3.9).

Secondary Talus

The secondary talus is observed on the lateral projection over the dorsum of the neck of the talus.

Os Sustentaculi

The os sustentaculi is found beneath the sustentaculum tali, and is best observed on an axial view of the calcaneus. It is a sesamoid bone (Fig. 3.10).

Os Intermetatarsium

Os intermetatarsium refers to either a small ossicle between the base of the first and second metatarsal bones on the dorsoplantar view, or to the very common sesamoids found either plantar or plantar medial to the lesser metatarsal heads (Fig. 3.11).

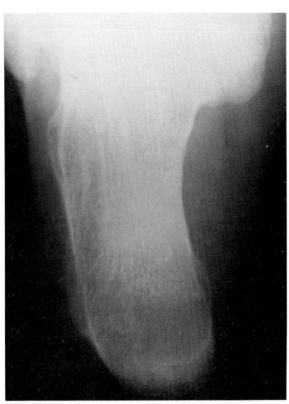

Figure 3.10.   A separate sustentaculum tali must be distinguished from an os sustentaculi.

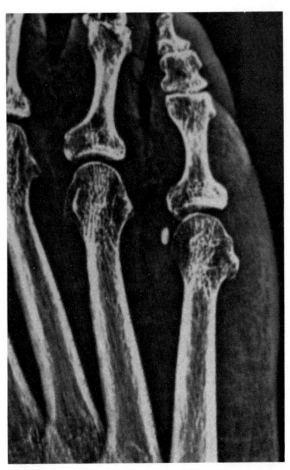

Figure 3.11.   Os intermetatarsium. Is a very common ossicle, and may be found next to any of the lateral metatarsal heads.

OSSIFICATION CENTERS

The feet of a newborn baby have all of the adult bones present at birth. However, a radiograph of an infant's foot will only show portions of a few of the bones that we would expect to see, because at this stage, the bones are mostly cartilagenous, and have not yet ossified. Only the ossified portion shows on the radiograph. The portion of the bones that begin to ossify first are termed primary centers of ossification. Certain bones, like the calcaneus, have more than one ossification center. These secondary centers of ossification usually are concerned with changing the shape of the bone, such as the tuberosity of the calcaneus.

When referring to ossification centers, the term epiphysis is used for a center that effects a change in length of a bone. Apophysis is a secondary growth center that is involved in changing the shape of a bone such as the calcaneal apophysis at the posterior portion of the calcaneus. The ossification centers are very important in determining the chronological age of a child. Some children do not develop properly and the bone age might be different from the birth age. This is especially true in premature infants. At birth, the primary centers of ossification that can be seen are the talus, the calcaneus, the cuboid, the shafts of the five metatarsals and the phalanges. Within the first months of growth, all of the phalanges, with a possible exception of the fifth digit, become ossified, and the lateral cuneiform appears. The navicular which is not observable at birth usually begins to ossify by the age of 3 years. Occasionally there is a delay in the ossification of the navicular that may be related to Köhler's disease. The delay in ossification of the navicular may be caused by excessive pronation, which causes pressure on the navicular from the abnormal position of the talus and interrupts the ossification by affecting circulation in the ossification center.

The sesamoids usually appear between the ages of 9 and 11. The second cuneiform appears between the ages of 9 months and 5 years, and the first cuneiform appears between the ages of 9 months and 4 years, and usually follows the second cuneiform in its ossification (Figs. 3.12 and 3.13)

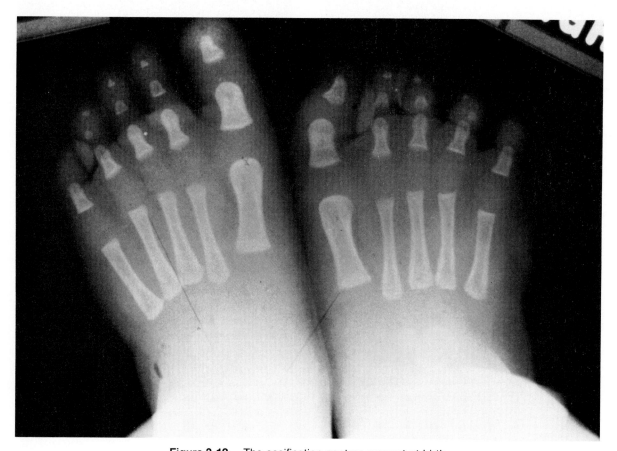

Figure 3.12.   The ossification centers present at birth.

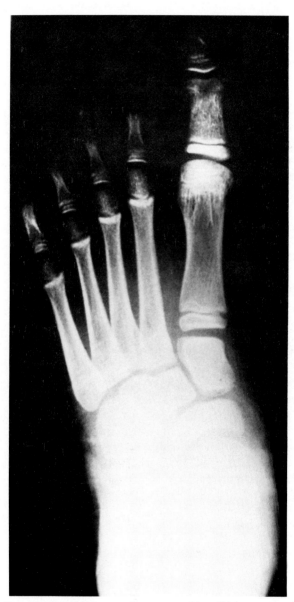

Figure 3.13. The ossification centers present in a thirteen-year-old patient.

SECONDARY CENTERS OF OSSIFICATION

The second through fifth metatarsals exhibit secondary centers of ossification in the head of these long bones. The first metatarsal shows a secondary center of ossification at its base and occasionally in the neck area. In the phalanges, the secondary centers of ossification are located at the base. The calcaneus is the only tarsal bone that has a constant secondary center for ossification. Long bones in general tend to have secondary centers of ossification, accounting for the growth in the length of the bones (Figs. 3.14 and 3.15).

REFERENCES

1. LEMONT, H.: Accessory navicular. J.A.P.A., **71**: 423, 1981.
2. CAMPBELL, W. C.: *Operative Orthopaedics*, 6th Ed, C. B. Mosby, St. Louis, 1980, vol. 2, p. 87.

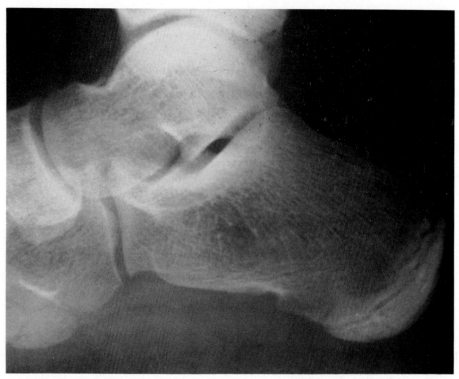

Figure 3.14. The calcaneal apophysis or secondary ossification center of the calcaneus.

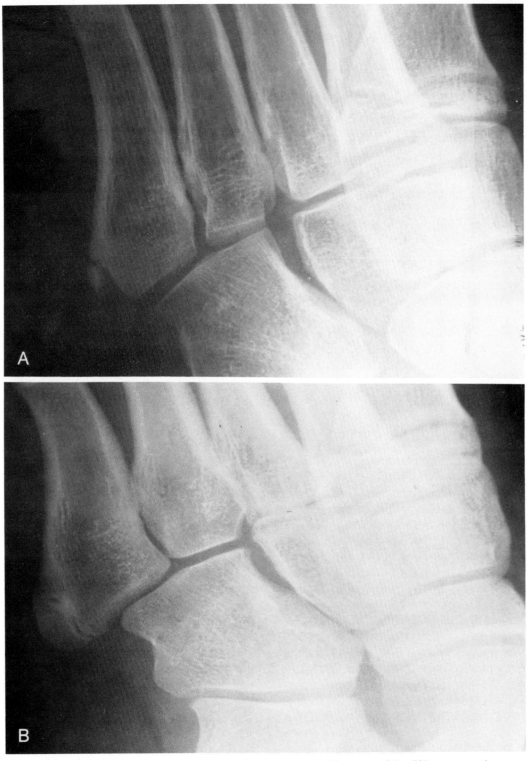

Figure 3.15.   *A* and *B*, secondary ossification center of the base of the fifth metatarsal.

CHAPTER 4

Biomechanically Acquired Foot Types

Over the years, orthopaedics of the foot has gone through many stages and phases, each of which has spawned a whole vocabulary of its own. Today we are in the biomechanical age, which represents a giant step forward in understanding the functions and mechanisms governing those functions of the lower extremity. A great deal of scientific research on the various foot types and pathological entities is now being performed.

From a radiographic point of view, a knowledge of certain angular relationships must be achieved before one can peform a "biomechanical evaluation." In order to validate the gross clinical findings, following an examination of a patient, a biomechanical evaluation can be performed on the radiographs taken. It must be remembered, however, that x-rays are never the sole means of making a diagnosis. They are just one of many findings that must be put together to arrive at a pertinent clinical assessment or diagnosis.

To facilitate this, the apparent positioning of the foot at the time the radiographs are taken is important. In 1967, Hlavac[1] first noted that, by changing the position of the foot when the radiograph was taken, the various angular relationships would change. A normal foot was made to appear pronated, normal, and supinated on three successive films by simply changing the position of the foot. This reinforced the development of the technique of angle and base of gait x-rays.[2]

Angle and base of gait x-rays are taken for a number of reasons. It is felt that by observing the patient in gait and trying to determine as closely as possible the appropriate angle and base of gait, and using this information to position the foot, it would allow the practitioner to place the foot in a position that most closely represents the average position of the foot in functioning. This would present the bones in their representative functional position.

Measurements taken in this position should have more relevance to an analysis of the structure of the foot than measurements taken with the feet placed randomly when the x-ray is taken. A study was performed in the late 1970s, in which this author participated, which definitively showed that there is a statistically significant difference in a number of angles that were measured of people whose feet were first placed in the angle and base of gait, and on a second x-ray were randomly placed on the x-ray films. (The patients placed their feet in a comfortable position before the x-rays were taken.) This study confirmed the earlier work of Hlavac and went on to quantify the normals for many of the angles that will be presented.[3]

Angle and base of gait radiographs offer another often overlooked advantage in that they allow the practitioner to take x-rays with the feet in a position that can very easily be reproduced from year to year. This can be of utmost importance when determining the results of a surgical procedure, or of any therapeutic measure. How can you place any dependance upon an analysis in which you do not control the position of the part being analyzed?[4]

MAJOR AXIS OF THE FOOT ON THE DORSOPLANTAR PROJECTION

Longitudinal Axis of the Rearfoot

The longitudinal axis of the rearfoot (Fig. 4.1) is defined as a line formed by two points: the bissection of the posterior surface of the calcaneus and the distal antero-medial corner of the calcaneus. If these points are available on an x-ray, they should be used to determine the longitudinal axis of the rearfoot. If they cannot be visualized, and very frequently the posterior aspect of the calcaneus cannot be visualized on a standard dorsoplantar film, then we are forced to use an alternate axis. If the lateral border of the calcaneus is relatively straight, we will use the distal portion of it as our longitudinal axis of the rearfoot. I recommend that this line be influenced by the trabecular pattern of the distal portion of the calcaneus. As a rough guide, most of the time the longitudinal axis of the rearfoot is roughly parallel to the long axis of the fourth metatarsal, although in many pathological instances this relationship does not hold true.[3,5,6]

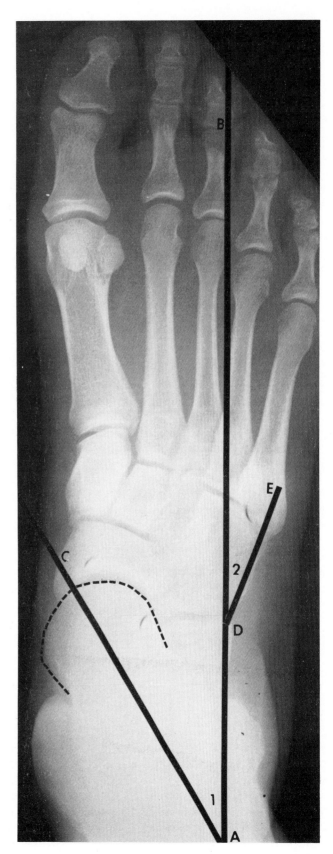

Figure 4.1. The longitudinal axis of the rearfoot (*line AB*) is constructed parallel to the lateral border of the calcaneus and is influenced by the trabecular pattern of the calcaneus. The head and neck of the talus are bisected, giving *line AC* the collum tali axis. *Angle 1,* or the talocalcaneal angle, is formed by the intersection of the longitudinal axis of the rearfoot and the collum tali axis. *Line DE* is parallel to the lateral border of the cuboid and intersects *Line AB* to form *angle 2*, the cuboid abduction angle.

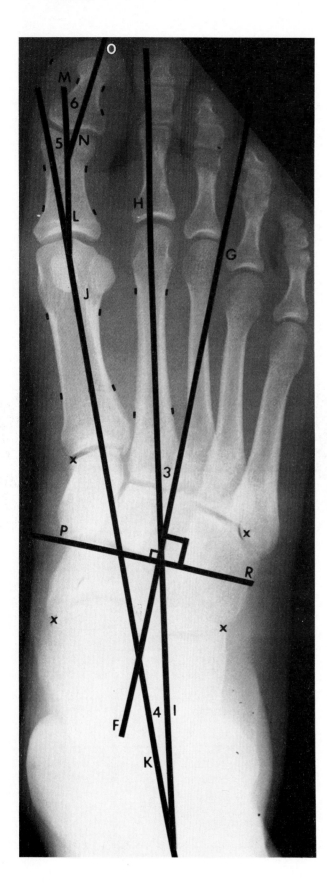

Figure 4.2.   The lesser tarsus is transected in the following manner. Point *P* is one-half the distance between the medial aspect of the talonavicular joint and medial aspect of the first cuneiform first metatarsal base joint, and point *R* is one-half the distance between the lateral aspect of the calcaneocuboid joint and the lateral aspect of the cuboid fourth metatarsal base joint. Connecting points *P* and *R* gives the transection of the lesser tarsus. A perpendicular is constructed to this line (*line FG*) which is the longitudinal axis of the lesser tarsus. The longitudinal axis of the metatarsus is represented by a bisection of the second metatarsal (*line HI*). The first metatarsal, first proximal phalanx, and the first distal phalanx all are bisected in a similar manner, giving *lines JK*, *IM*, and *NO*, respectively. The angle between the long axis of the lesser tarsus and the long axis of the second metatarsal, *angle 3*, is the metatarsus adductus angle. The angle between the axes of the first metatarsal (*line JK*) and the second metatarsal (*line HI*) is the metatarsus primus adductus or intermetatarsal angle (*angle 4*). The hallux abductus angle, or *angle 5*, is formed by *lines LM* and *JK*. The hallux interphalangeal angle (*angle 6*) is formed by the intersection of *lines LM* and *NO*.

Longitudinal Axis of the Lesser Tarsus

The longitudinal axis of the lesser tarsus (Fig. 4.2) is of use when comparing the positioning of the lesser tarsus to both the position of the metatarsus and the position of the greater tarsus. To find this, we must first transect the lesser tarsus. This is performed as follows.

The medial point is determined by taking one-half the distance between the medial aspect of the talonavicular joint and the medial aspect of the joint between the first metatarsal and first cuneiform. The lateral point is determined by taking one-half the distance between the lateral aspect of the calcaneocuboid articulation and the lateral aspect of the base of the first metatarsal. When determining this point in particular, we must be certain not to use the tip of the styloid process but the lateral aspect of the articulation between the cuboid and fifth metatarsal. If this point cannot be visualized, it will usually suffice to use the lateral proximal aspect of the base of the fourth metatarsal at its articulation with the cuboid. The two points thus determined should be connected, giving a transection of the lesser tarsus. A perpendicular to this transection yields the longitudinal axis of the lesser tarsus.[3,5,6]

Longitudinal Axis of the Metatarsus

The longitudinal axis of the metatarsus (Fig. 4.2) is constructed by bisecting the neck of the second metatarsal and the base end of the shaft (not the base) of the second metatarsal. Connecting these two points gives a longitudinal axis of the metatarsus. The second metatarsal is used because it would seem to be the stablest metatarsal.[3,5,6]

Longitudinal Axis of the Digits

A line passing longitudinally through the proximal phalanx of the second toe is considered to be the longitudinal axis of the digits (Fig. 4.2).[5,6]

ANGULAR RELATIONSHIPS ON THE DORSOPLANTAR PROJECTION

Talocalcaneal Angle

The talocalcaneal angle is formed by a line bisecting the head and neck of the talus, the collum tali axis, and the longitudinal axis of the rearfoot. Over the years, the method for constructing this angle has been changed many times; hence, the alternate names of Kite's angle and Harris and Beath angle.[5] The normal range for this angle is from approximately 17° to 21°. In pronation, the talocalcaneal angle will increase above the 21° point and in supination, it will decrease below 16°.

It is just as important to consider the total relationships in the rearfoot as it is to determine this number. Approximately 75% of the head of the navicular should articulate with the talus in the normal. When pronation occurs on x-ray, it would appear that the talus has moved in a medial direction away from the rest of the foot. What really does happen is that, because the talus is locked in the ankle mortise, it can move in a plantar direction, but cannot adduct, meaning that, the foot has moved in a lateral direction away from the talus, thus increasing the talocalcaneal angulation and causing the articulation between the talus and navicular to be less than 75%.[9] This motion will also change the relationship of the longitudinal axis of the talus with the head of the first metatarsal. In the normal, the axis of the talus should run through the center of the first metatarsal head. When pronation occurs, it will run medial to the first metatarsal head. And when supination occurs, it will project lateral to the first metatarsal head. In the pronated talocalcaneal relationship, a notch or talocalcaneal gap will be revealed between the head of the talus and the distal portion of the calcaneus on the dorsoplantar film.[3–8]

Cuboid Abduction Angle

The cuboid abduction angle (Fig. 4.1) is formed by a line representing the lateral aspect of the cuboid and the longitudinal axis of the rearfoot. The normal is from 0° to 5°. Above 5° is considered abnormal, and an adduction of the cuboid which would actually give a negative angle is also considered abnormal. When pronation involving the mid-tarsal joint occurs, the cuboid abduction angle tends to increase. When supination and adduction of the forefoot occurs, the angle can decrease past 0° into a negative angle.[3,5]

Talonavicular Angle

The talonavicular angle (Fig. 4.3) is constructed by using the collum tali axis and the transection of the lesser tarsus. (Perhaps a better name for this angle would be called the talo-lesser tarsus angle.) Normal should be in the 60° to 80° range. Pronation will bring the angle below 60° and supination will bring the angle above 80°. This seems to be a very vital angle in showing the relationship between the greater tarsus and lesser tarsus.

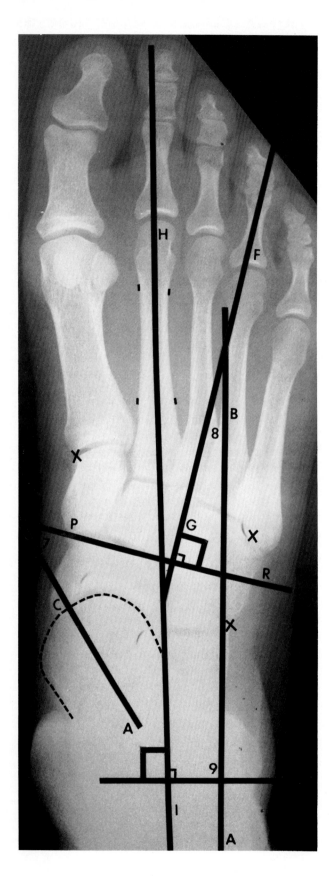

Figure 4.3.   The forefoot adductus angle is formed by the intersection of the longitudinal axis of the second metatarsal (*line IH*) and the longitudinal axis of the rearfoot (*line AB*). If these lines do not meet on the x-ray, the angle may be measured by constructing a perpendicular to *line IH* and measuring the angle that it forms with *line AB*, *angle 9*. 90° minus *angle 9* equals the forefoot adductus angle. The lesser tarsus angle, *angle 8*, is formed by the intersection of *lines FG* and *AB*. The talonavicular angle, *angle 7*, is formed by the intersection of *line AC*, the axis of the talus, and *line RP*, the transection of the lesser tarsus.

Lesser Tarsus Angle

The lesser tarsus angle (Fig. 4.3) is formed by the intersection of the longitudinal axis of the lesser tarsus and the longitudinal axis of the rear foot. This angle will tend to increase with pronation and can decrease with supination. It does not seem to be used as much in podiatry as the cuboid abduction angle and the talonavicular angle.[9, 10]

Forefoot Adductus Angle

The forefoot adductus angle (Fig. 4.3) is formed by the intersection of the longitudinal axis of the metatarsus (long axis of the second metatarsal) and the longitudinal axis of the rearfoot. This angle will tend to decrease as the forefoot abducts in pronation and will tend to increase when an adduction of the forefoot occurs. In pronation, when the forefoot is markedly abducted, this angle can actually become negative going below 0°. When the long axis of the second metatarsal is parallel to the long axis of the rearfoot, the angle is considered to be 0° (which is decreased). The ideal forefoot adductus angle is 8°. High normal is up to 12° to 14°. The forefoot is considered to be a rectus forefoot if the forefoot adductus angle is less than 12° to 14°. If it is above 12° to 14° degrees, the forefoot is said to be an adductus type of forefoot.[4–6]

Metatarsus Adductus Angle

The metatarsus adductus angle (Fig. 4.2) is formed by the intersection of the longitudinal axis of the metatarsus and the longitudinal axis of the lesser tarsus. The ideal metatarsus adductus angle is 8°, high normal is up to 12° to 14°. The metatarsus adductus angle does not change in pronation. It is considered to be a structural rather than a functional angle. Metatarsal adductus can be associated with a pronation of the foot.[5, 6, 11]

The metatarsus is considered to be a rectus metatarsus if the metatarsus adductus angle is less than 12° to 14°. If it is above 12° to 14°, the metatarsus is said to be an adductus type of metatarsus.

Metatarsus Primus Adductus Angle

The metatarsus primus adductus angle (Fig. 4.2), also known as the intermetatarsal angle, is formed by the intersection of the longitudinal axis of the first and second metatarsal shafts. The ideal intermetatarsal angle is 8°. If the forefoot and metatarsus are rectus then the intermetatarsal angle can normally go up as high as 14°. However, if the forefoot and metatarsus are adductus in nature, then the intermetatarsal angle can go up to a high of 12°. When we have an adductus in either the forefoot or metatarsus, it by nature makes the head of the first metatarsal more prominent medially, so the foot can only tolerate a lesser amount of intermetatarsal angle.[4–6, 12]

Hallux Abductus Angle

The hallux abductus angle (Fig. 4.2) is formed by the intersection of the longitudinal axis of the first metatarsal and the longitudinal axis of the proximal phalanx of the hallux. Normal is up to 15°. When the angle is increased above this level, it is said that there is a hallux abducto valgus deformity. In hallux varus or adductus, the angulation will be decreased below 0° to 5°.[4–6, 12]

Hallux Interphalangeal Angle

The interphalangeal angle of the hallux (Fig. 4.2) is formed by the intersection of the longitudinal axis of the proximal and distal phalanges of the hallux. Similar angulation can be measured between any two consecutive phalanges in the foot. The normal hallux interphalangeal angle is up to 8° to 10°. When this angle increases above this point, the distal portion of the hallux will be pointing in a lateral direction and may be impinging on the second digit.[5, 12]

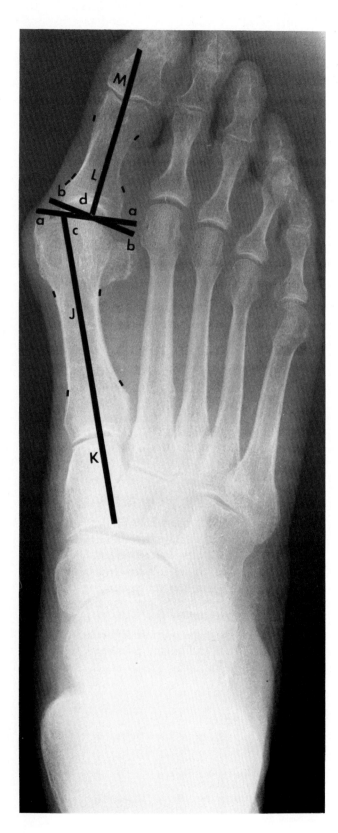

Figure 4.4.   The articular surface of the head of the first metatarsal is defined by *line aa* and the effective articular surface of the base of the proximal phalanx is defined by *line bb*. The proximal set angle is determined by subtracting *angle c*, the angle between *lines JK* and *aa*, from 90°. The distal articular set angle similarly is determined by subtracting *angle d*, the angle formed by the intersection of *lines bb* and *LM*, from 90°. The proximal articular set angle plus the distal articular set angle should add up to the hallux abductus angle.

Proximal Articular Set Angle

The proximal articular set angle (Fig. 4.4) is formed by a perpendicular to the effective articular surface of the first metatarsal head, and its intersection with the longitudinal axis of the first metatarsal. The normal for this angle is from 0° to 8°. In hallux abducto valgus, through bony adaptation and abnormal position, the proximal articular set angle will tend to increase above 8°, and is considered abnormal. The effective articular surface of the metatarsal head is determined by using the most lateral aspect of the articular surface of the first metatarsal head, and the most medial aspect of the functioning articular cartilage on the head of the first metatarsal. If a sagittal groove is present on the first metatarsal head, this point is used as the medial point.[12]

Distal Articular Set Angle

The distal articular set angle (Fig. 4.4) is formed by a perpendicular to the effective articular surface of the base of the proximal phalanx of the hallux, and its intersection with the longitudinal axis of the proximal phalanx. The normal for this angle is from 0° to 5° or 6°. This angle can tend to increase as the hallux enters an abductus position.[12]

MAJOR AXES OF THE FOOT ON THE LATERAL PROJECTION

Plane of Support

The plane of support (Fig. 4.5) on the lateral is determined by connecting two points. The first is the most plantar aspect of the tuberosity of the calcaneus, and the second is the most plantar aspect of the head of the fifth metatarsal.[5]

Calcaneal Axis

The axis of the calcaneus (Fig. 4.5) or calcaneal inclination axis is determined by connecting a point representing the most plantar aspect of the tuberosity of the calcaneus, with the most distal plantar aspect of the calcaneus (at the calcaneal cuboid joint).[5,13,14]

Collum Tali Axis

The axis of the head and neck of the talus (Fig. 4.5) or the collum tali axis is determined by performing a bisection of the head and neck (not to include the body) of the talus.[5,13,14]

First Metatarsal Declination Axis

The first metatarsal declination axis (Fig. 4.5) is determined by bisecting the neck and the base end (not the base) of the shaft of the first metatarsal and connecting these points.[4]

ANGULAR RELATIONSHIPS ON THE LATERAL FILM

Calcaneal Inclination Angle

The calcaneal inclination angle (Fig. 4.5) is the angle formed by the intersection of the plane of support and the calcaneal inclination axis. The normal is 18° to 22°. In a pronated foot, this angle can decrease significantly, and in a supinated foot, it can likewise increase significantly.[4,5,15,16]

Talar Declination Angle

The talar declination angle (Fig. 4.5) is the angle formed by the plane of support and the collum tali axis. This angle should be about 21°, and in the ideal foot, this axis will be co-linear with the first metatarsal declination axis. The first metatarsal declination angle is formed by the intersection of the first metatarsal declination axis and the plane of support. The normal should be approximately 21°.[4,5,15]

Cyma Line

The cyma line (Fig. 4.5) is another name for the mid-tarsal joint, or Chopart's joint. In the normal foot, the talonavicular and calcaneocuboid portions of Chopart's joint should be in line with each other to form a continuous S-shaped curve. In pronation, as the talus slides anteriorly, there will be an "anterior break" in the cyma line. The talonavicular portion will be located distal to the calcaneocuboid portion of this cyma line. When supination occurs, the talus moves posterior into the ankle mortise and the cyma line is said to have a "posterior break." The talonavicular portion of the cyma line in this state will be located proximally and superiorly to the calcaneocuboid portion of the cyma line.[4,5]

Sinus Tarsi

The sinus tarsi (Fig. 4.5) is seen on the lateral projection of the foot. It appears as an oval area of decreased bone density, separating the posterior from the middle subtalar facets. In a normal foot, it will appear to have an oval shape. When pronation occurs, as the talus rides anteriorly on the calcaneus and plantarflexes, the sinus tarsi is obliterated. The talar portion of the sinus tarsi will have moved anteriorly, and a portion of the body of the talus will be blocking the calcaneal portion of the sinus tarsi from view.[4] In a supinated foot, the sinus tarsi will take on the configuration of a "bullet hole."[4]

Lateral Talocalcaneal Angle

The lateral talocalcaneal angle (Fig. 4.5) is formed by the intersection of the calcaneal inclination axis, and the collum tali axis.[15]

BIOMECHANICAL RADIOGRAPHIC INTERPRETATION

Once all of the angles have been measured, they must be applied to the examination that has already been performed upon the foot. It must be emphasized that the radiographic interpretation can be quite helpful in analyzing the foot type and the symptomatology present, but it should not be used as the only means of making a diagnosis. It is only one of the inputs to be used in arriving at a diagnosis.

COMPENSATED REARFOOT VARUS

A rearfoot varus (Fig. 4.6) by definition is that condition in which when the subtalar and midtarsal joints are placed in their neutral positions and the midtarsal joint is loaded in a direction of dorsiflexion, the calcaneus is inverted with respect to the bissection of the lower one-third of the leg. It is obvious that, in this position, the calcaneus will be inverted. When it compensates, the calcaneus comes to the vertical position, and this becomes a mild to moderately pronated foot. On x-ray, we will see a normal to mildly increased talocalcaneal relationship on the dorsoplantar film. The amount of increase in this angle seems to depend upon the axis of the subtalar joint.[17] However, since the subtalar joint will be functioning in a pronated position, i.e., out of its neutral position, a certain degree of unlocking of the midtarsal joint will occur and this will be reflected as an increase in the cuboid abduction angle.

On the lateral film, the cyma line will be either normal or slightly broken in an anterior direction. The calcaneal inclination angle will vary between slightly increased to normal to slightly decreased. The talar declination angle will be within a relatively normal range, possibly slightly increased.

The sinus tarsi will be present to partially present. On occasions, when the amount of pronation in the rearfoot seems somewhat high for a rearfoot varus, a pseudosinus tarsi may be evident. In this instance, the posterior subtalar articulation seems wider anteriorly, and gives the appearance of a sinus tarsi. Observation of the calcaneal tuberosity in a normal or supinated foot will often show an apparent sclerotic line that represents the medial tubercle of the calcaneus. This is not visualized in a pronated foot.

COMPENSATED FOREFOOT VARUS

The next most severe form of pronation is the compensated forefoot varus (Fig. 4.7). By definition, a forefoot varus is that condition that exists when the subtalar joint and midtarsal joints are placed in their neutral positions and the midtarsal joint is locked in a position of dorsiflexion. The forefoot will be inverted with respect to the rearfoot. The rearfoot will usually be perpendicular to the ground unless a rearfoot varus is also present. If the patient were to walk in this position, the medial aspect of his foot would be off the ground.

Consequently, a compensation will occur which brings the medial side of the foot down to the ground. The usual compensation is via pronation in the rearfoot. If the rearfoot everts, it brings the forefoot down to the ground. In this instance, we will see a slight increase in the talocalcaneal angle above the normal 21°. The cuboid abduction angle will usually be increased as well. In some feet, there is a greater increase in the cuboid abduction angle with a lesser increase in the talocalcaneal angle, and vice versa. This seems to depend once again upon the direction of the axis of the subtalar joint. We notice, however, the axis of the talus will now be pointing medially to the first metatarsal head. There will be a talocalcaneal gap or notch and less than 75% of articulation of the head of the navicular with the talus. In the more severe variety, a wedge-shaped navicular will also be noted (the navicular usually is roughly rectangular). Frequently, in both forefoot and rearfoot varus conditions, there will be a short fifth metatarsal. This is possibly due to trauma on the epiphysis in the neck of the metatarsal. This extra trauma to the fifth metatarsal during gait due to the varus attitude results in early epiphyseal closure. In the more severe cases of compensated forefoot varus, the forefoot adductus angle will show a mild to moderate decrease.

On the lateral projection, there will be an anterior break in the cyma line and an absence of a

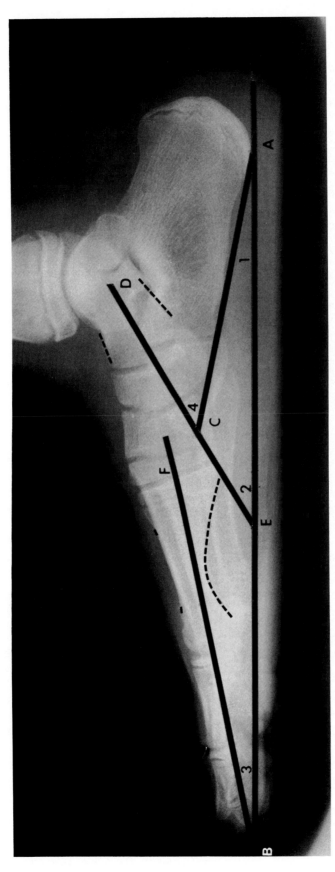

Figure 4.5. The plane of support is defined by connecting the most plantar aspect of the tuberosity of the calcaneus, point A, and the most plantar aspect of the head of the fifth metatarsal, giving *line AB*. The calcaneal inclination axis is formed by connecting point A with the most distal portion of the calcaneus plantarly, at the calcaneocuboid joint, giving *line AC*. *Angle 1*, the calcaneal inclination angle, is the intersection of *lines AC* and *AB*. The head and neck of the talus are bisected, yielding *line DE*, the collum tali axis. *Angle 2*, the talar declination angle, is the intersection of *lines DE* and *AB*. The first metatarsal declination axis is formed by bisecting the first metatarsal. It gives *line FB*. The first metatarsal declination angle, *angle 3*, is formed by the intersection of *lines AB* and *BF*. The lateral talocalcaneal angle, *angle 4*, is formed by the intersection of *lines AB* and *DE*.

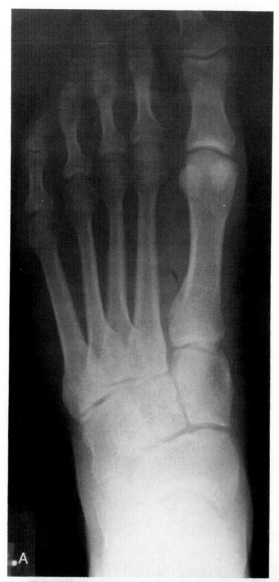

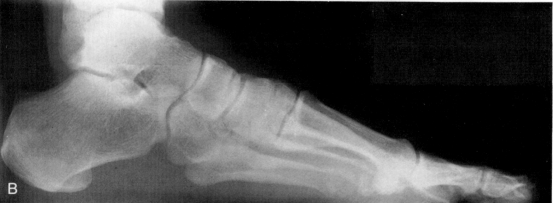

Figure 4.6.   *A* and *B*, in a compensated rearfoot varus the talocalcaneal angle is approximately normal, the cuboid abduction angle is normal to slightly increased, the calcaneal inclination angle is normal to slightly increased, and the talar declination angle is slightly increased. The cyma line may be normal or slightly broken anteriorly, and sinus tarsi may be present.

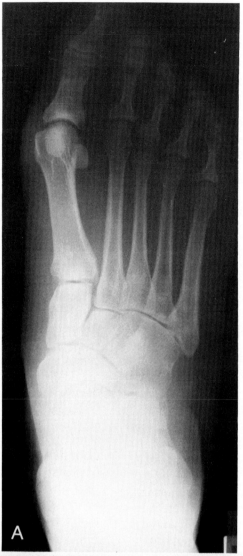

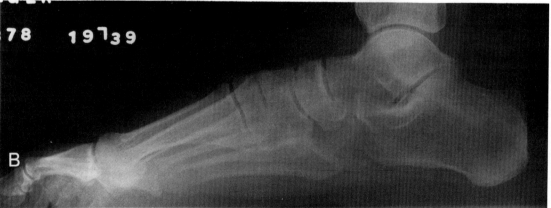

Figure 4.7. *A* and *B*, a compensated forefoot varus. In a compensated forefoot varus the talocalcaneal angle and cuboid abduction angles are increased. The navicular may be wedge-shaped. The forefoot adductus angle may be slightly decreased and hallux abducto valgus and hammer toe deformities are common. The calcaneal inclination angle may be normal to slightly decreased, the talar declination angle will be increased, and the sinus tarsi will be absent with an anterior break in the cyma line.

sinus tarsi. The calcaneal inclination angle will be normal to mildly decreased. When examining the tuberosity of the calcaneus, usually we can only see the lateral tubercle, due to the pronation. The medial tubercle is now rotated slightly out of the way, and it is invisible. The talar declination angle will usually be increased. In the normal, it seems to point through the first metatarsal head, and in this instance, it will be pointing below and proximal to the first metatarsal head. There will be a general sagging in the midtarsal area, producing a naviculocuneiform fault, and the first metatarsal declination angle will usually be decreased in this condition.

When hypermobility of the first ray is present, as in forefoot varus, there are two signs. The first sign is the naviculocuneiform fault, and the second sign is an abnormally wide split between the first and second cuneiforms on the dorsoplantar film. Hypermobility implies that there is motion at a time when there should be no motion.

EQUINUS

Equinus (Fig. 4.8) is that condition in which when the foot is maximally dorsiflexed (not pronated), there is a limitation of dorsiflexion of the foot upon the leg, such that the needed 5° to 10° of dorsiflexion is lacking. The equinus can either be due to a bony block or a "muscular" or soft tissue equinus. Either a gastrocnemius shortness or a gastrocnemius and soleus shortness can cause the soft tissue equinus. The implication that there is a limitation of **needed** dorsiflexion is important. In gait, the heel normally should remain on the ground for a certain period of time. If there is a lack of dorsiflexion or a shortness in the posterior muscle group, the heel cannot remain on the ground for an adequate amount of time, and normal gait cannot occur.

The foot reacts to this limitation of dorsiflexion in a number of ways. It cannot compensate at all, in which case the patient would be a toe walker. The heel would not be on the ground during gait. This seems to be most frequently seen in children. The more common compensation for this usually involves pronation and the development of an abducted gait. Pronation is a tri-plane motion involving dorsiflexion, eversion, and abduction (stated in the order of the greatest component first). The pronation can add some dorsiflexion to make up for a portion of the deficit. For this reason, equinus frequently compensates by a severe amount of pronation. There is a great deal of pronation available in the midtarsal joint, and

this joint will tend to sublux in the direction of the most force, consequently allowing dorsiflexion to occur.* Radiographically, there will be a very high talocalcaneal angle. On the dorsoplantar film in the severe cases of compensated equinus, the head of the talus will actually become somewhat pointed, the apex of the point being the most medial portion of the articulation between the talus and the navicular. On close examination, it can also be seen that the more medial non-articular portion of the head of the talus will appear somewhat atrophic. There will be a loss of trabeculation and of bone substance in this area.

A severe increase in the cuboid abduction angle, a very wedged-shaped navicular, and a marked decrease in the forefoot adductus angle will also ensue. Frequently, in this case, it will be abducted (the angle will be negative).

In the mild to moderate forms of flatfoot, patients will tend to develop bunions. In the *severely* compensated equinus, they will tend to not develop bunions, probably, because their gait becomes very apropulsive, and a major portion of the deforming force for a bunion and hallux abducto valgus is therefore absent.

On the lateral film, the calcaneal inclination angle will become quite low, sometimes as low as 8° to 10°. There will be an absence of the sinus tarsi, and a very high talar declination angle. A navicular cuneiform fault will be present, and a very low first metatarsal declination angle also will be seen. Frequently, in a severely pronated foot, a great deal of osteoarthritic spur formation will be noticed along the dorsal aspect of the tarsal joints, because of the constant microtrauma, and pinching of the dorsal aspects of these joints, from the dorsally directed stresses in this condition.

In the partially compensated equinus, there will frequently be a retrocalcaneal spur observed on the lateral film. There must be a great deal of stress at the insertion of the tendo achilles in the patient with an uncompensated or partially compensated equinus. If, because of the strong architecture of the foot, the foot is able to resist the deforming pull, eventually, the tendo achilles will pull away from its insertion into the posterior portion of the calcaneus. As it pulls away from the calcaneus (very slowly over a period of time), a mild inflammation occurs at its insertion, and this causes reactive new bone formation produced by the periosteum at the insertion of the tendo achilles. In effect, it ends up slightly lengthening the tendo achilles.

---

*Other forms of compensation can occur, such as genu recurvatum and early heel lift during midstance.

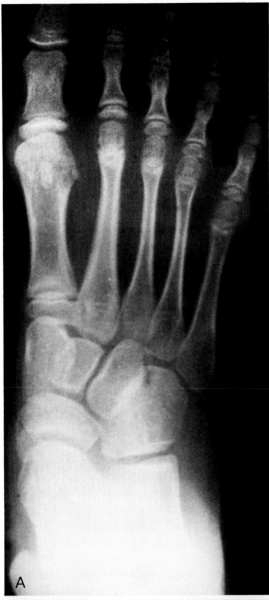

Figure 4.8.   *A* and *B*, compensated equinus. In a compensated equinus the talocalcaneal angle will be severely increased as will the cuboid abduction angle. The navicular will usually be wedge-shaped and the forefoot adductus angle will range from decreased to a negative value. In children the medial aspect of the head of the talus will be somewhat flattened and will show osteoporosis due to lack of use. On the lateral film, the calcaneal inclination angle will be quite low and the talar declination angle will be severely increased. The cyma line will be severely broken anteriorly and the sinus tarsi will be obliterated. On this lateral, a forefoot supinatus can also be observed. The metatarsals are piled one behind the other so that each one cannot be individually distinguished as in the normal. The soft tissues appear quite lacking in volume and are atrophic.

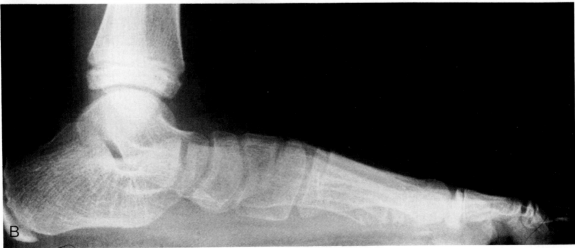

FOREFOOT SUPINATUS

Forefoot supinatus (Fig. 4.8) is not a cause of pronation, but is a result of pronation. It seems to occur mostly in very severe pronation. The rearfoot pronates so much that the forefoot assumes a relatively inverted or supinated position with respect to the rearfoot. This is primarily a soft tissue deformity. If the forefoot did not relatively invert with respect to the rearfoot, it would not remain flat on the ground during gait. There is controversy about whether this is a proper descriptive name and if in fact it is a relative supination that occurs as opposed to a dorsiflexion of the forefoot.

On physical examination, these patients will seem to have a forefoot varus that is extremely high, usually in the 12° to 18° range.

On the normal lateral film, all five of the metatarsals can be distinguished, and each has its own relative height. The first is the highest and the fifth is the lowest. In the patient with forefoot supinatus, all of the metatarsals will now have the same height. On visualization, you will not be able to distinguish any of the metatarsals from each other, because they are all piled up, one behind the other. The foot is exceptionally everted, abducted, and very flat. The intrinsic musculature in this foot will be atrophic. Therefore, on the lateral film, the foot will appear very thin, as though it has a loss of soft tissue mass.

FOREFOOT VALGUS

By definition, a forefoot valgus is when the subtalar and midtarsal joints are placed in their neutral positions, and the midtarsal joint is loaded in a direction of dorsiflexion. The forefoot will be everted with respect to the rearfoot. A forefoot valgus can compensate in either of two ways: flexible or rigid. A consideration of the sagittal plane relationships of the first ray is very important in considering the forefoot valgus. Some authorities have stated that flexible forefoot valgus is one of the most common forefoot deformities. This is somewhat debatable, and depends on the definition used by the observer. There are many feet in which the first metatarsal is lower than the remaining metatarsals. It is quite important to determine the amount of rigidity in the first ray, however.

In the non-weight-bearing position, we should be able to dorsiflex the first metatarsal approximately as much above the level of the second metatarsal head as we can plantarflex it below the

level of the second metatarsal head. If we find that the range of motion is normal, but the first metatarsal still seems to assume a plantarflexed position, this foot can be called a flexible forefoot valgus. It can also be called a forefoot varus (since usually the second through fifth metatarsals are in varus in this condition), with a flexible plantarflexed first ray. This foot, for all intensive purposes, will function as a forefoot varus would, because in gait, the flexible first ray will dorsiflex and the foot will sag into pronation as would a typical forefoot varus. Radiographically, it will appear the same as a forefoot varus.

In some cases, we can only dorsiflex the first metatarsal a limited amount. Usually it will dorsiflex some, but will not extend just as much above the level of the second metatarsal head as it will go below. In these cases, usually, the amount of motion of the first ray is normal, but it seems to be displaced in a plantarward direction. This foot can be referred to as a semi-rigid form of forefoot valgus (Fig. 4.9). In functioning, this foot will take on some of the characteristics of the rigid forefoot valgus, and some of the manifestations of the compensated forefoot varus. There will be a partial supinatory rock during gait, but with some pronation occurring after this aborted first supinatory rock occurs. Radiographically, this is a very difficult foot to determine. The talocalcaneal angle usually appears mildly increased, as will the cuboid abduction angle. The first metatarsal sometimes appears somewhat shortened in this foot. On the lateral film, the calcaneal inclination angle will be mildly increased usually in the 22° to 25° range. The first metatarsal declination angle may be from normal to slightly increased, and there will be a very mild posterior break in the cyma line. The talar declination axis will usually still point through the first metatarsal head, but the angle may be slightly increased.

In those cases in which the first metatarsal is rigidly plantarflexed, the diagnosis of rigid forefoot valgus is made (Fig. 4.10 and 4.11). In this case, usually, the first metatarsal at its most dorsal position is still well below the head of the second metatarsal. On examination it may be found to have a further range of plantarflexion available. This is one of the forms of a cavus foot. Some people refer to this as a local cavus, meaning that the first metatarsal and sometimes the fifth metatarsals are in a plantarflexed position, but the remaining metatarsals generally are not. There is a nucleated lesion present beneath the first and fifth metatarsal heads in this condition.

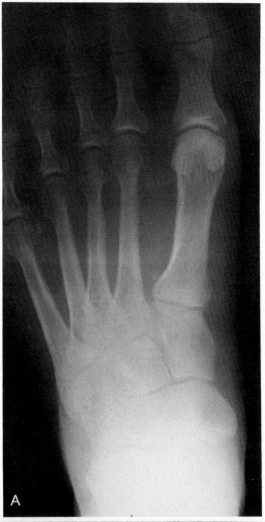

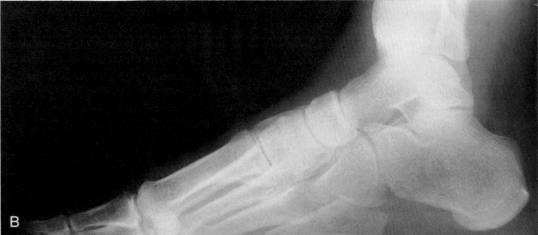

Figure 4.9.   *A* and *B*, semi-rigid forefoot valgus. In a semi-rigid forefoot valus the talocalcaneal angle will be normal to slightly increased, and the cuboid abduction angle will usually be somewhat increased. On the lateral film, the calcaneal inclination angle will be mildly increased, the talar declination angle will be increased, but the talar declination axis will still point through the head of the first metatarsal. The cyma line will be normal to slightly posteriorly broken. The sinus tarsi will be normal. Frequently, an exostosis of the neck of the talus will be seen (bony ankle equinus).

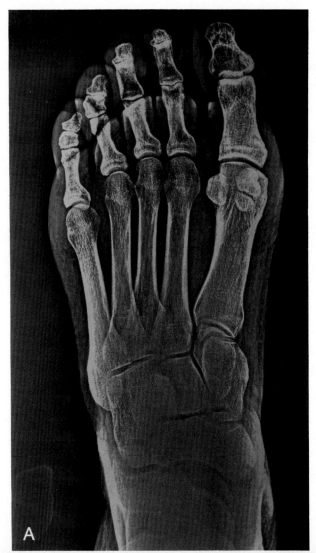

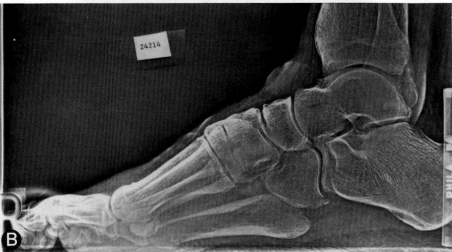

Figure 4.10.   *A* and *B*, rigid forefoot valgus. In a rigid forefoot valgus the talocalcaneal angle is decreased, the cuboid abduction angle usually is normal to slightly adducted or negative in value. The fifth metatarsal frequently is too short and frequently the first metatarsal is too short. There is mild lateral bowing of the fifth metatarsal on the dorsoplantar projection. On the lateral film, the calcaneal inclination angle is moderately increased, the talar declination angle is increased, but still points through the head of the first metatarsal. There will be a posterior break in the cyma line, and a normal sinus tarsi and ankle equinus usually is present.

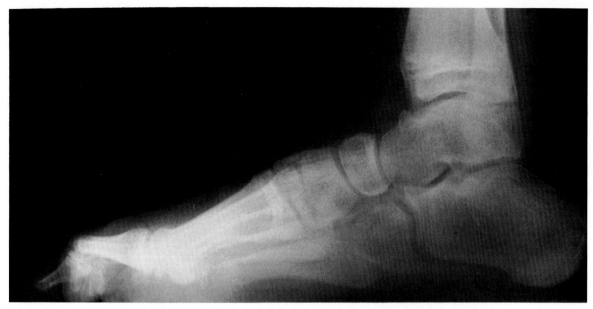

Figure 4.11.   Semi-rigid forefoot valgus with a much more pronounced ankle equinus. Note the exostosis on the dorsal aspect of the talus and on the distal anterior aspect of the tibia in this teenager.

On gait, the patient will tend to have a normal heel strike, but will not be able to pronate thereafter. There will be a supinatory rock as the progression of forces reaches the point where they should go through the first metatarsal head. They are not able to because of the plantarflexed position, and so the body shifts the weight to the lateral portion of the foot to get "around" the rigidly plantarflexed first ray. As this happens, it must be remembered that the fifth metatarsal does have a range of motion of its own, and it will usually dorsiflex and evert in response to the abnormal weight thrown on it at this point. On x-ray, the talocalcaneal angle will be decreased; the cuboid abduction angle will be normal to possibly slightly decreased. Very frequently, there will be a short first metatarsal, possibly due to early closure of the epiphysis, due to trauma. There will be lateral bowing of the fifth metatarsal and possibly the fourth metatarsal. This lateral bowing is due to the fact that the fifth metatarsal (and also the fourth at times) will dorsiflex and evert in response to the position of supination. As they evert, we begin to see a portion of the plantar contour of the metatarsal giving it a bowed appearance. On the lateral projection, the calcaneal inclination angle will be moderately increased. This gives a measurement of from 25° to 30°. The first metatarsal declination angle will be increased, the talar declination angle will be increased, and very frequently the first metatarsal declination axis and the collum tali axis will be colinear. A posterior

break in the cyma line will be seen, and a bony or ankle equinus will be present.

The bony or ankle equinus manifests itself as a dorsal exostosis on the neck of the talus, and an exostosis on the distal anterior aspect of the tibia. In the normal foot, the neck of the talus is placed so that, in extreme dorsiflexion, the distal anterior aspect of the tibia fits into the neck of the talus preventing trauma. When micro-trauma occurs in the form of a bony impingement of the talus upon the tibia, exostosis formation will eventually ensue, and can thus be observed on x-ray.

The posterior break in the cyma line probably results because of two basic mechanisms. As the subtalar joint supinates, there is a mild screw-like motion that occurs so that the talus moves slightly posteriorly with respect to the rest of the foot. Also, there must be a retro-grade force from the ground pushing up along the medial ray of the foot. This will tend to push the talus further back into the ankle mortise, giving both a posterior break in the cyma line and also causing the bony impingement known as ankle equinus or bony equinus.

UNCOMPENSATED REARFOOT VARUS

Uncompensated rearfoot varus (Figs. 4.12 and 4.13) usually manifests itself as a true cavus foot. When the subtalar joint is in its neutral position, the calcaneus is inverted with respect to the ground. The compensation that occurs frequently

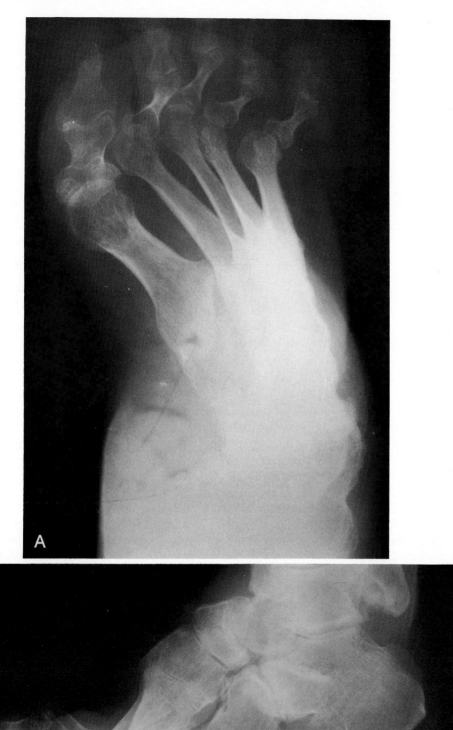

Figure 4.12. *A* and *B*, cavus foot. The true cavus foot shows a very low talocalcaneal angle and a normal to adducted cuboid abduction angle. The metatarsals will be in either an adducted or varus position. The calcaneal inclination angle will be quite high, and there may be a secondary equinus in which the calcaneus will be lifted off the ground. The talar declination angle is very low and there may be a plantarflexion of the forefoot, as seen in this post-polio spastic foot.

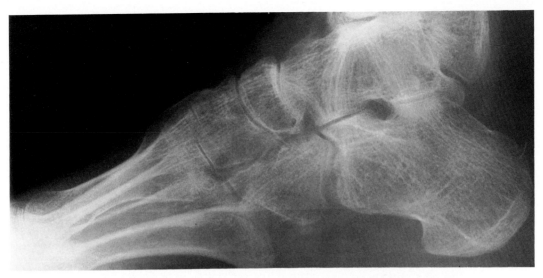

Figure 4.13. A lateral projection in an uncompensated rearfoot varus type of cavus foot.

is by a plantarflexion of the first ray, which can tend to further exentuate the inversion in the rearfoot. This foot will tend to have a hyperdeclination of all the metatarsals, and a thickened callus across the entire submetatarsal head area of the forefoot. On the dorsoplantar film, it will be seen that the talus articulates 100% with the navicular, and the talar axis points lateral to the first metatarsal head. The cuboid abduction angle will either be normal to somewhat decreased. Very frequently, the metatarsals will be in a varus position. This foot type frequently represents the untreated or unsuccessfully treated talipes equino varus. The metatarsals will overlap considerably at their bases, and the mid-foot region will appear very narrow when compared to the normal and the pronated foot. Usually, all the lesser digits will be contracted into a claw-toe configuration. On the lateral projection, the calcaneal inclination angle will be quite high from 28° to 30° and much higher. The talar declination angle will be decreased, and the collum tali axis will usually point dorsal to the first metatarsal head. The first metatarsal declination angle will usually be increased. There will be a normal cyma line and sinus tarsi will have a "bullet hole" configuration.

In this foot type, there can be observed an intersection of the collum tali axis and the first metatarsal declination axis. The location of this intersection can be used to classify the foot as an anterior, middle, or posterior cavus. In the anterior cavus, the intersection would be in the vicinity of the first metatarsal cuneiform articulation. In the middle cavus, it would be located in the vicinity of the naviculocuneiform articulation,

and in the posterior cavus, it would be located posterior to that point.

TARSAL COALITIONS

A number of conditions exist in which there is either a bony or a cartilaginous bridge or coalition between two or (more) of the tarsal bones (Fig. 4.14). The most commonly seen tarsal coalitions are the talocalcaneal, calcaneonavicular and talonavicular. These coalitions cause a limitation of motion or an absence of motion of the involved joint and this can obviously affect the entire foot in gait. This limitation of motion tends to cause two of the pathognomonic signs of tarsal coalition, i.e., peroneal spasticity and talonavicular beaking. The most common muscle spasticity is that of the peroneals, which leads to a rigid flatfoot deformity. On very rare occasions, the anterior muscle group has been known to be spastic, in which case a supinated foot occurs.

On the lateral x-ray film, a large exostosis at the dorsal aspect of the talonavicular articulation is considered to be talonavicular beaking, which can be observed as early as 6 to 8 years of age. It seems to develop first as a small point at the dorsal aspect at the head of the talus, the navicular being affected later on in the progression. It must be recognized that the beaking is a degenerative arthritic manifestation and can also be seen in all of the intertarsal articulations. In cases of talocalcaneal coalition, occasionally a "halo sign" can be observed on the lateral projection. The halo is seen around the sinus tarsi.

When evaluating the foot for a tarsal coalition, certain standard views must be taken: the Isher-

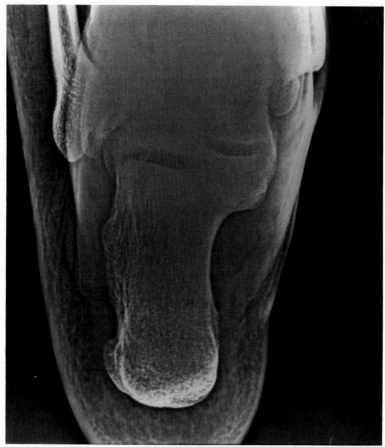

Figure 4.14.   Normal Harris and Beath projection. Both the posterior and middle subtalar facets should be present; they should be parallel to each other and parallel to the bottom of the film. The facets must be complete.

wood views, consisting of a 45° and 60° lateral oblique projection; and the Harris and Beath or ski-jump views. The 45° oblique is used to check for a calcaneonavicular bar. The 60° oblique is used to observe the anterior subtalar joint facet to determine if it is coalesced. The ski-jump views will allow for an examination of the posterior and middle subtalar joint facets.

These facets should be parallel to each other, parallel to the ground, and should both be present and complete. If they are present and complete, but are not parallel to each other, a functional coalition occurs. This indicates that because of the excessive angulation between these two facets, the normal range of subtalar joint motion cannot occur. On the lateral film, the posterior and middle subtalar joint facets should be parallel to each other, and should not exhibit signs of degenerative arthritis, including bony sclerosis and narrowing (Figs. 4.15 to 4.18).[18–24]

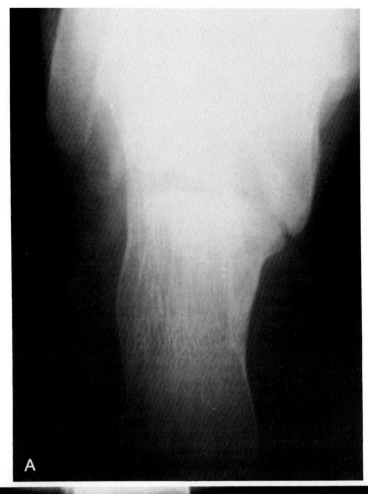

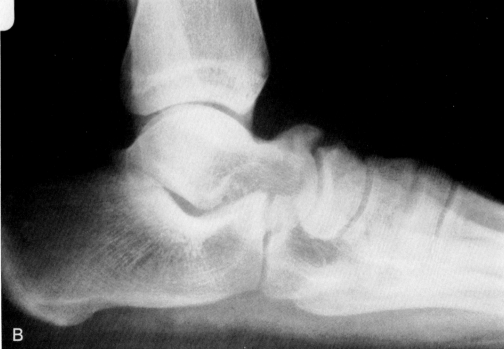

Figure 4.15.   *A* and *B*, a functional subtalar coalition. This Harris and Beath view reveals that the subtalar joint facets are neither parallel to each other nor are they parallel to the bottom of the film. The joint spaces are quite uneven and arthritic. On the lateral projection, beaking of the talonavicular articulation is present.

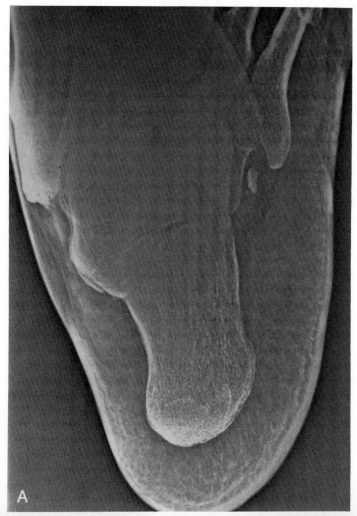

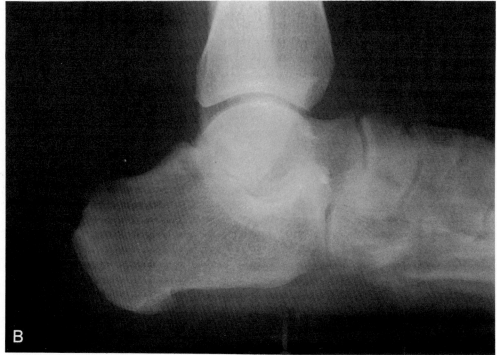

Figure 4.16. (*A* and *B*)

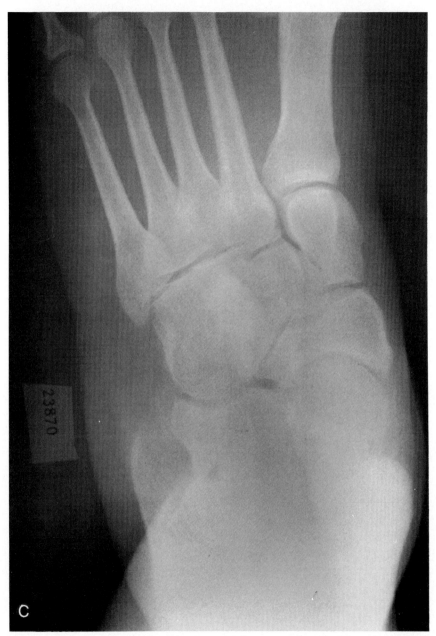

Figure 4.16. *A* to *C*, subtalar coalition. The middle subtalar joint facet is completely absent on the Harris and Beath projection. The lateral film shows early beaking of the talonavicular articulation while the dorsoplantar film merely shows severe pronation with wedging of the navicular.

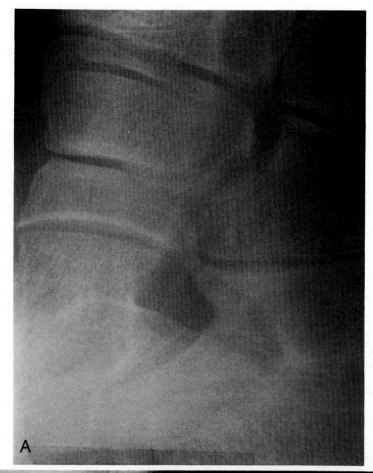

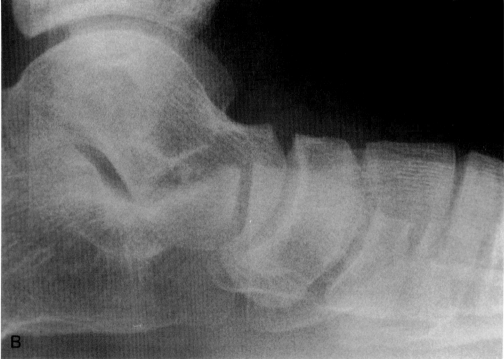

Figure 4.17.   *A* and *B*, calcaneonavicular coalition. A calcaneonavicular bar is noted on the oblique projection; early beaking of the talonavicular articulation is seen.

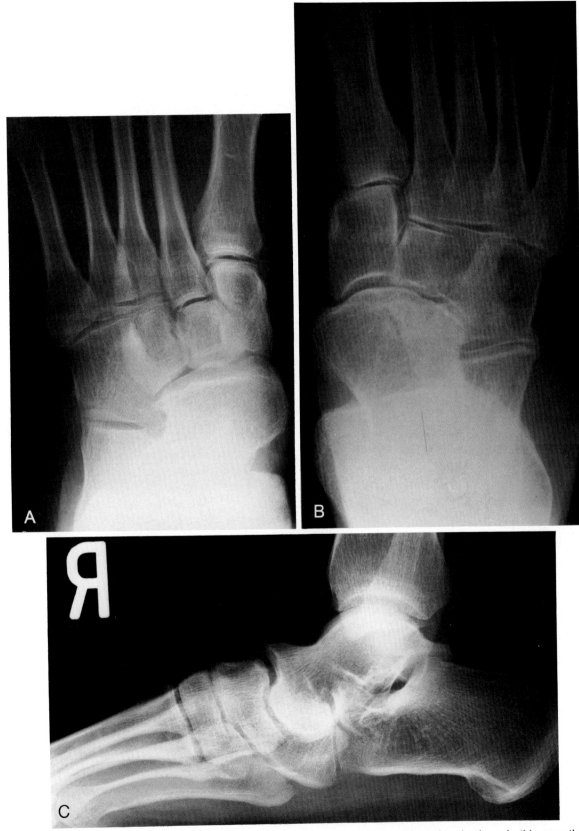

Figure 4.18. *A* to *C*, a talonavicular bar is observed on the dorsoplantar and lateral projections. In this case there was pain in the midtarsal joint area, and arthritic changes of the naviculocuneiform joint can be seen.

REFERENCES

1. HLAVAC, H. F.: Differences in x-ray findings with varied positioning of the foot. J.A.P.A., **57:** 465, 1967.
2. SGARLATO, T. E.: The angle of gait. J.A.P.A., **55:** 645, 1965.
3. GREEN, D., WEISSMAN, S. D., ET AL.: Roentgenologic analysis: Angle of base of gait versus random positioning in relation to reducing x-ray exposure. Study performed at Pennsylvania College of Podiatric Medicine, 1977.
4. GAMBLE, F. O., AND YALE, I.: *Clinical Foot Roentgenology*, 2nd Ed, Krieger, Huntington, NY, 1975.
5. SGARLATO, T. E.: *A Compendium of Podiatric Biomechanics*, California College of Podiatric Medicine, San Francisco, 1971.
6. ROOT, M. L., ORIEN, W. P., WEED, J. H., AND HUGES, R. T.: *Biomechanical Examination of the Foot*, Clinical Biomechanics, Los Angeles, 1971, Vol 1.
7. KITE, J. H.: *The Clubfoot*, Grune & Stratton, New York, 1964.
8. HARRIS, R. I., AND BEATH, I.: Hypermobile flatfoot with short tendoachilles. J. Bone Jt. Surg., **30A:** 116, 1948.
9. GIANNESTRAS, N. J.: *Foot Disorders*, Lea & Febiger, Philadelphia, 1976.
10. GIANNESTRAS, N. J.: Flexible valgus flatfoot resulting from naviculocuneiform and talo-navicular sag. *Foot Science*, ed by J. E. Bateman, WB Saunders, Philadelphia, 1976, pp. 67–105.
11. PONSETI, I., AND BECKER, J.: Congenital metatarsus adductus: The results of treatment. J. Bone Jt. Surg., **48:** 705, 1966.
12. LaPORTA, G., MELILLO, T., AND OLINSKI, D.: X-ray evaluation of hallux abducto valgus deformity. J.A.P.A., **64:** 544, 1974.
13. ALTMAN, M. I.: Sagittal plane angles of the talus and calcaneus in the developing foot. J.A.P.A., **58:** 463, 1968.
14. WHITNEY, A. K.: *Radiographic Charting Technique*, Pennsylvania College of Podiatric Medicine, Philadelphia, 1978.
15. DiGIOVANNI, J. E., AND SMITH, S. D.: Normal biomechanics of the adult rearfoot: A radiographic analysis. J.A.P.A., **66:** 812, 1976.
16. LEWIS, M. R.: *Atlas of Foot Roentgenology*, Edwards Brothers, Ann Arbor, 1967, pp. 301–325.
17. MANTER, J. T.: Movements of the subtalar and transverse tarsal joints. Anat. Rec. **80:** 297, 1941.
18. CONWAY, J. J., AND COWELL, H. R.: Tarsal coalition: Clinical significance and roentgenographic demonstration. Radiology, **92:** 799, 1969.
19. HARRIS, R. I., AND BEATH, T.: John Hunter's specimen of talocalcaneal bridge. J. Bone Jt. Surg., **32B:** 203, 1950.
20. GOLD, G. S.: Tarsal coalitions: Clinical significance, diagnosis and treatment. J.A.P.A., **61:** 11, 1971.
21. HEATS, T. E., AND HARRISON, R. B.: *Hypertrophy of the Talar Beak*, International Skeletal Society, 1979, pp. 37–39.
22. GOLD, G. S.: Tarsal coalitions: Clinical significance, diagnosis and treatment. **61:** 409, 1971.
23. GREEN, D. R., SGARLATO, T. E., AND WITTENBERG, M.: Clinical biomechanical evaluation of the foot. J.A.P.A., **65:** 732, 1975.
24. JACOBS, A. M., SOLLECITO, V., ET AL.: Tarsal coalitions: An instructional review. J. Foot Surg., **20:** 239, 1981.

CHAPTER 5

Radiology of the Foot in Pediatrics

RICHARD JAY, D.P.M.

A proper evaluation of the pediatric foot is of utmost importance in podiatric medicine. Most major deformities are present at birth, or develop shortly thereafter, and are more easily correctable in the pediatric patient. It makes sense to begin treatment at the earliest possible date. If the major problems are corrected in childhood, then in adulthood the patient will not be plagued with the usual static forefoot deformities that we see so often.

THE NORMAL FOOT

From birth to approximately 2 years of age there is a large space seen on x-ray between the talus and calcaneus. Actually, the two bones are articulating with each other, but on x-ray only the calcified portions can be observed. These spaces are completely filled with cartilagenous bone. On the lateral film the talus will appear distal to the calcaneus even though its position is probably completely normal. This is strictly due to the location of the ossification centers. The navicular does not usually appear on x-ray until age 3 to 5. It is usually the last bone to appear. In a very young child most of the phalanges are present; all of the metatarsals are present, as are the talus, calcaneus, cuboid, and often the lateral cuneiform. The first and second cuneiforms and navicular are not present at this time.

In the age group 2 to 5 years old, first the middle cuneiform will begin to calcify, followed by the medial cuneiform. The navicular finally will begin to ossify between the ages of 3 to 5. The appearance of the navicular may be delayed past the normal time, usually due to excessive pronation.

From the 5th through 12th years, not much change in the foot occurs. Most of the bones have appeared with the exception of the sesamoids.

They ossify between the years 9 and 11. The calcaneal apophysis appears at approximately the age of 8 years, and usually fuses with the body of the calcaneus by 12 or 13. It should be stressed that an epiphysis is involved in the growth of the length of a bone. An apophysis is involved in changing the shape of a bone. The calcaneal apophysis becomes the calcaneal tuberosity.

Foot problems that are present in adults are usually present during childhood, but often go undiagnosed because the patients are not seen by a podiatrist early enough. Frequently, parents are told by other practitioners that the child will outgrow the deformity, but this rarely, if ever, occurs.

As the child grows older, the angles between the different metatarsals increase, until they reach the normal adult spacing.

CLUB FOOT

The word "talipes" comes from the Latin *tal*, meaning "talus," and *pes*, meaning "foot." Talipes is usually used together with a second word describing the abnormal position of the talus and foot. There are six different positions that are described when discussing a club foot. These positions are: dorsiflexion, plantarflexion, inversion, eversion, adduction, and abduction. The dorsiflexed position is referred to as calcaneus, the plantarflexed position is referred to as equinus. Inversion is called varus, eversion is called valgus. Adduction is described by adducto- and abduction is described as abducto-. When the term "club foot" is used alone without any descriptive term following, it usually refers to the condition equino varus ("equino-," meaning the toes are lower than the heel or plantarflexed, and "varus-," meaning the fixed position of the foot in inversion).

When describing a club foot, it is important to remember, that the abnormal position should be

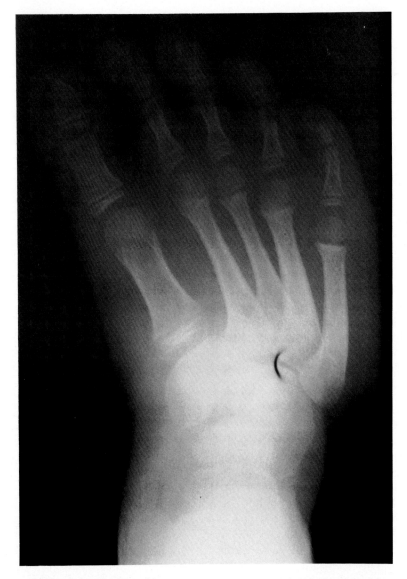

Figure 5.1. Equino-adducto-varus. Equino-adducto-varus on x-ray must be distinguished from metatarsus adductus. In this condition, the talocalcaneal angle is very low, the metatarsus is adducted, and in a varus position.

described in all three planes, so the usual equino varus really should be talipes equino-adducto-varus. The club foot may be either a soft tissue or an osseous deformity. Probably the abnormal position comes first, followed by a change in the shape of the bones and soft tissues to conform to the abnormal position.

There are many theories that have been developed over the years to explain why club feet develop. Included among these are:

(1) Arrested anomalus development of the extremities in the embryo. Certain bones continue to show normal growth, while in others the growth becomes arrested. The end result of this will be an abnormal position of the foot at birth.

(2) Abnormal position of the extremities which occurs because of the failure of certain preplanned motions or torsions to occur. This theory seems more believable than the prior theory. Certain preplanned motions should occur to the embryo *in utero*. At the 3rd month of gestation, for example, the foot is normally in an equino-adducto-varus position. As the fetus develops, an inward rotation of the leg occurs so that by the 7th month of gestation, the foot is usually in a normal position. If the preplanned rotation fails to occur, the foot will remain in an equino-varus position.

(3) A number of other factors have been implicated, including a small-size uterus, tight amniotic membranes, a large child, and a breach or transverse lie of the fetus.

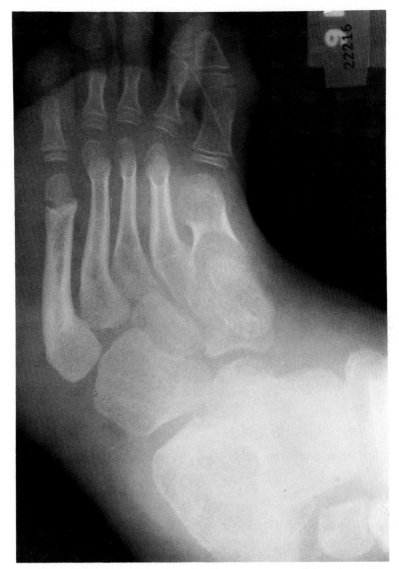

Figure 5.2. Equino-adducto-varus with deformity in the shape of the talus and metatarsals.

Talipes Equino-Adducto-Varus

The equino-adducto-varus club foot is twice as common in males as it is in females, and is more common in one foot than it is bilateral. It seems to run in families, probably being due to the patient's genetic makeup.

In talipes equino varus, the achilles tendon becomes shorter secondary to the plantarflexion (Figs. 5.1 and 5.2). The anterior and posterior tibial tendons become contracted, also secondary to the abnormal inversion of the foot. The ligaments and capsules on the medial side of the foot become shortened, thickened, and contracted, and the opposite occurs on the lateral side of the foot; the capsules and ligaments being elongated,

thinned, and stretched. The neck of the talus becomes shortened and deviated medially and plantarly. The subtalar articular surfaces are in a varus and equinus position. The calcaneus is at times shortened and wider than normal, and the posterior portion of the talus may become wedge-shaped from top to bottom as it is squeezed between the calcaneus and the tibia.

Radiographically, the angle between the talus and calcaneus on the dorsoplantar film will become decreased as the calcaneus moves further beneath the talus in this condition. A torsion of the tibia and fibula can occur, and this will be visualized as an abnormal position of the fibula on the lateral film. The talus will appear plantar-flexed, as will the entire foot on the lateral film.

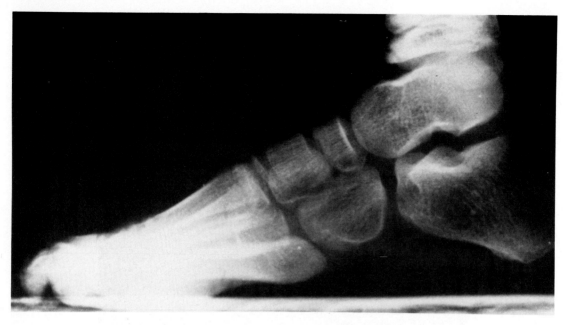

Figure 5.3. Cavus in a 7-year-old boy. There is increased calcaneal inclination and the bisection of the talus runs superior to the first ray. Marked heel varus is noted.

The metatarsals on the dorsoplantar film will be in an adducto-varus position. This must be distinguished from metatarsus-adductus.

Equinus (Spastic Deformities)

The spastic equinus foot results from a neurologic condition which causes a spastic plantarflexed position of the foot at the ankle. The deformity may be caused by any one of several interactions: the gastroc-soleus complex can be partially or entirely spastic, or a weakness of the anterior muscles can result in relative overpowering by the posterior muscles (Figs. 5.3 to 5.7).

When we compare the anterior and the posterior muscles in a normal person's gait pattern, we find that the triceps surae begin to function soon after heel contact. The soleus itself becomes active when the leg moves forward, causing a stabilizing plantarflexory force. As the forward movement of the leg continues, it promotes a stretch reflex in the gastrocnemius muscle, which fires and transmits a force that plantarflexes the foot at the ankle. This continues through toe-off. The anterior muscles are active mainly during "swing phase."

It must be remembered that in normal gait dorsal flexors are not antagonists to the gastroc-soleus complex, since they do not function during the same interval of the gait cycle. This, however, is not true in the presence of a spastic equinus. The gastroc-soleus complex is spastic throughout the gait cycle. The gait is no longer that of heel-to-toe; the pattern becomes one of a toe-to-toe with the spastic condition of the triceps surae being so tight that not even the child's weight can force the rearfoot down. If the triceps spasticity is of a lesser quality, the heel may come down after the toe touches or the entire foot may strike in a plantargrade fashion. This depends upon the degree of spasticity of the gastroc-soleus complex in relation to the function of the anterior muscles.

Considering the above, we see that the primary cause of the equinus deformity is the unequal balance between flexor and extensor muscles.[2]

Calcaneovalgus (Talipes Calcaneo-Abducto-Valgus)

This form of club foot represents the superpronated foot. Frequently in children with this deformity it is possible to dorsiflex the foot until the dorsum of the foot touches the anterior aspect of the leg. It is a triplane deformity as described in the name.

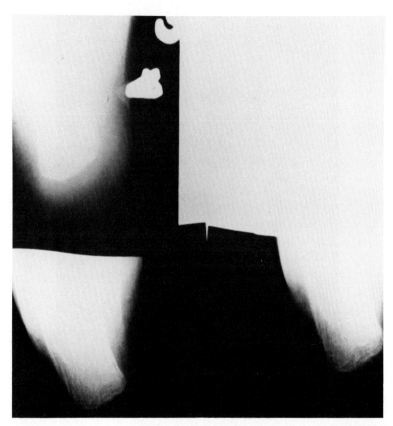

Figure 5.4.   Cavovarus in a 7-year-old boy. A tight tendo-achilles exterts a medial pull on the calcaneus causing a marked rearfoot varus. A 0° projection of the heel comparing a normal foot (*top*) with heel varus (*bottom two projections*). Due to the constant pull of the tight tendo-achilles medially, torquing the bone inward, the bone has adapted.

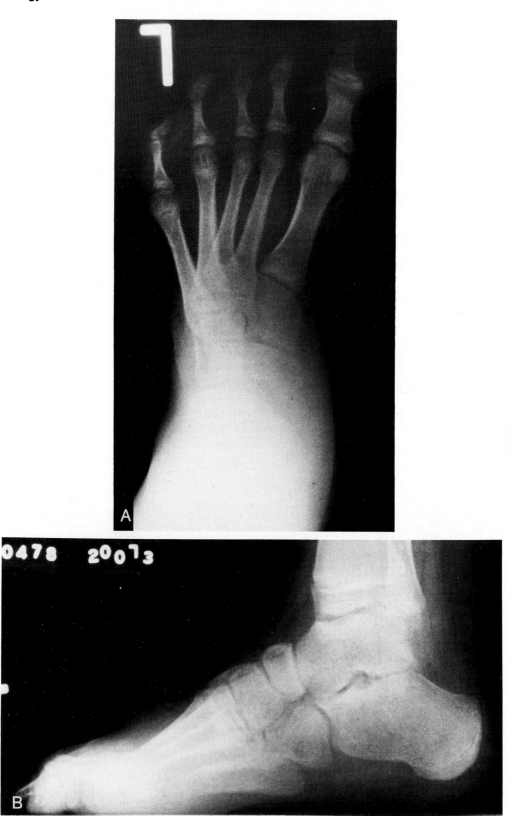

Figure 5.5.   Neurological cavus. *A*, neurological cavus in a 15-year-old male. A narrow talocalcaneal angle and marked supination of the subtalar joint with adductus of the forefoot is present. *B*, high calcaneal inclination and low talar declination are seen with the talus pointing superior to the plantarflexed first ray. The talus has rotated laterally, giving an x-ray appearance of a flat-topped talus.

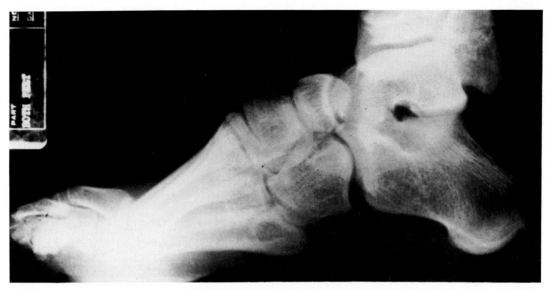

Figure 5.6.   Cavus deformity, secondary to Charcot Marie Tooth disease in a 15-year-old female who was a chronic ankle sprainer. Heel varus, subtalar varus, and a rigid forefoot valgus were noted.

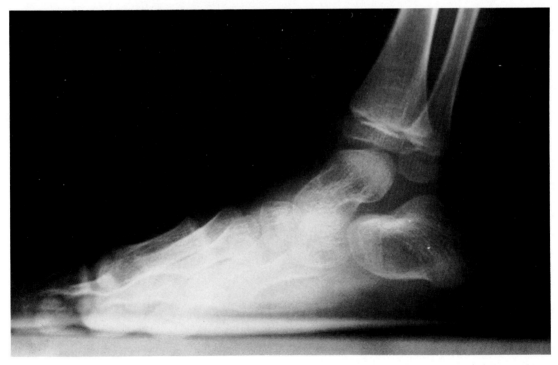

Figure 5.7.   Spastic equinus. A tight gastroc-soleus complex yields an equinus deformity. The foot is plantarflexed with respect to the leg. The talar dome is starting to flatten due to compression, causing a decrease in endochondral bone growth.

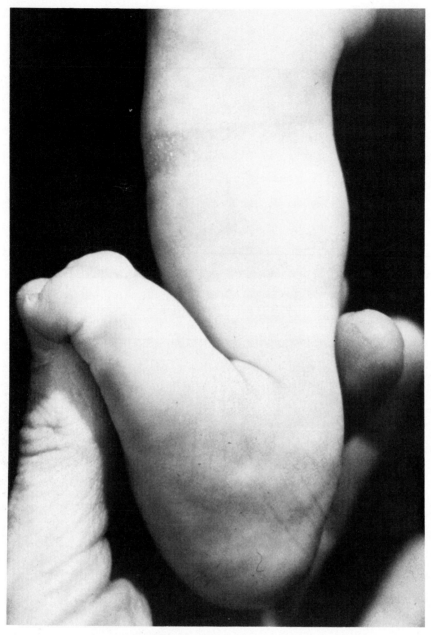

Figure 5.8. The dorsum of the foot lies in close proximity with the anterior aspect of the tibia in calcaneovalgus.

CLINICAL SIGNS

The foot is in an up and out position, relative to the leg (Figs. 5.8 to 5.10). This dorsiflexed position leaves the foot in calcaneus. There exists a limitation of plantarflexion and inversion and an increase in dorsiflexion and eversion. These ranges of motion vary, depending on the degree of the deformity. With the calcaneovalgus deformity, the dorsum of the foot lies in close proximity to the anterior aspect of the tibia. If the foot is rapidly shaken and then released, the foot will still assume a dorsiflexed everted position relative to the leg. The normal foot assumes a plantarflexed (or at least a right angle) attitude to the leg. Increased skin folds are commonly seen along the lateral border of the foot in the area of the sinus tarsi. When these are present, they blanch when the foot is plantarflexed and inverted.

ETIOLOGY

Factors that affect the position of the calcaneovalgus foot can be attributed to and aggravated by

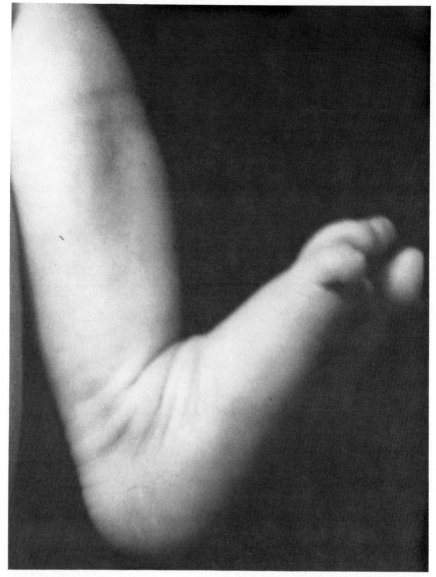

Figure 5.9. The resting position of the foot remains in a dorsiflexed and everted attitude.

(in order of severity) the following:

a. Small uterus;

b. Tight amniotic membranes;

c. Breech or transverse lie fetus;

d. Large child;

e. Sitting and sleeping positions that force the foot outward. This is seen in children sleeping in a prone position with the foot outward and also in a reverse tailor sitting position with the feet forced outward. These conditions aggravate the deformity;

f. Muscular imbalances. Certain muscles overpower the weaker muscles and drive the foot into an outward position. Strong peroneus brevis and strong tibialis anterior commonly cause this pronation;

g. Weak ligaments. A bone will follow in a course of least resistance. If an abnormal force is applied to a loose joint, the bone will deform in the direction of the applied force.

Close examination of the infant with this deformity will reveal that when the calcaneus is manipulated back into a normal position beneath the talus and the foot is then dorsiflexed, there is a limitation of true dorsiflexion of the foot upon the leg. In an adult this could be called a compensated equinus type of foot. In the infant this diagnosis does not seem proper, however, since a compensation should not have occurred in a foot that really has never borne weight in gait. Probably the limitation of dorsiflexion has occurred as a secondary contracture in the posterior muscle group, secondary to the abnormal position of the bones.

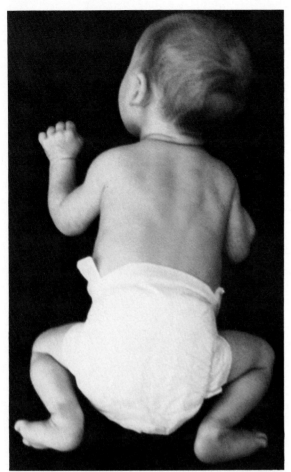

Figure 5.10. Sleeping in a prone position applies an external abductory force to the foot.

RADIOLOGY

With an understanding of the clinical signs and etiology, the osseous malposition is well understood. The ankle joint is a strong mortise that primarily allows the talus a sagittal motion (dorsiflexion and plantarflexion). If one were to move the foot in an abductory direction at the metatarsals, very little twist would take place in the ankle joint (Figs. 5.11 to 5.16). The net result is that the calcaneus will move outward or rather abduct and pivot under the talus. Since the calcaneocuboid joint is a strong, locked joint, when the calcaneus moves outwardly so does the cuboid. The entire lateral column abducts. The talus in the meantime remains locked within the ankle joint mortise. The navicular moves laterally on the talar head along with everything else. One must remember that the spring ligament (the plantar calcaneonavicular ligament) spans between the calcaneus and navicular and this ligament supports the talus. With the navicular moving laterally and bringing with it the spring ligament, the talus plantarflexes. We are now left with a foot that is in an abducted position due to an abductory force. This sequence of events is attributed to the etiology and aggravated by the previously mentioned factors.

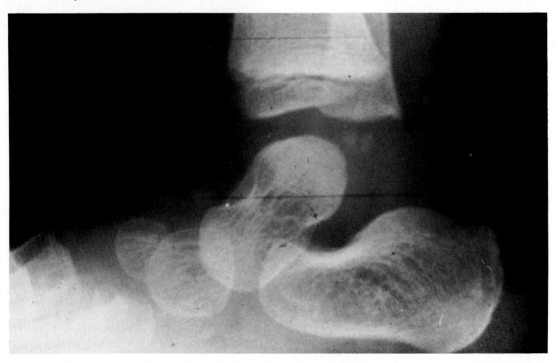

Figure 5.11. Calcaneovalgus. Talar plantarflexion with calcaneal abduction and a decrease in the calcaneal inclination angle are present. The talus bisects the cuboid in its lower one-third.

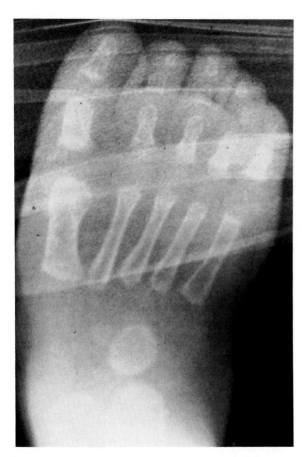

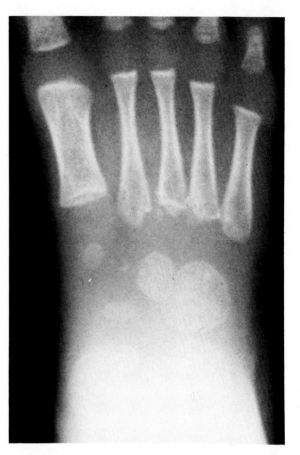

Figure 5.12. Calcaneovalgus. Abduction of the fore-foot is visible with abduction of the calcaneus. The cartilagenous navicular rides laterally due to pull of the calcaneonavicular ligaments with a resultant loss of support to the talar head. The talus appears to abduct, actually plantarflexing, and the calcaneus abducts in relation to the talus which is locked in the ankle mortise.

Figure 5.13. Calcaneovalgus. The entire foot is abducted in relation to the talus. The navicular articulates with the lateral surface of the talar head. Note the visual appearance of the ossification center of the navicular.

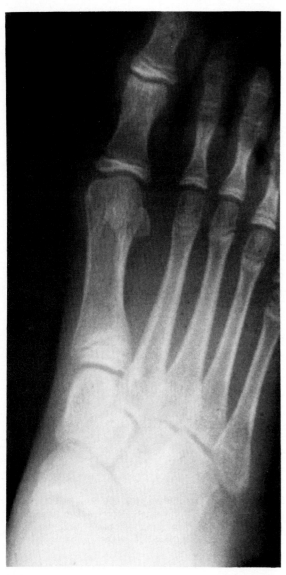

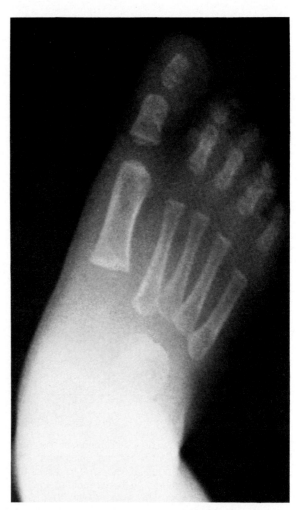

Figure 5.14. A 16-year-old patient with a rigid calcaneovalgus. Marked abduction of the forefoot is present. The talus lies within the ankle mortise and the remainder of the foot abducts. The navicular is wedge-shaped and rides lateral to the talar head. Cuboid abduction is present with midtarsal joint pronation.

Figure 5.15. Calcaneovalgus. The calcaneocuboid joint is stable. The metatarsal, cuboid, and calcaneus are all abducted and there is a high talocalcaneal angle.

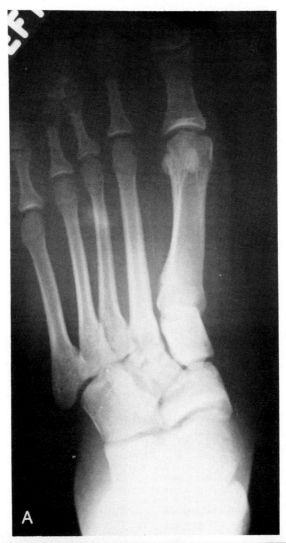

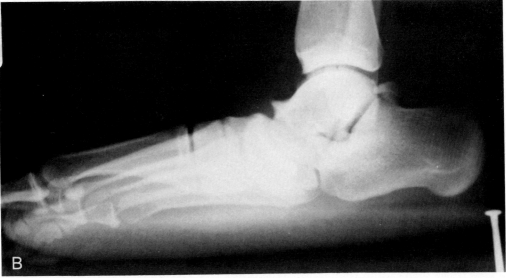

Figure 5.16.   Calcaneovalgus. *A*, long-standing severe calcaneovalgus. *B*, long-standing severe calcaneovalgus with a secondary contracture of the tendo-achilles. Dorsal lateral changes in the talar head are seen.

Equinus

Equinus is a limitation of dorsiflexion of the foot on the leg. By definition, 10° of dorsiflexion of the foot on the leg with the knee joint fully extended and the subtalar joint in its neutral position, with the midtarsal joint maximally pronated and locked, is necessary for normal foot function. We utilize 10° of dorsiflexion because at 50% of the midstance phase of normal gait, the following takes place:

1. The subtalar joint is in its neutral position.
2. The midtarsal joint is maximally pronated and locked due to the reactive force of gravity on the ground. The thigh is extended 10° to the pelvis with the knee joint fully extended, thus causing the ankle joint to be in 10° of dorsiflexion.

With a limitation of dorsiflexion when the knee joint is extended, the foot must attain more dorsiflexion. This is accomplished, somewhat, at the subtalar joint, but more importantly and more significantly, it is accomplished at the midtarsal joint. Here, the dorsiflexory component of the triplane motion comprises the major motion. Therefore, increased dorsiflexion occurs at the midtarsal joint (Figs. 5.17 and 5.18).

Equinus is a severe pronatory force when it is of a congenital or primary nature. Primary or congenital gastrocnemius equinus produces a severe pronatory force upon the foot, probably the most severe of all pronatory forces and equaled only by internal torque. The subtalar joint does not have a great dorsiflexory range of motion while the midtarsal joint around the oblique axis has dorsiflexion and abduction as the major components of its range of motion. With the midtarsal joint using its oblique axis, a compensation for the deformity can occur and causes significant changes around the midtarsal joint. An equinus deformity is considered a midstance pronator.[1]

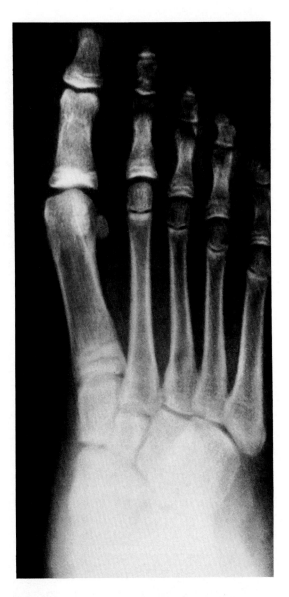

Figure 5.17. Equinus. Flattening of the head of the talus with a wedge-shaped navicular is seen. There is a pronated midtarsal joint and the cuboid is abducted on the calcaneus.

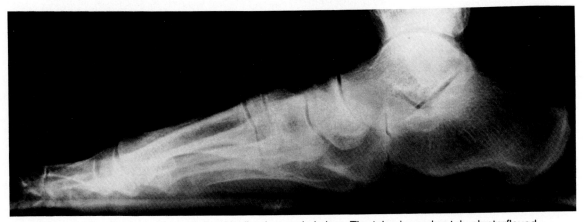

Figure 5.18. Equinus. The calcaneal inclination angle is low. The talus is moderately plantarflexed.

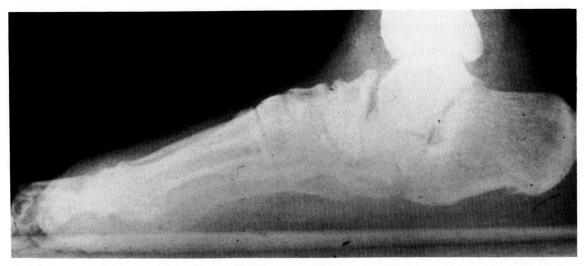

Figure 5.19. Vertical talus in a 16-year-old-male. The navicular is dorsally dislocated on the talus with a limitation of dorsiflexion at the ankle, and atrophy of the posterior leg muscles.

Flatfoot Secondary to Transverse Plane Abnormality

Transverse plane abnormalities in the lower extremity yielding in-toe and out-toe deformities constitute a large percentage of pediatric problems. A greater problem that exists with these axial deviations is the compensatory effect it has on the foot. With an internal drive on the lower extremity, the foot will compensate with the talus remaining locked in the ankle mortise, thus rotating medially with the leg. As a result of tibial internal rotation, the subtalar joint undergoes its triplane motion of pronation. With an increase in transverse plane deformities, transverse plane motion in the subtalar joint will increase.

VERTICAL TALUS

The primary deformity of a congenital vertical talus is a dorsal dislocation of the navicular. The navicular sits on the dorsal aspect of the neck of the talus. There can also be present a subluxation of the talocalcaneal joint. There is an eversion of the midtarsal joint with the forefoot dorsiflexed and abducted. The talus and the calcaneus are fixed in equinus and cannot be reduced. Clinically, the appearance in a newborn is that of a rigid deformity. The sole of the foot is convex and it too cannot be reduced. The calcaneus appears to be plantarflexed and the forefoot is dorsiflexed on the rearfoot at the midtarsal joint. There appear to be deep skin creases on the dorsum in the area of the sinus tarsi similar to that of calcaneal valgus. The talar head is prominent plantarly and medially (Figs. 5.19 to 5.21).

PATHOLOGICAL FINDINGS

In a congenital vertical talus, in addition to the navicular being dorsally dislocated on the neck of the talus, the pathology includes the talus developing an articular facet on its neck for the articulation of the navicular. The head and neck of the talus start to develop a spheroidal shape, similar to that of an hourglass. The anterior facet on the calcaneus is not present and there is hypoplasia of the middle facet.

RADIOGRAPHIC FINDINGS

The radiographic findings on a dorsoplantar view include a talocalcaneal angle that can exceed 40°. The lateral views demonstrate a vertically positioned talus which may appear in an hourglass shape. The talar-declination angle falls below the cuboid between the calcaneus and the cuboid. Normally, the talar-declination lies within the upper one-third of the cuboid. A differential diagnosis must be made between vertical talus and calcaneovalgus. A calcaneovalgus foot is very similar in appearance, however, to a vertical talus, but the vertical talus is a rigid deformity. In a true vertical talus, a forced plantarflexion of the forefoot on the rearfoot will not relocate the navicular on the talus. This is an important diagnostic radiographic maneuver.

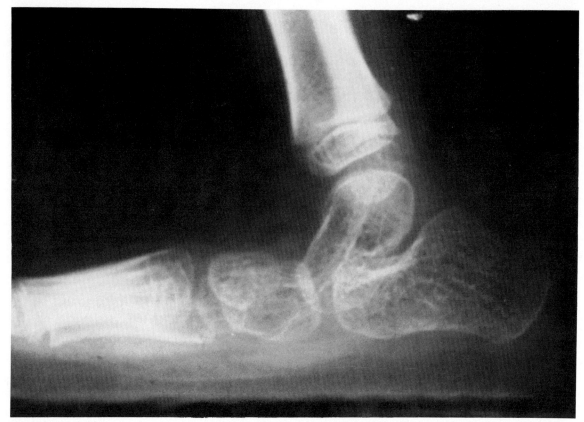

Figure 5.20.   Vertical talus in a 7-year-old male. The talar declination angle falls below the cuboid. Normally, the long axis of the talus passes through the upper one-third of the cuboid.

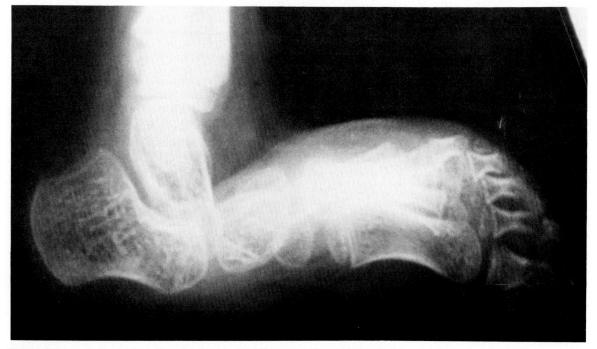

Figure 5.21.   Vertical talus. The forefoot is dorsiflexed at the midtarsal joint, and there is a convex appearance clinically.

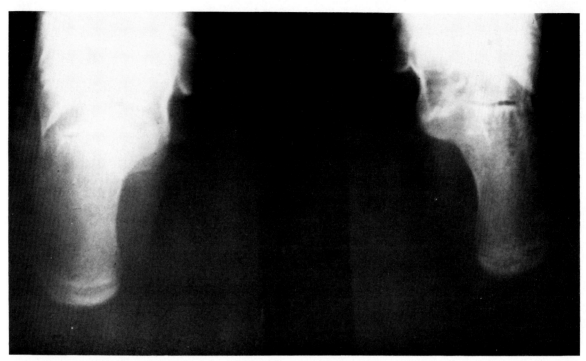

Figure 5.25.   Talocalcaneal coalition of the middle facet: Harris-Beath axial projections. No subtalar range of motion is present. A loss of the parallel posterior and middle facet relationship has occurred with irregularity of the cortex above the sustentaculum tali, indicative of a fibrous coalition in the right foot. A solid osseous coalition is on the left.

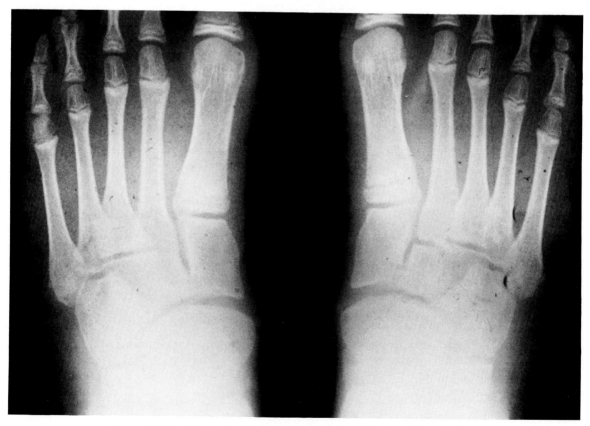

Figure 5.26.   Talonavicular fusion in a 15-year-old male, AP projection.

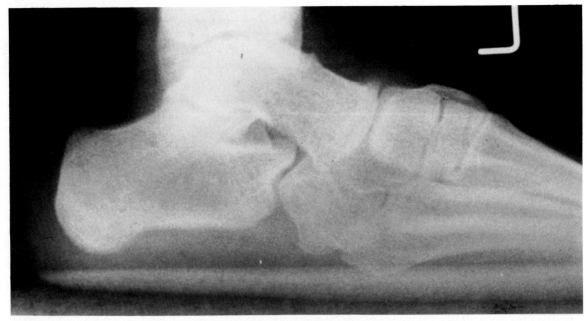

Figure 5.27.   Talonavicular coalition in a 15-year-old male, lateral projection. Pain was demonstrated on the dorsum of the naviculocuneiform joints. The start of beaking on the talonavicular head is seen.

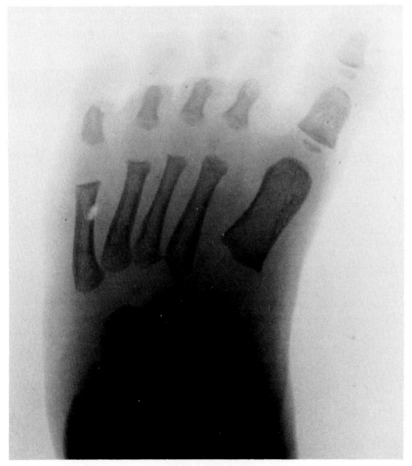

Figure 5.28.   Metatarsus adductus in an 18-month-old boy. The metatarsals are adducted at Lisfranc's (the tarsometatarsal) joint. The soft tissue shows a medial concavity with a lateral convexity.

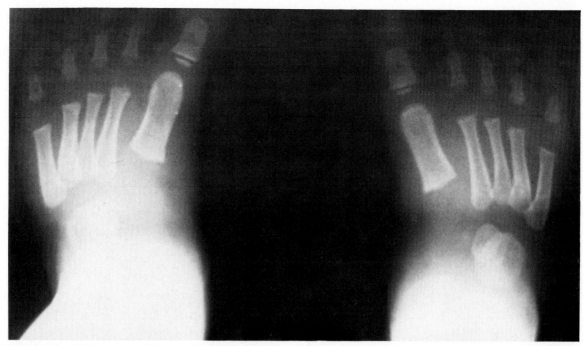

Figure 5.29. Metatarsus adductus in a 2-year-old boy. The metatarsal bases are rounded and the deformity is flexible. The talocalcaneal angle is increased.

METATARSUS ADDUCTUS DEFORMITIES

Metatarsus adductus can be described as an osseous transverse plane deformity that occurs at the tarsometatarsal articulation (Lisfranc's joint). It has been described as a skew or serpentine foot. Dr. Hiram H. Kite[4] termed metatarsus adductus as one-third of a clubfoot deformity; however, this is not exactly accurate. In metatarsus adductus, the navicular rides lateral to the talar head, whereas in the clubfoot deformity, the navicular rides medially to the talar head. The etiology of metatarsus adductus is not fully understood at this point, but it is possibly due to intrauterine pressures that are present with the first born or children that are born within a tight uterus. It is also possible that the malpositioning of the fetus and lack of ontogeny has a deterring effect on the metatarsus. With this resultant malpositioning, certain muscles become more powerful, or gain in mechanical advantage. Possibly, the abductor hallucis can become overactive, maintaining a metatarsus adducts deformity. In addition, with weak peroneal muscles, the tibialis anterior and tibialis posterior muscles can gain a mechanical advantage to supinate and adduct the fore part of the foot (Figs. 5.28 to 5.33).

One must remember that the diagnosis of metatarsus adductus is predominantly a clinical diagnosis. The following five criteria can be ob-served either with the feet weightbearing or non-weightbearing:

1. The foot maintains an inward position when you stroke the lateral border of the foot. The foot may twist outward for a moment, but it returns to its normal inward position.

2. The foot develops a medial concave border and a lateral convex border with a prominent base of the fifth metatarsal. The prominence of the fifth metatarsal base becomes more evident after the child loses some of its fat in that area. Also, the fifth metatarsal base becomes more prominent as the apophysis to the fifth meta-tarsal base becomes ossified. Also, note that the lateral C-shaped border is seen to be greater when the foot is viewed in a non-weightbearing attitude.

3. The metatarsus adductus foot can attain a high arch. The foot appears as though it were a cavus foot in the newborn.

4. One should observe a marked separation of the great toe from the lesser toes. This foot type develops a metatarsus primus adductus that can be greater than the metatarsus adductus.

5. When the metatarsus adductus foot is viewed in a nonweightbearing attitude, look at the plantar aspect of the foot and construct two imaginery lines. One line should bisect the heel longitudinally and the other line should bisect the forefoot area longitudinally. In a metatarsus

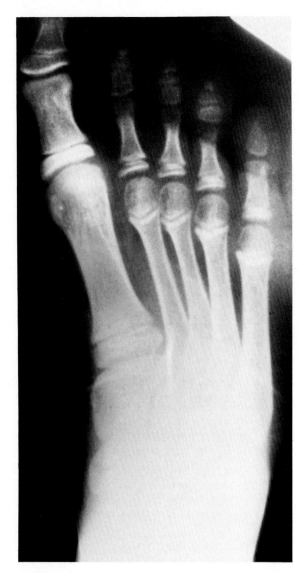

Figure 5.30. Metatarsus adductus in an 8-year-old boy, with a 30° metatarsus adductus angle.

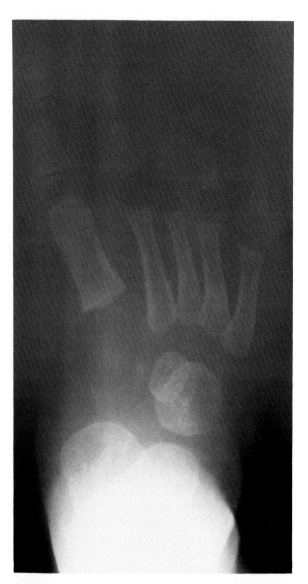

Figure 5.31. Metatarsus adductus in a 2-month-old child. The talocalcaneal angle is increased and the metatarsals are severely adducted.

adductus foot these two lines will not combine to form a straight line.

Three types of metatarsus adductus can be demonstrated: 1) a *total metatarsus adductus* in which the entire metatarsus one through five, are adducted relative to the lesser tarsus with a mild to moderate degree of pronation at the subtalar and midtarsal joints; 2) an *Atavistic form* or metatarsus primus adductus type of deformity is that condition in which the first ray is adducted so that the intermetatarsal angle is increased above fifteen degrees. The hallux stays in a varus attitude or stays in line with the metatarsal and the lesser metatarsals remain normal or slightly adducted; 3) the third type is skewfoot or *serpentine S-*

shaped foot. Here, one sees a severe metatarsus adductus with all five metatarsals being adducted and compensated for by an increased amount of subtalar and midtarsal joint pronation. Also, the hallux goes into a valgus deformity due to the foot pronation. An uncontrolled total metatarsus adductus can develop into this type of metatarsus adductus deformity.

Radiographs are not needed to establish a diagnosis of metatarsus adductus. It is a clinical diagnosis. Radiographs are an aid in confirming your accurate diagnosis, and quantifying the number of degrees of the deformity. Radiographs will help to confirm the presurgical plan and to accurately demonstrate the area of deformity. The

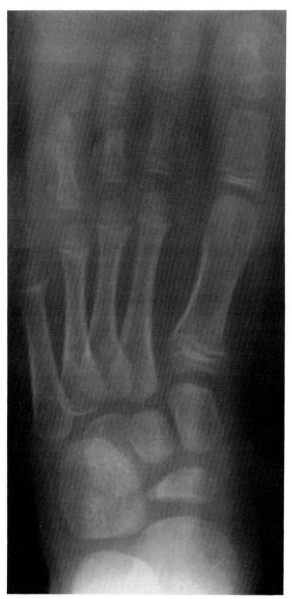

Figure 5.32. Metatarsus adductus in an 8-year-old child.

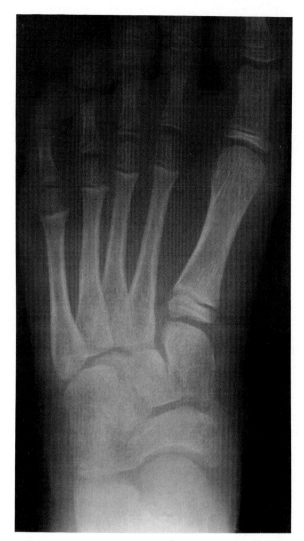

Figure 5.33. Metatarsus adductus in a 16-year-old child.

angle of metatarsus adductus as seen on radiographs should be less than 22°. Anything greater than 22° to 23° is considered to be a pathological adduction of the metatarsals.

When determining which procedure to do surgically, one notes the appearance of the metatarsal bases. During developmental years, the bases start as rounded in shape and wind up squared and securely placed in Lisfranc's articulation.

After casting procedures, it is a good technique to x-ray the foot to determine the position of the cuboid relative to the calcaneus. In a normal total metatarsus adductus, the calcaneocuboid angle should be nearly parallel or equal to 0°. With

midtarsal joint pronation and supination taking place about the oblique axis of the midtarsal joint, cuboid abduction can either increase or decrease. Cuboid abduction represents a midtarsal joint pronation. Cuboid adduction represents or signifies midtarsal joint supination. If the cuboid points laterally after your casting procedure has been in progress, this indicates that either you have pronated the foot and abducted it about the midtarsal joint oblique axis or you have not corrected the concomitant rearfoot pronation. This means you have done nothing to correct the tarsometatarsal articulation, and instead, you have left the child with a pronated or flatfoot. Therefore, you must monitor the progress of treatment with x-rays that are taken before, during, and after treatment.

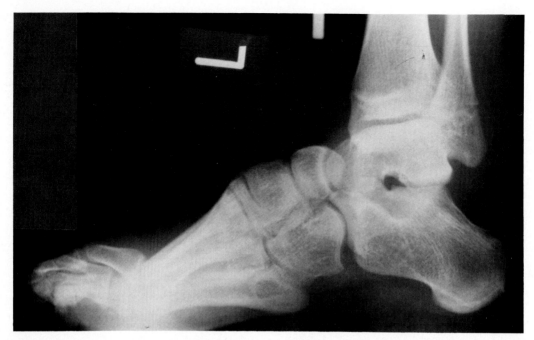

Figure 5.34.   Cavus deformity in a 15-year-old female. The subtalar joint is supinated with plantarflexion of the first ray and an increase in the calcaneal inclination angle.

CAVUS DEFORMITIES

It has been well documented that many forms of cavus deformity are associated with neuromuscular disease and the incidence of association may be as high as 60–70% and could be as high as 95% if our methods or neurologic evaluation could be refined. Associated with or without established neurologic disease, cavus deformity is often progressive and the structure of the foot and its function significantly change with time. With the progression of the deformity, numerous mechanical and functional changes occur, including contracted digits and increased supination of the subtalar joint.

Commonly associated with this deformity are a rearfoot varus and a rigid forefoot valgus. The rearfoot varus may be primary and, if of an uncompensated for or partially compensated nature, it will cause a secondary forefoot valgus by plantarflexion of the first ray. On the other hand, the rearfoot varus may be secondary to a total forefoot valgus, which will cause a rapid supination of the subtalar joint in gait with the development of subtalar and ankle instability and an increasing position of varus within the subtalar joint (Fig. 5.34).

Forefoot Valgus

It is now recognized that forefoot valgus is a common deformity and may be even more common than forefoot varus. Also, forefoot valgus can develop secondary to an uncompensated or partially compensated forefoot varus either as a primary deformity or associated with rearfoot varus. When a foot remains in a varus position, there is a greater tendency for stability laterally which will enhance the pull of the peroneus longus with resultant plantarflexion of the first ray. Initially, the first ray may be hypermobile with evidence of lesion formation more laterally. But in time, the first ray becomes more rigid with the lesion subtibial sesamoid and markedly intractable. As the first ray increases its plantarflexion, it prevents subtalar pronation and, eventually, via retrograde force, increases the varus position of the subtalar joint.

The rigid forefoot valgus demonstrates an everted forefoot to rearfoot relationship when the subtalar joint is in neutral position and the midtarsal joint is maximally pronated and locked. The entire forefoot may be everted or only metatarsals one and five may be everted. Metatarsals two through five may be in a varus attitude or perpendicular to the bisection of the calcaneus.

The plantarflexed first ray is probably the most common type of forefoot valgus and is associated usually with uncompensated or partially compensated rearfoot varus or compensated or partially compensated forefoot varus. With the latter, the relationship of metatarsals two through five, relative to the calcaneus, is in a position of varus; but metatarsals one through five demonstrate a perpendicular relationship. It is proposed that the first ray has plantarflexed because of an increased pull by the peroneus longus which has an increased force because of a stable cuboid.

The flexible cavus foot, which on weightbearing flattens significantly, is another type of forefoot valgus. This foot is very unstable and develops a significant forefoot symptomatology, including severe hallux abductus and submetatarsal lesion patterns. In the non-weightbearing attitude, the structural forefoot to rearfoot relationship is one of valgus, but when weight is superimposed, the forefoot collapses. In gait, the forefoot is not locked against the rearfoot and, therefore, instability exists.

REFERENCES

1. SCHOENHAUS, H. D., AND JAY, R. M.: A modified gastrocnemius lengthening. J.A.P.A., **68:** 31, 1978.
2. JAY, R. M., AND SCHOENHAUS, H. D.: Further insights into anterior advancement of tendo-achilles. J.A.P.A., **71:** 73, 1980.
3. SCHOENHAUS, H. D., AND JAY, R. M.: Cavus deformity: Conservative management. J.A.P.A., **70:** 235, 1980.
4. KITE, J. H.: *The Clubfoot.* Grune and Stratton, New York, 1964, p. 170.

CHAPTER 6

Metatarsal and Digital Deformities

Analysis of abnormalities in the digits and forefoot is very important to the practice of podiatric medicine and surgery. The vast majority of static deformities of the foot involves this area. Consequently, the student must become proficient at examining the forefoot, paying special attention to the analysis of first ray abnormalities. In this chapter, the analysis of first ray abnormalities will be covered by each body plane separately, beginning with the transverse plane.

DEVELOPMENT OF NORMAL OSSIFICATION

At birth, the ossification centers of the metatarsals and most of the phalanges are present. The proximal epiphysis of the first metatarsal usually appears between the ages of 2 and 4 years. The epiphyses in the neck of the second through fifth metatarsals also appear at approximately the same age. The proximal epiphyses of the phalanges appear between the ages of 1 through 4. Occasionally, there is an epiphysis in the neck of the first metatarsal, which appears in late childhood. The sesamoids usually do not appear until the age of nine to eleven. When examining the foot of the child, after trauma has occurred, it is important to remember that the epiphysis of the first metatarsal is at its base whereas in the other metatarsals they are in the neck. There is a separate epiphysis that is occasionally present in the styloid process of the fifth metatarsal. When present, it is usually bilateral, and must not be mistaken for a fracture. This epiphysis will run in a longitudinal direction. The first metatarsal epiphysis has usually completed growth by approximately the age of 16 years (see Figs. 3.12 and 3.13).

TRANSVERSE PLANE ANALYSIS

The bulk of the analysis of the first ray deformities occurs in this plane. When considering hallux-abducto-valgus and bunion deformity, it is very important to know the forefoot adductus

angle, the metatarsus adductus angle, the intermetatarsal angle, the hallux abductus angle, the hallux interphalangeal angle, and the sesamoid position (see Chapter 4). All are pertinent in evaluating the first ray.

First, it is important to determine if the metatarsus and forefoot are rectus or adductus. If the metatarsus adductus angle is 13° or lower, the metatarsus is considered to be rectus. If it is 14° or higher, it is considered to be adductus. Similarly, if the forefoot angle is 13° or below, the patient is considered to have a rectus forefoot, and if it is 13° and above, the patient is considered to have an adductus foot type. If the patient has an adductus foot type or metatarsus, then he can maximally tolerate a lower IM angle than if he has a rectus forefoot. To clarify: An adduction of the metatarsals will automatically make the medial aspect of the head of the first metatarsal more prominent than will a rectus position of the metatarsals. Therefore, the patient can tolerate only a 12° IM angle to maintain a normal first ray. In a rectus foot type, the high normal for an IM angle is 14°. In an adductus forefoot, the high normal is only 12° (Fig. 6.1).

The ideal hallux abductus angle is approximately 10°. The high normal for this angle is 15°. An increase in the hallux abductus angle is a compensation for an increase in the intermetatarsal angle. The ideal intermetatarsal angle is approximately 8°. An increase in the proximal articular set angle is a reaction to an increase in the intermetatarsal angle. These two angles will usually increase together. The body is attempting to straighten out the ray, and this is why the compensation occurs. The patient therefore ends up with a sort of zig-zag pattern to his first ray. The high normal for the proximal articular set angle is up to 8°. The high normal for the distal articular set angle varies from 5° to 8° (see Figs. 4.2 and 4.4).[1,3]

Hallux varus is a condition that can occur either

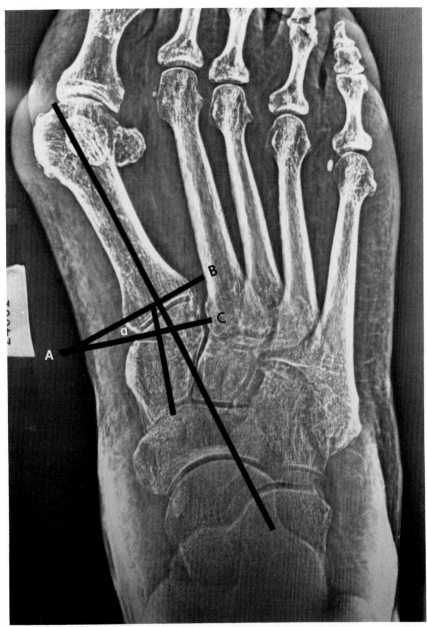

Figure 6.1.   Hallux-abducto-valgus deformity. The hallux abductus angle, intermetatarsal angle, and forefoot adductus angles are increased. The sesamoids are in a position 5 and the first metatarsophalangeal joint is subluxed. A valgus rotation of the hallux is also present. The first metatarsal cuneiform angle is constructed by drawing *line AB* perpendicular to the longitudinal axis of the first metatarsal and *line AC* perpendicular to the longitudinal axis of the first cuneiform. The first metatarsal cuneiform angle is *a*.

congenitally or iatrogenically. The congenital cases seem to consistently be associated with metatarsus adductus and metatarsus primus adductus in particular. The iatrogenically caused hallux varus usually follows hallux-abducto-valgus surgery in which the hallux abductus was overcorrected. It has been implicated in those cases in which the medial aspect of the joint capsule is shortened too much, and in cases in which the

sesamoid apparatus has been grossly altered (Figs. 6.2 and 6.3).

Positional versus Structural Deformities

A structural deformity is a deformity in the shape of a bone. A positional deformity is merely a deformity in the position of the bones. If either the proximal articular set angle or the distal articular set angle is increased above its high normal, then a structural deformity is said to occur.

In the normal, the hallux abductus angle (HAA) equals the proximal articular set angle (PASA) plus the distal articular set angle (DASA).[3] If this relationship is unequal, it means that a positional deformity has occurred. A positional deformity is usually considered to be caused by a contracture in the soft tissues which then holds the bones in an abnormal position. After the bones function in an abnormal position for a while, adaptive bony changes will occur, and eventually a structural deformity will also develop. It is possible to have both a structural and a positional deformity at the same time.[3, 10]

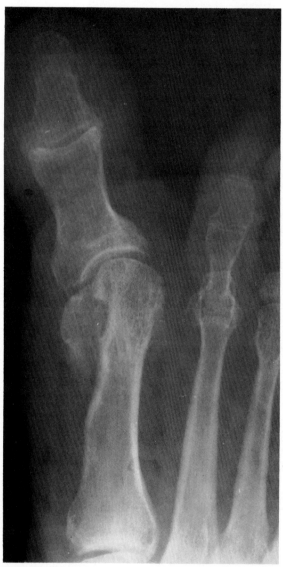

Figure 6.2. Hallux-adducto-varus. Secondary to surgical procedure.

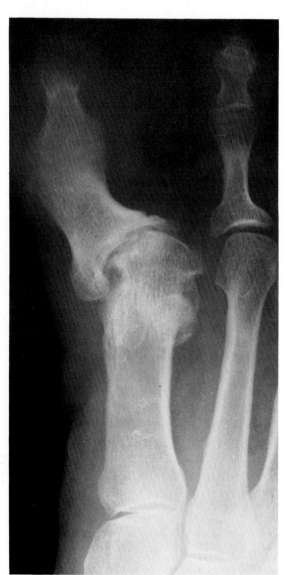

Figure 6.3. Hallux-adducto-varus. Secondary to surgical procedure.

The First Metatarsal First Cuneiform Angle

This angle is measured by constructing two lines: one is a perpendicular to the longitudinal axis of the first metatarsal, drawn at the base; and the second line is a perpendicular to the longitudinal axis of the first cuneiform and is drawn near the distal end of the cuneiform. These two lines will form an angle on the medial side of the foot, which should range from 0° to 25°. If this angle is from to 0° to 25°, and the intermetatarsal angle is going to be corrected, the procedure can be easily done by osteotomy at the metatarsal base, and including soft tissue realignment. However, if the angle is greater than 25°, resection of bone should probably be done more proximally.[7,8] This angle is also influenced by the shape of the distal portion of the cuneiform, and if it is greatly angulated, it is referred to in podiatric literature as an atavistic cuneiform (Fig. 6.4).

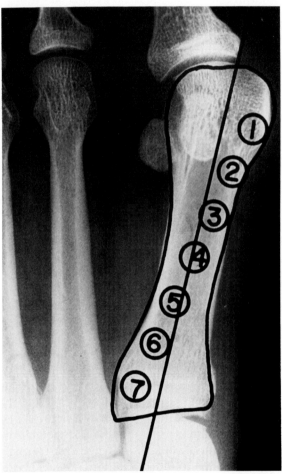

Figure 6.4. Schematic representation of sesamoid position. The sesamoid in this x-ray is in a position *6*.

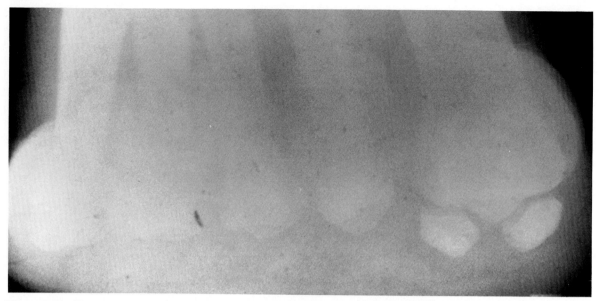

Figure 6.5.   The crista. An axial sesamoidal view showing the articulation of the seamoids with the first metatarsal head and the crista.

Sesamoid Position

The sesamoid position is determined by the relative position of the tibial sesamoid with respect to the longitudinal axis of the first metatarsal (Fig. 6.4). If the tibial sesamoid is completely medial to the long axis of the metatarsal, and is not touching the axis, the sesamoid position is number one. If the tibial sesamoid is completely medial to the long axis, but is touching the long axis, then it is said to be in position number two. If the tibial sesamoid is overlapping the long axis of the first metatarsal, but most of the body of the sesamoid is medial to the axis, then it is in position number three. In sesamoid position number four, the tibial sesamoid is exactly bisected by the long axis of the first metatarsal. When the tibial sesamoid is overlapping the long axis of the metatarsal, but most of the body of the sesamoid is lateral to the long axis, it is said to be in position number five. When the tibial sesamoid is completely lateral to the long axis of the first metatarsal, but touches the long axis, it is in position number six. In position number seven, the entire tibial sesamoid is lateral to the long axis to the first metatarsal and is not touching the long axis of the metatarsal. This staging of the sesamoid position is important in determining whether the fibular sesamoid should be removed. Some authorities feel that when the sesamoids have moved into a position four or greater, that the fibular sesamoid may be moving dorsally into the intermetatarsal space and increasing the intermetatarsal angle and deformity of the first metatarsophalangeal joint. This examination should be combined with an axial sesamoidal view to determine if the crista has been injured. When the sesamoids have moved into a position four or greater, the tibial sesamoid has crossed over the crista, and probably has worn the crista away from the planter aspect of the first metatarsal head (Figs. 6.5 to 6.7).[1,6]

When considering the sesamoid position, it is important to realize that the sesamoids really have not moved, they have stayed in their normal place within the soft tissues, and it is the first metatarsal that has moved medially away from the sesamoids.

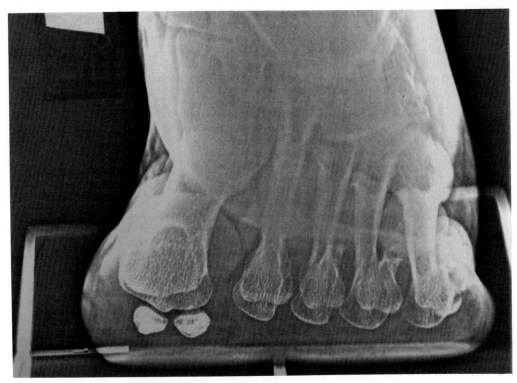

Figure 6.6. The tibial sesamoid has now moved into a position 3, and is seen to be partially overriding the crista in this axial sesamoidal projection.

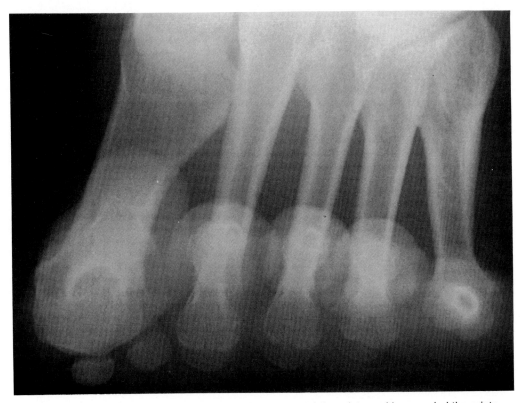

Figure 6.7. The tibial sesamoid now is riding on top of the crista and has eroded the crista.

Alignment of the First Metatarsophalangeal Joint

It is important to determine if the first metatarsophalangeal joint has a normal or abnormal alignment. A congruous joint is one in which the articular surfaces are parallel to each other and wholly articular with each other. A deviated joint is one in which the articular surfaces are no longer parallel, but the bones are still wholly articulating with each other. A subluxed joint is one in which the articular surfaces are no longer parallel and the bones are no longer wholly articular.

The lines used to determine the proximal and distal articular set angles may be used in determining if the joint is congruous, deviated, or subluxed. In a congruous joint, the proximal and distal set lines should be parallel (Fig. 6.8). In a deviated joint, they will cross each other outside and lateral to the first metatarsophalangeal joint (Fig. 6.9). When the joint is subluxed, they will cross each other within the joint (Figs. 6.10 and 6.11).[8]

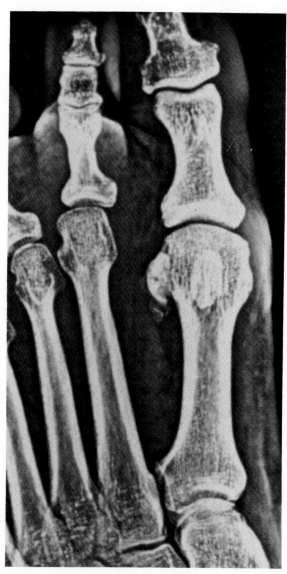

Figure 6.8.   Congruous joint. The first metatarsophalangeal joint is congruous. It is evenly spaced and the articular surfaces are parallel. Note the enlargement of the fibular sesamoid and the short first metatarsal.

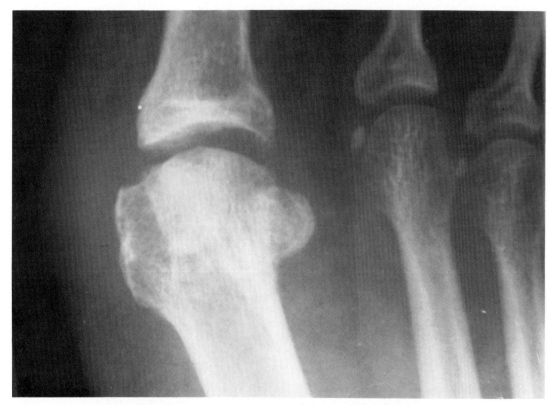

Figure 6.9.   Deviated joint. This first metatarsophalangeal joint is somewhat uneven. There is an erosion present in the center of the first metatarsal head and there is a medial exostosis on the head of the first metatarsal. The sesamoids are beginning to drift laterally. The proximal articular set angle is increased.

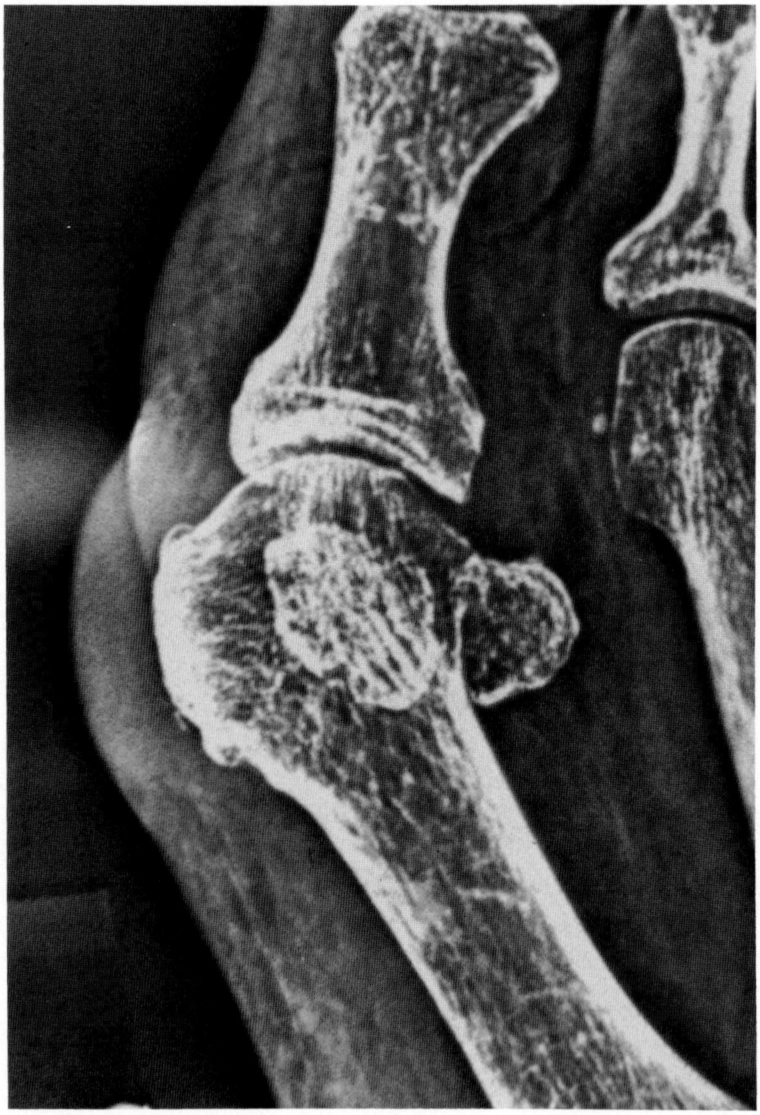

Figure 6.10. Subluxed joint. The lateral portion of the base of the proximal phalanx of the hallux is now nonarticulating with the head of the first metatarsal. There is a valgus rotation of the hallux, the sesamoids are in a position 5, and there is medial enlargement of the head of the first metatarsal. The proximal articular set angle is increased.

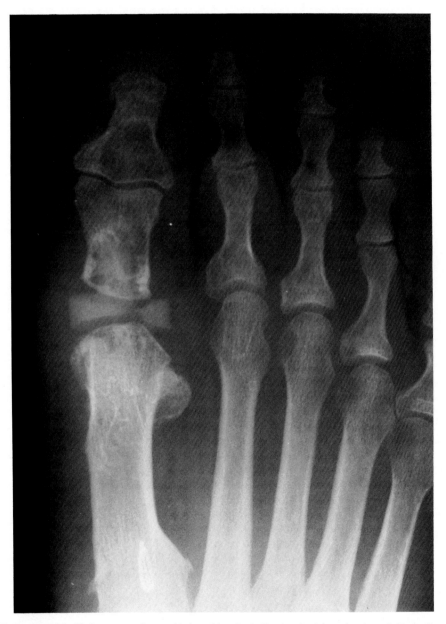

Figure 6.11.   Following this Keller procedure with hemi-implant, the implant has fractured. Note the wire suture in the base of the first metatarsal.

The Hallux Interphalangeal Angle

The normal for the hallux interphalangeal angle has been variously described as from five to ten degrees. In this author's opinion very few are found to be below five degrees. Therefore, the normal should be in the eight to ten degree range. When the angle is found to be above the eight to ten degree normal, it must be taken into account when determining which type of osteotomy should be performed, and where it should be located (Fig. 6.12).[3, 6, 10]

The Relative Metatarsal Protrusion Pattern

In considering hallux-abducto-valgus deformities, it is important to consider the relative lengths of the first and second rays. This is accomplished by placing the point of a compass at the apex of the angle formed by the longitudinal axes of the first and second metatarsals. First, draw an arc with the pencil point placed at the tip of the first metatarsal head, then draw a second arc with the pencil placed at the tip of the head of the second metatarsal (Fig. 6.13). The distance between the two arcs is measured to determine the relative length. In the normal, the length of the first and second metatarsals should be approximately equal plus or minus 2 mm.[6] If the first metatarsal is found to be too long, then it would be normal to perform a closing osteotomy which would shorten the bone somewhat. Conversely, if the first metatarsal is found to be too short, this must be considered in planning the osteotomy. Should the bone be lengthened?[6]

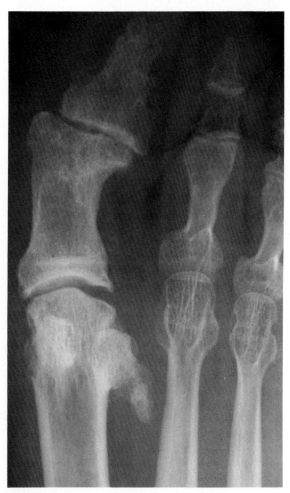

Figure 6.12. High hallux interphalangeal angle. The hallux interphalangeal angle is severely increased in this radiograph. The interphalangeal joint shows signs of arthritic degeneration, as well as similar changes in the first metatarsophalangeal joint. Note the hyperplastic fibular sesamoid.

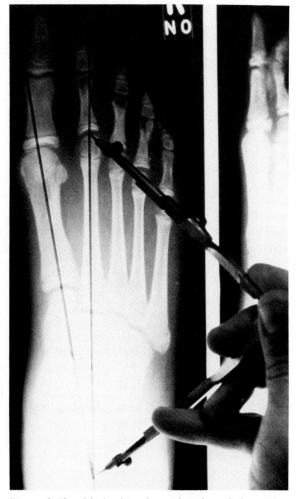

Figure 6.13. Method to determine the relative metatarsal protrusion length.

CONSIDERATIONS IN THE SAGITTAL PLANE

The next most important considerations about the first ray are in the sagittal plane. The first metatarsal declination angle must be measured. The normal for this angle is approximately 21°. When this angle changes, it changes the total relationship of the first metatarsal with the first toe. A decreased first metatarsal declination angle, for whatever reason, changes the range of dorsiflexion of the great toe upon the metatarsal decreasing it. This leads to a hallux limitus and hallux rigidus deformity. Hallux limitus refers to a limitation of dorsiflexion of the great toe upon the first metatarsal, and hallux rigidus refers to a complete lack of motion that can occur in the end stages of this condition, in which severe degenerative arthritic changes and osteophyte proliferation have occurred.

Hallux limitus is classified according to the manner in which the first metatarsal declination angle became lowered. It is considered to be a structural hallux limitus if the head of the first metatarsal is raised as in a metatarsus primus elevatus. It is considered to be a functional hallux limitus if the first metatarsal declination angle became lowered because the base of the first metatarsal has dropped. This tends to occur when pronation is present, as the entire medial column of the foot sags (Figs. 6.14 and 6.15).

If the first toe cannot dorsiflex during toe-off, then a jamming of the joint occurs, the base of the proximal phalanx jamming into the head of the first metatarsal. This constant microtrauma erodes the cartilage in the joint, leads to flattening of both articular surfaces, and causes extensive osteophyte proliferation on the medial, lateral, proximal, distal, and dorsal aspects of the first metatarsophalangeal joint.

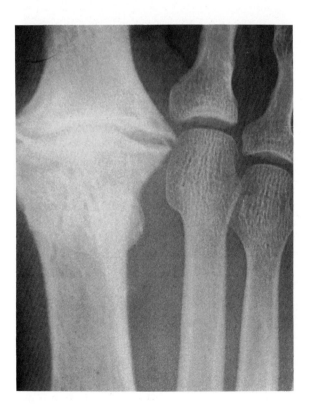

Figure 6.14. Hallux rigidus. There is flattening of the head of the first metatarsal and base of the proximal phalanx. Osteophytic changes are present on the medial, lateral, and dorsal aspects of the joint both proximally and distally. Note the bony sclerosis secondary to the arthritic condition.

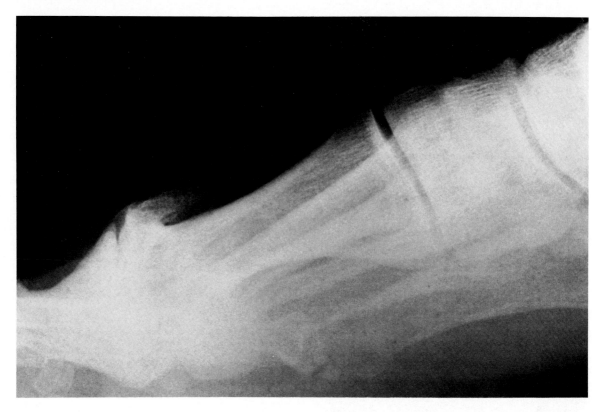

Figure 6.15. Hallux limitus. Lateral projection showing the large dorsal exostosis and arthritic changes present within the first metatarsophalangeal joint in hallux limitus and rigidus. The first metatarsal is in an elevated position.

Hypermobility of the First Ray

Radiographically, there are two signs of hypermobility of the first ray. One is on the sagittal plane x-rays (lateral projection) and the second is on the transverse plane x-rays (the dorsoplantar films). On the dorsoplantar films, when there is an abnormally large gap between the bases of the first and second metatarsals and the first and second cuneiforms, it is referred to as a cuneiform split and is a sign of hypermobility of the first ray. The second sign of hypermobility of the first ray is seen on the lateral film and is referred to as a naviculocuneiform fault (see Figs. 6.16 and 6.17).

FRONTAL PLANE EVALUATION OF THE FIRST RAY

Frontal plane evaluation of the first ray is very difficult to perform radiographically. The only component of a hallux-abducto-valgus deformity that occurs in the frontal plane is the valgus portion of the deformity. This refers to the rotation of the great toe in a valgus direction. Usually the toenail will end up facing in a dorsomedial direction rather than in a straight dorsal direction as in the normal. This can be interpreted from the dorsoplantar film in which when a valgus rotation has occurred, the proximal phalanx of the hallux will become asymmetrical in shape. In the normal, both the medial and lateral contours of the shaft of the phalanx are symmetrical. When the rotation has occurred, a portion of the plantar aspect of the shaft rotates into a lateral position causing the lateral side (on the DP view) to have a greater curvature, and the medial side (really the dorsal aspect of the phalanx) to have a lesser curvature (Fig. 6.18).

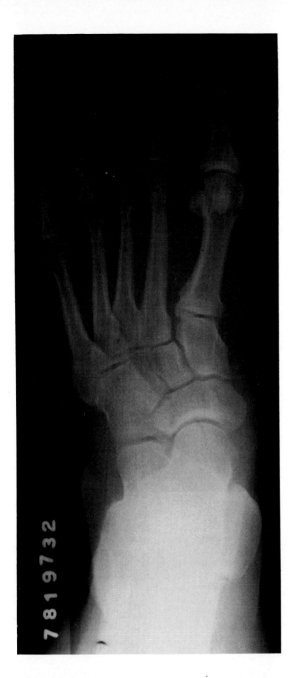

Figure 6.16.   There is an abnormally wide joint space between the base of the first and second metatarsals and first and second cuneiforms. This "cuneiform split" is a sign of hypermobility of the first ray.

Figure 6.17.   *Below*, naviculocuneiform fault. The naviculocuneiform joint is deviated on this lateral projection and there is abnormal dipping of the dorsal aspect of the both bones toward the center of the joint.

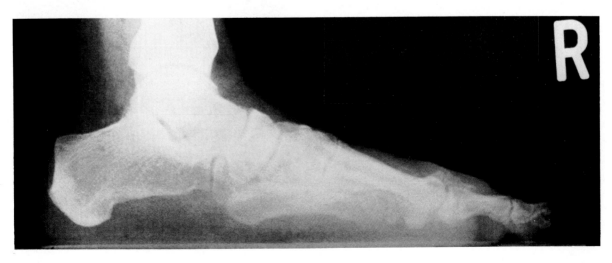

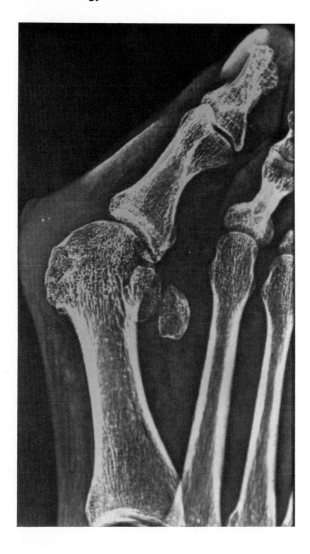

Figure 6.18. Valgus rotation of the hallux. The curvature of the medial and lateral aspects of the proximal phalanx of this hallux are now grossly asymmetrical due to the valgus rotation that has occurred. The toenail is now facing in a medial direction. There is medial enlargement of the first metatarsal head, a high intermetatarsal angle, a sesamoid position of 7, and soft tissue thickening medial to the first metatarsal head.

INTRACTABLE PLANTAR KERATOSIS

Intractable plantar keratosis refers to a plantar callus, the treatment of which is resistant to any form of conservative therapy. Frequently these lesions are caused by a dropped, prolapsed, or plantarflexed metatarsal or metatarsals. This diagnosis must be made combining clinical and radiographic signs.

Clinically, the examiner should be able to palpate the plantarflexed metatarsals. Radiographically, the examiner should place a wire marker around the callus before taking the x-rays so that the exact location of the callus is known. Examination of the dorsoplantar view will aid in localizing the exact extent of the callus with respect to bony markers. Some authorities feel that an axial sesamoidal view should be taken to determine if the metatarsals are in fact plantarflexed or if there is hypertrophy of the plantar condyles of the metatarsal heads (Figs. 6.19 and 6.20).

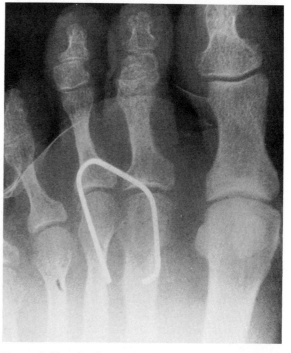

Figure 6.19. A wire marker has been placed around the intractable plantar keratosis, revealing that it is beneath both the second and third metatarsal heads.

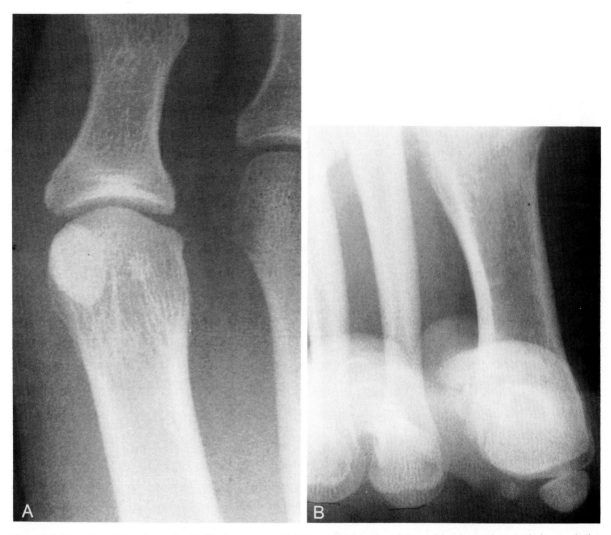

Figure 6.20.   *A* and *B*, a hypoplastic fibular sesamoid. This patient had an intractable plantar keratosis beneath the tibial sesamoid due to abnormal pressure.

DIGITAL DEFORMITIES

The normal lesser digits should be roughly straight with interphalangeal joints that are parallel and equally spaced. Deformities in the digits are classified by which joints become affected.

Hammer Toes

In a hammer toe deformity there is a dorsal contracture of the metatarsophalangeal joint, with a flexion deformity of the proximal interphalangeal joint, and a extension deformity of the distal interphalangeal joint (Fig. 6.21).

Claw Toes

In the claw toe deformity, the metatarsophalangeal joint is extended, the proximal interphalangeal joint has a flexion deformity, and the distal interphalangeal joint also exhibits a flexion deformity. This is most commonly seen in cavus and neurologically induced cavus foot types (Fig. 6.22).

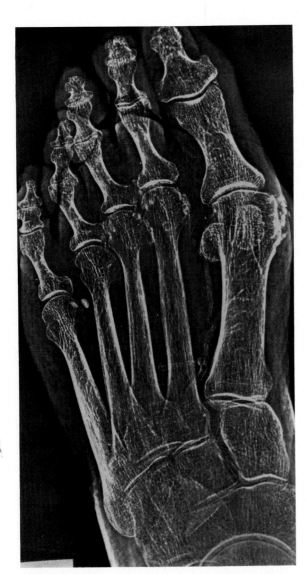

Figure 6.21. Hammer toe deformities. There are hammer toe deformities present in the second, third and fourth digits of this foot. A mild hallux abducto valgus is present with medial enlargement of the first metatarsal head. These hammertoes are typical in that there is an extension deformity at the metatarsophalangeal joint, a flexion deformity at the proximal interphalangeal joint and an extension deformity at the distal interphalangeal joint.

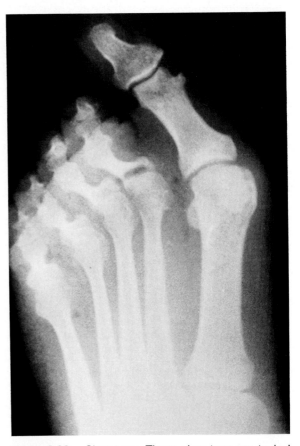

Figure 6.22. Claw toes. These claw toes are typical in that there is an extension deformity of the metatarsophalangeal joints with a flexion deformity of both the proximal distal interphalangeal joints.

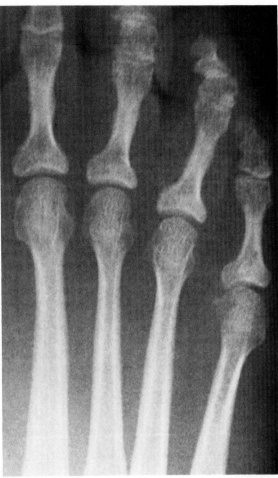

Figure 6.23. Mallet toe deformity of the fourth toe. The metatarsophalangeal joint appears normal, the proximal interphalangeal joint is normal, and there is a flexion deformity of the distal interphalangeal joint. Typical of a mallet toe deformity.

Mallet Toe

In a mallet toe deformity, the metatarsophalangeal joint and proximal interphalangeal joints usually are normal and there is a flexion deformity of the distal interphalangeal joint (Fig. 6.23).

Digital Excrescences

One of the more common foot problems involves corns on the lesser digits. A heloma durum is a corn on the dorsal aspect of the digit and a heloma molle is a soft corn between two digits. It is very helpful to place a wire marker around these lesions when x-raying the patient to determine the exact location and etiology of the lesion. Hammer toe, claw toe, and mallet toe deformities of the second, third, and fourth digits usually will result in a heloma durum on the dorsal aspect of the involved joint. The head of the involved phalanx will frequently be enlarged dorsally, and this can be determined on the dorsoplantar film, and occasionally on the lateral oblique films. When a heloma durum is present on the fifth digit, frequently the digit will be found to exhibit a varus rotation. In these instances, a lateral oblique projection is needed to demonstrate the widening that frequently is present in the head of the proximal phalanx of this toe (Fig. 6.24).

Subungual Exostoses

Subungual exostosis is most frequently seen on the distal phalanx of the hallux. It frequently follows a crush injury to the dorsal aspect of the involved toe. An exostosis develops and extends usually in the dorsal direction putting pressure on the nail plate. On occasions, dorsal subungual exostoses are the result of an osteochondroma (see Chapter 12) (Fig. 6.25 to 6.28).

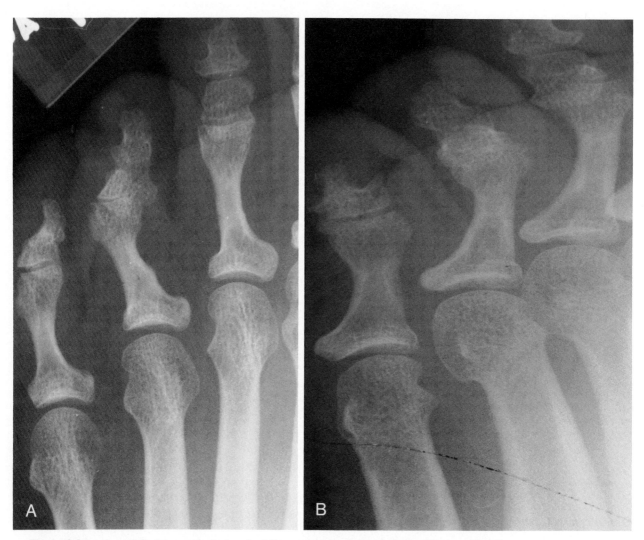

Figure 6.24. *A* and *B*, hyperostosis head of the proximal phalanx of the fifth toe. The dorsoplantar projection typically does not show the widening that occurs in the head of the proximal phalanx of the fifth digits due to the varus rotation of the digit. The lateral oblique projection exemplifies the widening of the head of the proximal phalanx in *B*. The head of the fifth proximal phalanx appears wider than that of the fourth and third.

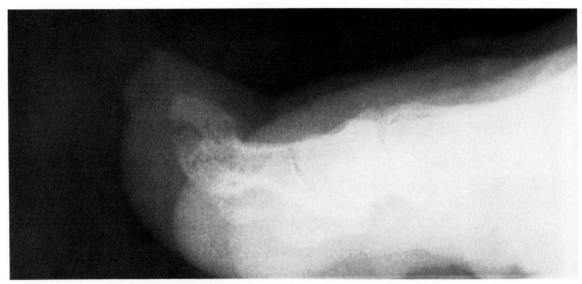

Figure 6.25.   Subungual exostosis of the hallux.

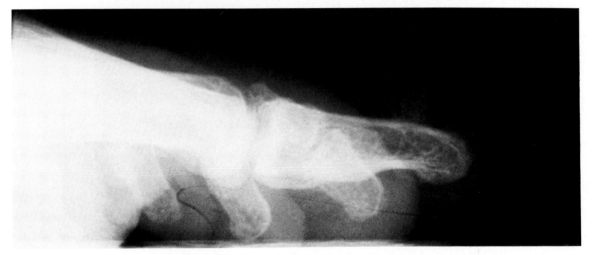

Figure 6.26.   Subungual exostosis of the hallux.

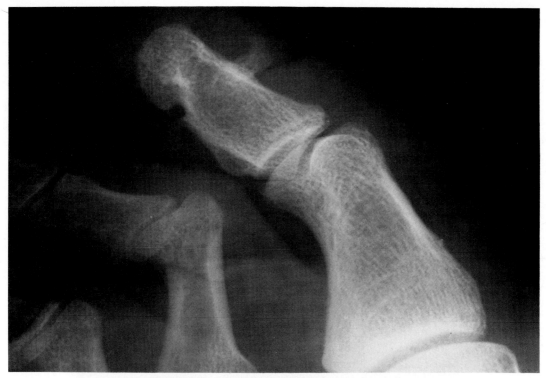

Figure 6.27.   Subungual exostosis of the hallux.

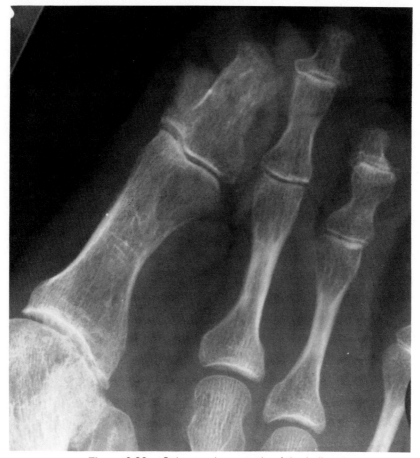

Figure 6.28.   Subungual exostosis of the hallux.

Adduction Deformity of the Second Toe

In cases of severe hallux-abducto-valgus, the second toe frequently will end up overlapping the great toe. When the hallux-abducto-valgus deformity is corrected, the deformity of the second toe must be taken into account. Usually, the second toe will have become adducted and dorsally contracted at the metatarsophalangeal joint, and also will have a flexion deformity of the proximal interphalangeal joint. An arthroplasty of the proximal interphalangeal joint and lengthening of the dorsal soft tissue structures in the vicinity of the metatarsophalangeal joint will usually not correct the adduction deformity of the second toe. A closer examination of this deformity will usually reveal an alteration in the proximal articular set angle of the second metatarsal head. This must also be corrected to realign the digit (Fig. 6.29 and 6.30)[11]

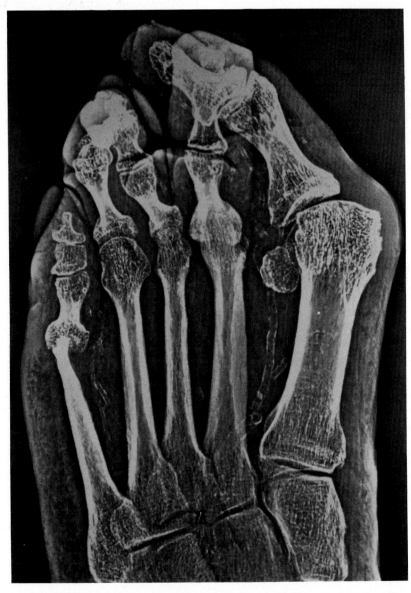

Figure 6.29. Overlapping second digit. There is a hallux-abducto-valgus deformity with the sesamoids in a position 6. Medial enlargement of the first metatarsal, a mild increase in the intermetatarsal angle, and a valgus rotation of the hallux is present. The second digit is now overlapping the first digit and is adducted. Note the vascular calcifications and osteolysis of the fifth metatarsal.

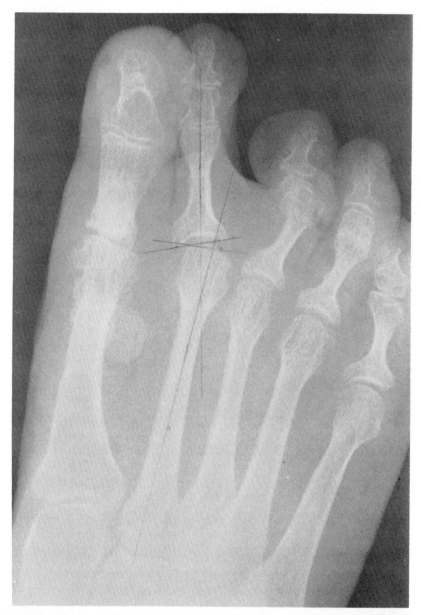

Figure 6.30.   Adduction deformity of the second toe. The great toe is now in a straightened position, but a soft corn has developed between the first and second digits due to failure to correct the adduction deformity of the second digit. It will be noted that the proximal articular set angle of the second metatarsal head is increased.

CONGENITAL DIGITAL DEFORMITIES

Digiti Quinti Varus

This terminology is used to describe the congenital digital deformity in which the fifth digit is overlapping the fourth digit and is rotated into a varus position. The digit usually will be flattened and sometimes is called a paddle toe (Fig. 6.31).

Macrodactyly

Macrodactyly refers to a congenital deformity in which a single or multiple digits are abnormally enlarged (Fig. 6.32).

Microdactyly

Microdactyly refers to that deformity in which a digit is smaller than the remaining normal digits.

Polydactylism

Polydactylism is a condition in which there are extra toes. Frequently there will also be more than the normal five metatarsals. The polydactylic digits may be complete and appear as a normal extra digit or may be combined with another digit (a syndactylism) in some cases the extra bones are found within the soft tissue structures, and do not take the form of a digit (Figs. 6.33 to 6.35).

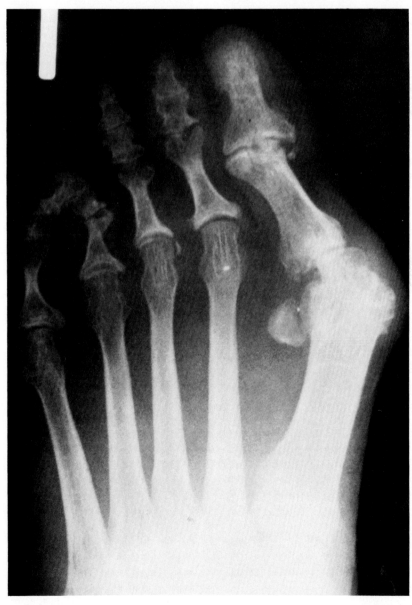

Figure 6.31. Digiti quinti varus. This fifth digit is in a severe varus rotation and is overlapping the fourth digit. Note the severe hallux-abducto-valgus and arthritic changes present throughout the forefoot area.

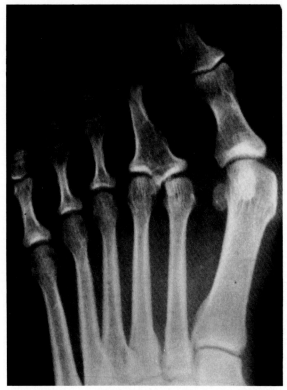

Figure 6.32. Macrodactylism second digit and polydactylism. There are six metatarsals present. The enlarged second digit is articulating with both the second and third metatarsal heads. There appear also to be four cuneiforms.

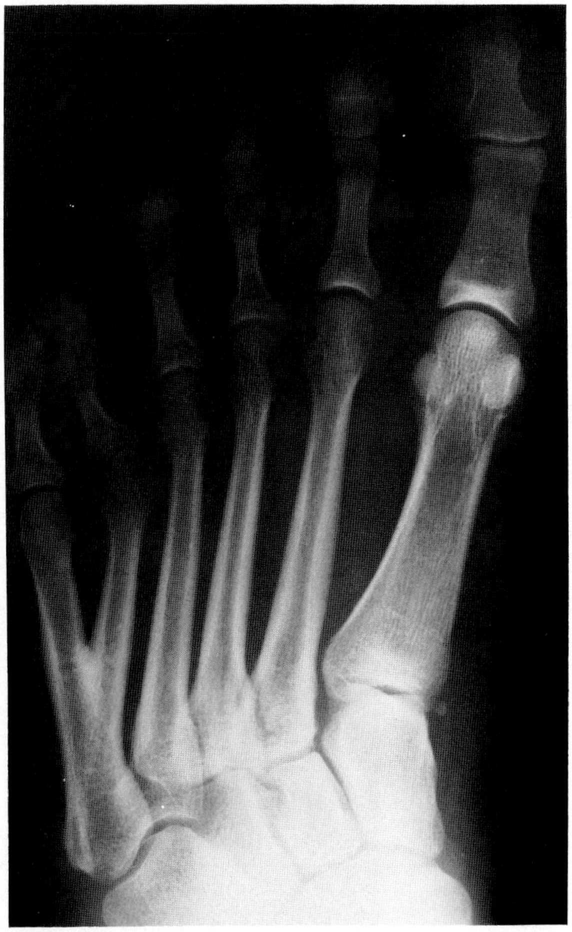

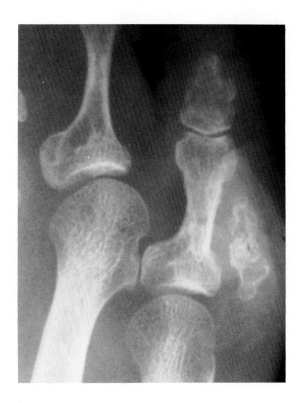

Figure 6.33. Polydactylism. There is a bifid fifth metatarsal with a sixth digit. This was a bilateral deformity.

Figure 6.34. Polydactylism and syndactylism. The sixth digit in this case was not a complete digit, and was found within the soft tissues of the fifth digit.

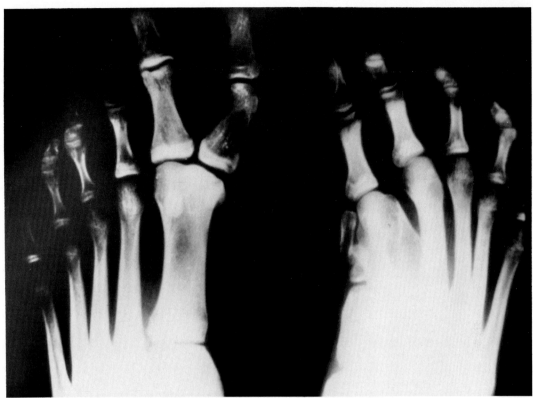

Figure 6.35. The left foot exhibits polydactylism with two complete digits articulating with the first metatarsal. The right foot has an enlarged shortened first metatarsal with a sixth digit extending medially from the metatarsal shaft. This x-ray courtesy of Dr. Richard Jay.

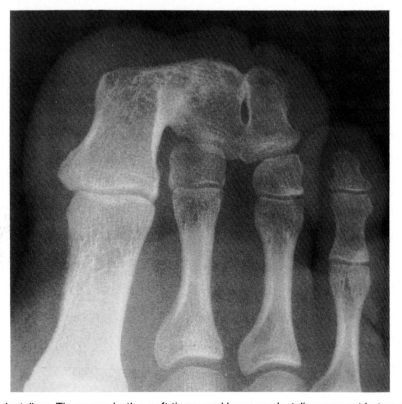

Figure 6.36. Syndactylism. There was both a soft tissue and bony syndactylism present between the first, second, and third digits.

Bradymetapody

Bradymetapody refers to an abnormally short-ened metatarsal. Another name for this is brach-ydactyly. While this is usually a congenital anom-aly, it may be associated with other congenital anomalies. In 1952, Albright described a syn-drome in which multiple congenital defects occur, but without any biochemical findings. Brachy-metapody may also be associated with pseudohy-poparathyroidism and with a genetically related disorder called pseudopseudohypoparathy-roidism (Figs. 6.35 to 6.40).[2]

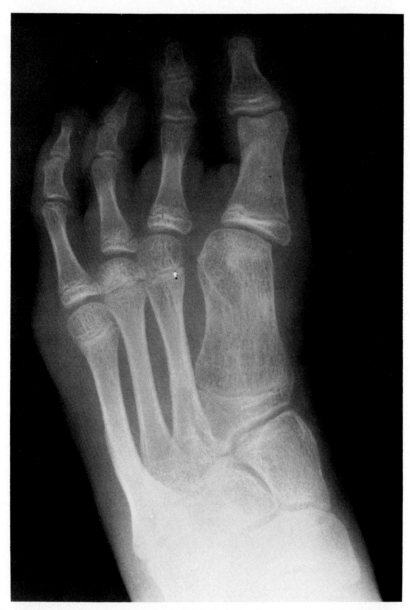

Figure 6.37.   This patient had only three digits congenitally. The first metatarsal is quite deformed and probably represents a fusion of the first and second metatarsals.

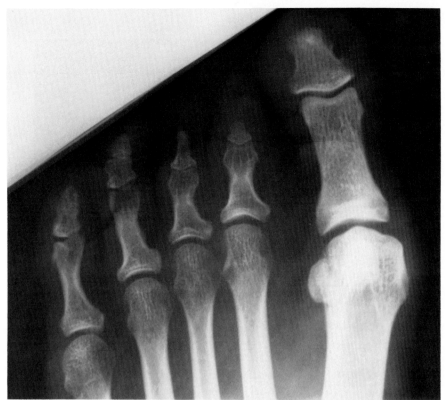

Figure 6.38. The second and third digits exhibit an absence of the middle phalanx. The first, fourth, and fifth digits are normal.

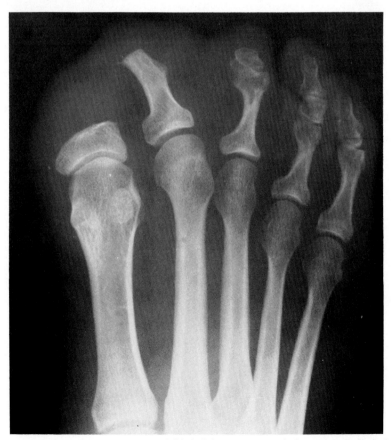

Figure 6.39. The deformity of the first, second, and third digits are congenital, not surgically induced, in this patient.

129

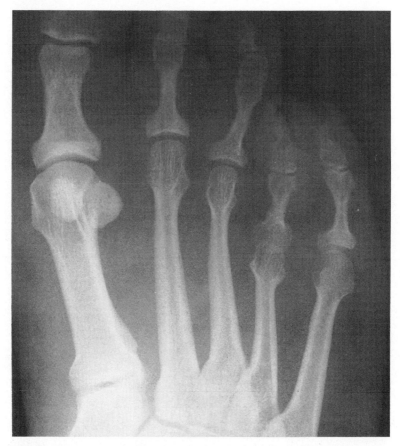

Figure 6.40.   Congenitally short fourth metatarsal is very common and in some families it is congenital. Occasionally it is associated with pseudohyperparathyroidism and with pseudopseudohyperparathyroidism.

REFERENCES

1. HARDY, R. H., AND CLAPHAM, J. C.: Hallux valgus (predisposing anatomical causes). Lancet, **53:** 1180, 1952.
2. HADJIPOVLU, A., ET AL.: Metatarsalgia in pseudo-pseudo-hypoparathyroidism: A case report. Acta Orthop. Belg., **45:** 209, 1979.
3. LAPORTA, G., MELILLO, T., AND OLINSKY, D.: X-ray evaluation of hallux abductus deformity. J.A.P.A., **64:** 544, 1974.
4. KELIKIAN, H.: *Hallux Valgus, Allied Deformity of the Forefoot,* W. B. Saunders, Philadelphia, 1965.
5. SHAW, A. H., AND PACK, L. G.: Osteotomies of first ray for hallux abducto valgus deformity. J.A.P.A., **64:** 567, 1974.
6. GERBERT, J., MERCARDO, O. A., AND SOKOLOFF, T. H.: *The Surgical Treatment of the Hallux-Abducto-Valgus and Allied Deformities,* Futura, Mt. Kisco, NY, 1973, vol. 1.
7. GOLDNER, J. L., AND GAINES, R. W.: Adult and juvenile hallux valgus: Analysis and treatment. Orthop. Clin. North Am., **7:** 863, 1976.
8. GIANNESTRAS, N.: *Foot Disorders Medical and Surgical Treatment,* 2nd Ed, Lea & Febiger, Philadelphia, 1973.
9. VENN-WATSON, E. A.: Problems in polydactyly of the foot. Orthop. Clin. North Am. **7:** 909, 1976.
10. SGARLOTTO, T. E.: *A Compendium of Podiatric Biomechanics,* California College of Podiatric Medicine, San Francisco, 1971.
11. WEISSMAN, S. D., AND DONLEY, K.: Application of the reverdin correction for hallux-abducto-valgus in deformities of the lesser metatarsophalangeal joints. A case report. J. Foot Surg., **18:** 110, 1979.

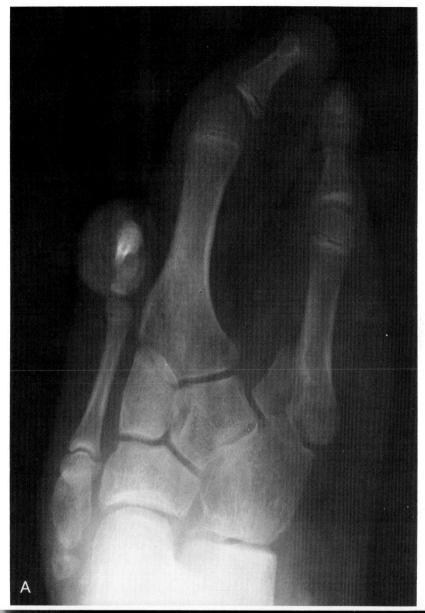

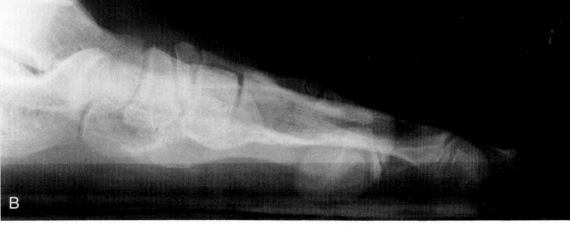

Figure 6.41.   *A* and *B*, claw or cleft foot.

CHAPTER 7

Physiologically and Pathologically Induced X-ray Changes

X-RAY EVALUATION OF THE SOFT TISSUES

Proper evaluation of the soft tissues is a very useful tool in arriving at a final diagnosis following trauma, when masses are present, and can be of help in determining vascular pathology in a patient.

X-rays of the soft tissues must be evaluated for soft tissue volume, soft tissue atrophy, soft tissues tumors, soft tissue calcifications, and foreign bodies.[20]

Edema of Soft Tissue

Edema within the soft tissues can usually be attributable to one of three main etiologies, including trauma, infection, and due to circulatory conditions.

Static or posttraumatic edema can be seen following sprains, blows, or other types of trauma. Following these injuries, it is of importance to examine the soft tissues. There is too great a tendency to minimize injuries when we do not see an apparent bone injury. The location and extent of the edema is an excellent indication of the type of soft tissue damage that has occurred. It is important to remember the anatomy of the area that exhibits the posttraumatic edema for consideration of which structures may possibly have been injured.

In posttraumatic swelling, the fascial planes are visible and the increase in density of the soft tissue is clear rather than hazy. The principle soft tissue swelling will be located over the most traumatized structure.[20]

Infectious Edema

In infectious or reactive edema, we usually see obliteration of the fascial planes. The edema will be an indistinct increase in the density of the soft tissues. In this type of edema, we will have a coarsened reticular pattern, occasionally with prominence of the fibrous septa. The soft tissue edema of pyogenic infections of bone is the only change seen early in this disease. By the time the osseous changes appear, the disease is fairly well along and the changes may be permanent at this time (Fig. 7.1).

TRAUMATIC OR CIRCULATORY (STATIC) EDEMA

Edema found after a traumatic incident or as a result of circulatory insufficiency can be distinguished from infectious edema on a clear, sharp radiograph. It presents an increase in thickening of the soft tissue with fascial planes that are visible. The increased density is clear rather than hazy, and the increase in soft tissue volume will be diffused not delineated or circumscribed or encapsulated (Fig. 7.2).[27]

Soft Tissue Tumors

An increase in soft tissue volume may be indicative of a soft tissue mass. All soft tissue tumors are of a unit or water density except:
(1) fat tumors (more radiolucent);
(2) masses with hemosiderin content (more radiodense);
(3) longstanding tophi (may calcify);
(4) masses with calcification or ossification.

A definitive diagnosis on x-ray is rarely possible. The location, size, and distribution can be determined radiographically, however, as well as the behavior of the tumor with respect to bone. It is important to know if the tumor has caused saucerization, erosion, invasion of bone, or sclerotic reaction of bone.

The soft tissue masses will appear clear, circumscribed, or as an elongated increase in density of soft tissues. There is a definite outline to the mass or increase in density different in texture from the adjacent normal soft tissues. Deliniation and demarkation are obvious. Deformity is noted when a mass is present and an abnormal skin contour can be observed (Figs. 7.3 to 7.6).

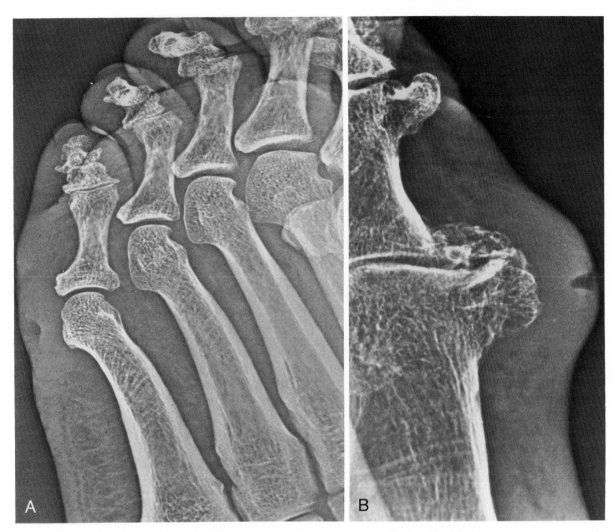

Figure 7.1. *A,* infectious edema. An ulceration in the skin lateral to the fifth metatarsal head can be seen in this xeroradiograph. Infectious edema is present on the lateral aspect of the fifth metatarsal head. *B,* ulcer with sinus tract over the first metatarsal head. Note the hazy soft tissue edema about the entire joint. *C,* ulceration over the medial malleolus with induration of the skin surrounding the ulceration. *D,* large defect is present in the soft tissues lateral to the fifth metatarsal. The defect extends down to the shaft of the metatarsal. Note the increased stromal markings about the area.

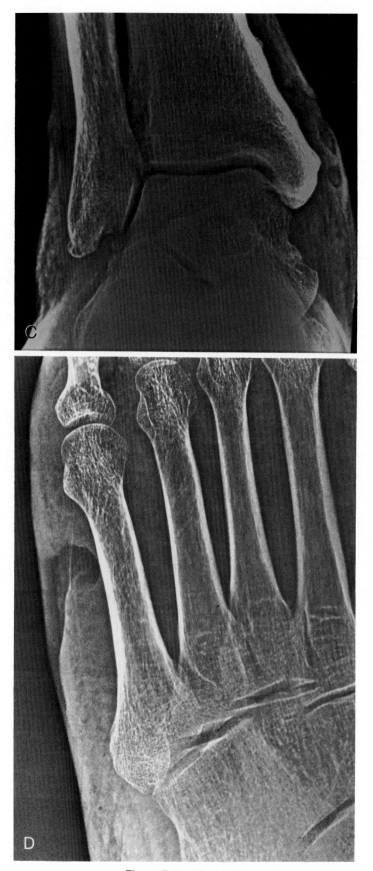

Figure 7.1.   (*C* and *D*)

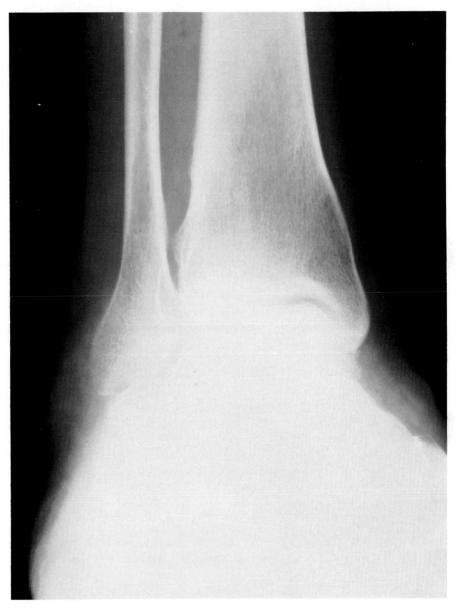

Figure 7.2.   Traumatic edema. In traumatic edema the fascial planes remain visible and become attenuated.

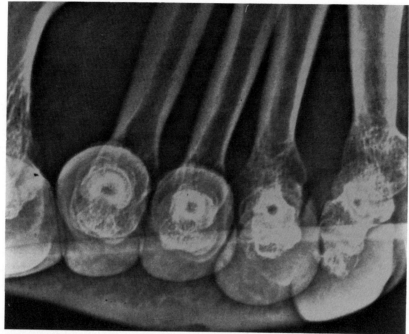

Figure 7.3.   A mass can be seen in the soft tissues beneath the third metatarsal head on this sesamoid axial projection. The lucent area in the skin superficial to the mass was due to a callus that had been debrided prior to the x-ray.

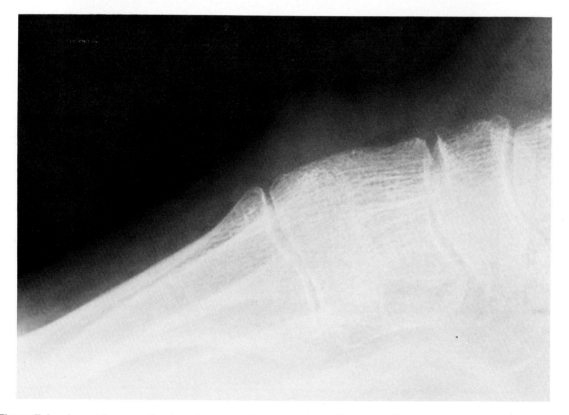

Figure 7.4.   A ganglion over the dorsal aspect of the second cuneiform is well circumscribed in the soft tissues.

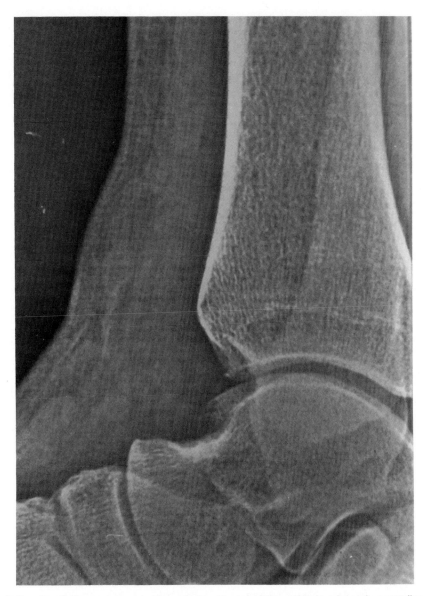

Figure 7.5.   A soft tissue mass on the anterior aspect of the ankle in a lateral xeroradiograph.

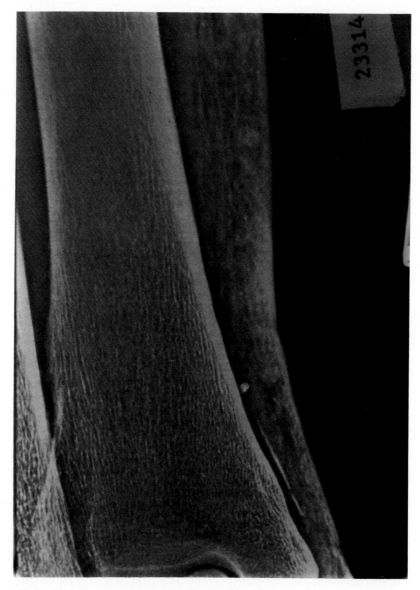

Figure 7.6. Cutaneous induration. Thickening of the skin on the medial aspect of the lower leg can be seen on this xeroradiograph. This was due to a localized area of acute cellulitis.

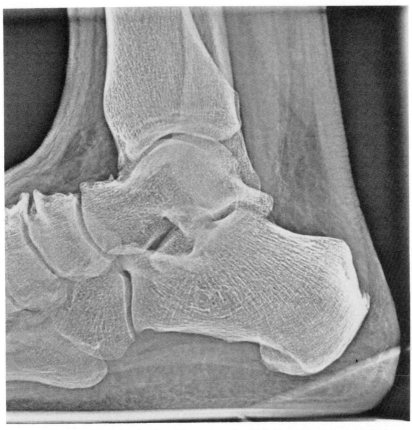

Figure 7.7. Toygar's or Kager's triangle. A triangular area of radiolucency is noted posterior to the normal ankle. This area is bounded by the tendo-achilles, the flexor hallucis longus, and the dorsal aspect of the calcaneus. It is absent when edema occurs in the area.

Toygars' Triangle

Toygar's or Kager's triangle is a radiologically clear area found in the soft tissue posterior to the ankle on lateral films. In the normal patient, the triangle will be clear, while in infection, posttrauma, and connective tissue disease, it tends to be obliterated. The boundaries of Kager's triangle are as follows: anteriorly, the flexor hallucis longus; posteriorly, the tendo-achilles; inferiorly, the dorsal surface of the calcaneus (Figs. 7.7 and 7.8).[2]

Soft Tissue Atrophy

Soft tissue atrophy can occur as the result of either local disturbances or systemic manifestations. It can be either from atrophy of a previously developed structure or from a lack of development. It may be localized or generalized, unilateral or bilateral. A knowledge of the normal anatomy and contour of the extremities will lead to a diagnosis of soft tissue atrophy. The etiologies may be nutritional, i.e., malnutrition, cachexia, etc.; neurologic, i.e., muscular dystrophies, post-paralytic atrophy, polio-myelitis, etc.; or disuse as in the treatment of a fracture post-plaster cast, etc. (see Fig. 7.30).

Soft Tissue Emphysema

Soft tissue emphysema is defined as air in the soft tissues.[3] The etiology can be two-fold, the first being posttrauma and the second as a result of gas-producing organisms within the soft tissues. It will appear radiographically as an increased radiolucency in the soft tissues in circular bubbles. Examination of these tissues can produce a crackling sound as the air moves around and escapes (Fig. 7.9).

Acromegaly

An increase in soft tissue volume is a clinical characteristic of acromegaly. In this endocrine disorder, the skin becomes coarse, thick, and leathery. The mean skin thickness increases from 1–1.7 mm in the normal female and 1.1–1.8 mm in the normal male, up to 1.75–2.8 mm in acromegaly. A non-weightbearing lateral film will be of use in determing if the heel pad sign is present.

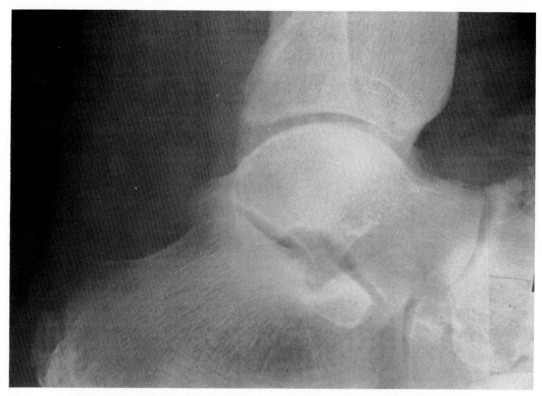

Figure 7.8. Toygar's triangle is absent. It is obliterated by posttraumatic edema secondary to a ruptured tendo-achilles.

The thickness of the fat pad of the normal heel is 13–21 mm with a mean of 17.8. In acromegaly, the heel pad will be from 17–34 mm thick. This soft tissue thickness can be measured using the method of Kho. It is important to realize that the heel pads frequently are slightly thicker in black people, obese people, and, of course, after injury and any form of edema.[4, 23]

SOFT TISSUE CALCIFICATION

There are three main categories of soft tissue calcification. These are 1) metastatic calcification, 2) calcinosis, and 3) dystrophic calcification. These calcifications must first be distinguished from ossification. Ossification implies a deposition of calcium salts in soft tissues with an organization into trabeculae and with a cortex. Calcification simply implies a deposition of calcium salts without organization, trabeculation, or cortex.[5, 6, 21]

DYSTROPHIC CALCIFICATION

Dystrophic calcification indicates calcium deposition in damaged tissues without generalized metabolic derangement. Because of the damage to the tissues, which can be from many different etiologies, including peripheral vascular disease, the tissue becomes devitalized and, therefore, has a lower metabolic rate. This implies a decreased carbon dioxide concentration in the tissues which leads to a local alkalinity. Calcium and phosphorous salts are less soluble in alkaline medium and, therefore, precipitate in this area of devitalization. Examples of dystrophic calcification are ehlers danlos syndrome, pseudoxanthoma elasticum, fibromatosis, tumors, cysts, hematomas, postinflammatory foci, posttrauma, arteriosclerosis obliterans, Mönkeberg's medial sclerosis, and hyperparathyroidism.

Peripheral Vascular Disease

Arteriosclerosis obliterans is a chronic obliterative disease of the lower portion of the aorta, its main branches, and the arteries of the extremities, especially in the lower extremity. Although it primarily concerns the intima, it can also include the media of the vessels. The alterations of the involved artery are progressive and segmental in nature and usually non-reversable. The intima generally displays widespread atherosclerotic changes, including obstructions that completely occlude the arteriole. The changes are usually also both proximal and distal to the obstruction. Ath-

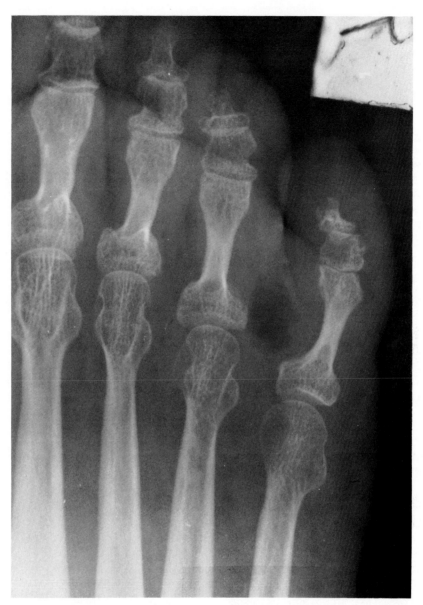

Figure 7.9. Soft tissue emphysema. Gas in the soft tissues between the base of the fourth and fifth proximal phalanges causes a circular radiolucent area. This infection was due to a gas-forming bacterium.

eromas affect those parts of the vasculature where there is a high mean pressure, especially the areas near the bifurcations of large vessels.

The symptoms include all of the cardinal symptoms of interruption of arterial flow, including intermittant claudication, trophic changes, decrease in temperature, decrease in pulses, and low oscillometric readings. Because of the progressive nature of the alterations in the arterial tree, the maintenance of tissue viability usually depends upon collateral circulation. A resultant decrease in lumenal size of a vessel of up to 60% induces only blood pressure changes. A 60–70% decrease causes symptoms distal to the occlusion. The most significant change in the wall of the vessel is an

atheromatus plaque in the intimal and subintimal tissues. This plaque is associated with a deposition of excess fibrous material and collagen and leads to a thickened intima. At a later stage, calcium deposition may occur along with thrombus formation within the arteriole. Associated with the calcium deposition will be atrophy and necrosis of the medial muscle fibers with replacement by collagen and then calcium deposition can occur in the media as well.

Radiographically, the only sign of arteriosclerosis obliterans that can be observed would be the patchy calcification that occurs in the later stages of the disease within the intima and media (Figs. 7.10 to 7.13).[5, 7, 8, 21]

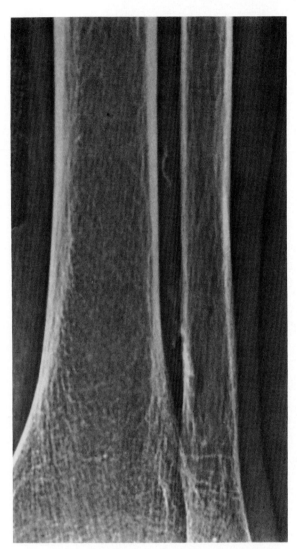

Figure 7.10.   Arteriosclerosis obliterans. Patchy calcification is present in the posterior tibial artery and must be differentiated from Mönkeberg's medial sclerosis.

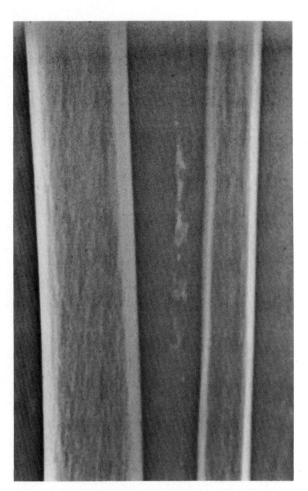

Figure 7.11.   Arteriosclerosis obliterans causing an almost complete blockage of the posterior tibial artery.

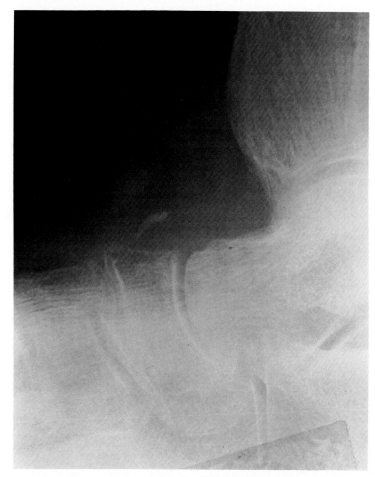

Figure 7.12. Arteriosclerosis obliterans of the dorsalis pedis.

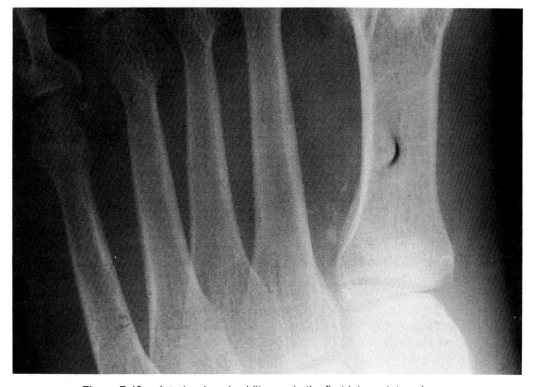

Figure 7.13. Arteriosclerosis obliterans in the first intermetatarsal space.

143

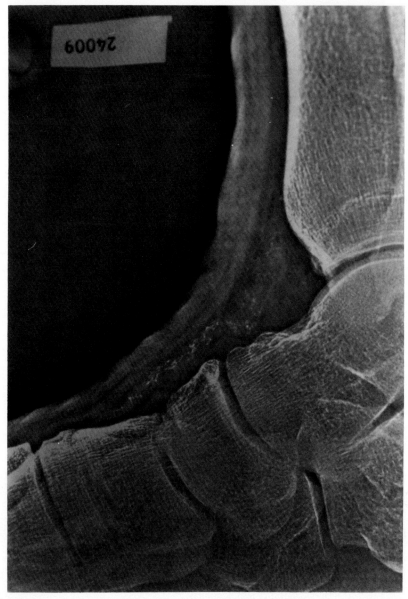

Figure 7.14. Mönkeberg's medial sclerosis of the dorsalis pedis forming a characteristic gooseneck appearance.

Mönkeberg's Medial Sclerosis

A popular misconception among practitioners is the significance attributed to the deposition of calcium in the media of large arteries and medium-size arterioles on x-ray.

Unfortunately, little attempt is usually made to differentiate this type of benign arteriosclerosis from thromboangitis obliterans or arteriosclerosis obliterans. This disease affects the muscular arteries in the lower extremities of young and middle-aged people and is unassociated with signs or symptoms of impaired arterial circulation. Usually the calcific changes are discovered by accident on an x-ray taken for other purposes. The calcification is totally within the medial coat of the arteriole and leads to a decreased distensibility of the vessel. Palpation of the pulses will reveal that they are slightly reduced when palpated manually and that oscillometric readings are mildly decreased. This disease does not interfere with movement of blood and therefore the patient suffers no

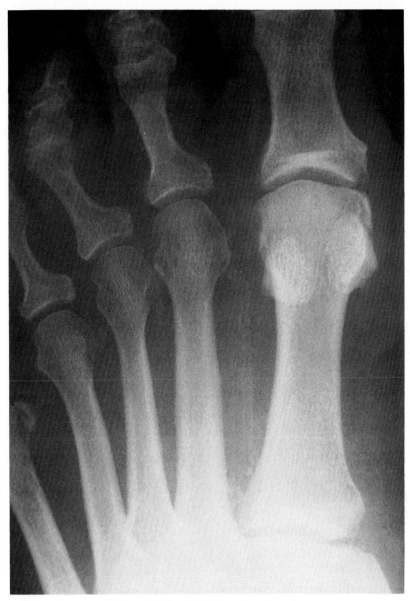

Figure 7.15.   Mönkeberg's sclerosis.

reduction of circulation into the tissues. Mönke-berg's sclerosis may possibly be associated with arteriosclerosis in the older individual.

The diagnosis is made radiographically by a consistent series of findings, including: two thin straight lines of calcium a few millimeters apart with a fine granular haze between them. The calcification will be segmental and will have many gaps. This deposition of calcium forms a chain of rings giving a "gooseneck lamp" appearance out-lining the arteries and their branches. These cal-cifications will run along the axis of the vessels, as opposed to arteriosclerotic-type calcifications which will be at the site of plaques and run transverse to the long axis of the vessels.[7,8,5]

Occasionally, sclerosis of the medial coat of the vessels is seen in infants and children and is referred to as the calcification of Baggenstoss and Keith. In this case the etiology is infection, con-genital syphilis, renal disease, hypervitaminosis-D, or hyperparathyroidism (Figs. 7.14 to 7.17).[7,21]

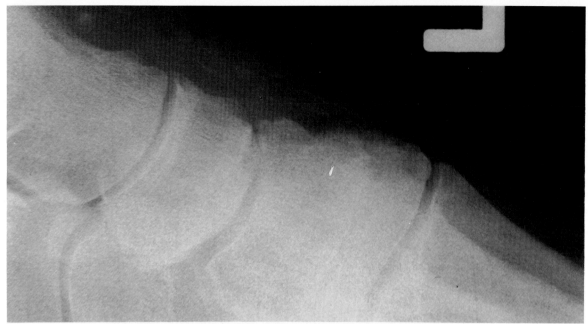

Figure 7.16. Mönkeberg's sclerosis.

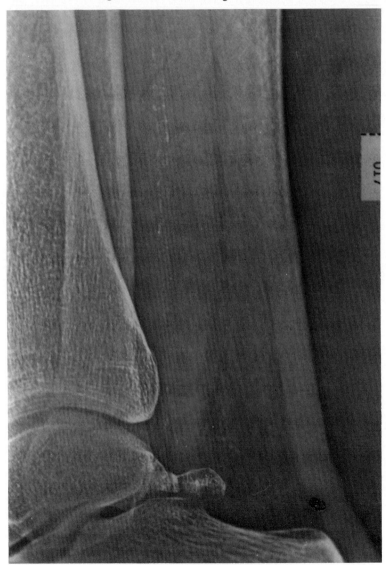

Figure 7.17. Mönkeberg's medial sclerosis of the posterior tibial artery in a young adult of 25 years of age.

Phleboliths

The histological examination of veins reveals that they have very little if any muscular coat. The media, therefore, is quite thinned and calcification is extremely rare in this coat. When calcific lesions of veins are observed on x-ray they are called phleboliths and usually represent calcified thrombae within the vein. Extensive venous calcification may be palpated as segments possibly several inches long which are subcutaneous and can be moved as a unit. Radiographically they appear as small rounded calcific structures following the course of a vein (Figs. 7.18 and 7.19).[7]

Calcinosis

Calcinosis refers to the deposition of calcium in the subcutaneous skin tissues and connective tissues in the presence of normal calcium metabolism. Included within this heading is subcutaneous calcinosis, calcinosis circumscripta, tumoral calcinosis, and scleroderma with calcinosis (Thibierge-Weissenbach syndrome).

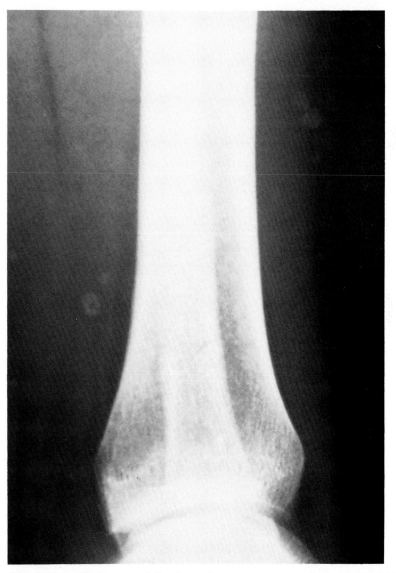

Figure 7.18. Phleboliths in the soft tissues of the lower leg appear as small rounded calcified structures and represent a calcified thrombus in the vein.

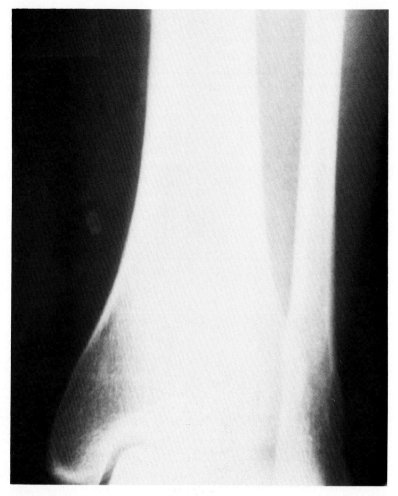

Figure 7.19.

Subcutaneous Calcinosis

This is a relatively infrequent complication of long-standing varicosities, kidney disease, or hyperparathyroidism. It involves the deposition of calcium both inside and outside the involved veins. These calcifications may penetrate the cutis, thus tending to initiate a stasis ulcer. They can be very extensive, including the entire circumference and length of a segment (Figs. 7.20 and 7.21).

Tumoral calcinosis (Calcifying Collagenolysis)

This entity is of unknown etiology. Usually no other abnormalities are found in the patient and it usually occurs in blacks. Masses of discrete calcification are found in the extremities in the vicinity of joints. They are firm, rubbery and gritty, multilocular cystic masses. These juxta-articular lesions are usually painless, but edema and disability can occur in extreme cases. The patient will have a slow-growing calcific mass in the periarticular tissues. X-ray examination will show small, calcified nodules which grow into large, lobulated tumors with a linear, lacy calcific distribution (Fig. 7.22).[9, 10, 11, 26]

Other Forms of Calcinosis

A common form of calcinosis is the calcified bursa. They will appear in an area next to the bone, usually not attached, and are in the area of a known bursa. On examination, they are slightly flocculant. They must be distinguished from chronic bursitis (Figs. 7.23 and 7.24), gout, pseudogout, calcinosis circumscripta, and hypervitaminosis-D. On x-ray, they have a fluffy calcific appearance.[5]

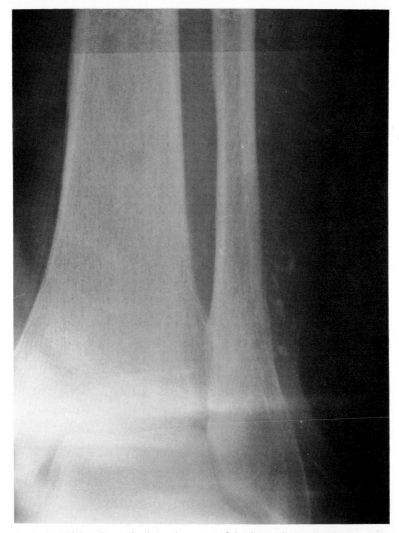

Figure 7.20. Subcutaneous calcinosis on the lateral aspect of the lower leg secondary to venous stasis ulceration.

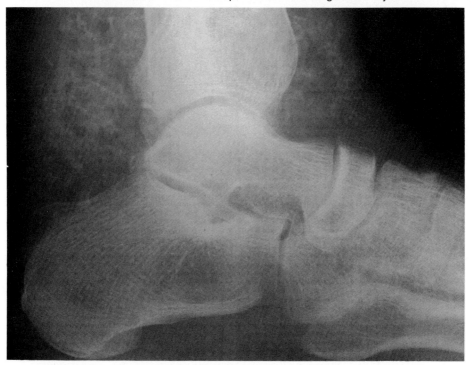

Figure 7.21. Subcutaneous calcinosis due to long-standing venous stasis.

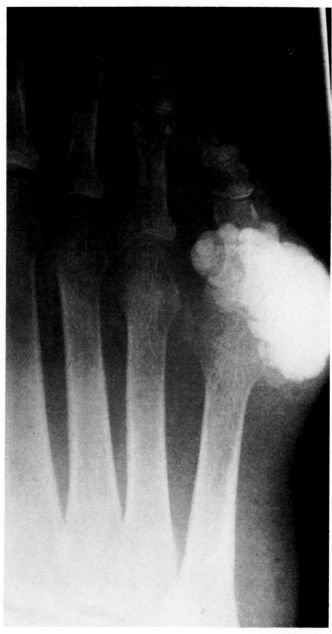

Figure 7.22.   Tumoral calcinosis. A conglomeration of small calcified lobulated tumors with a linear calcific distribution in the area of a joint.

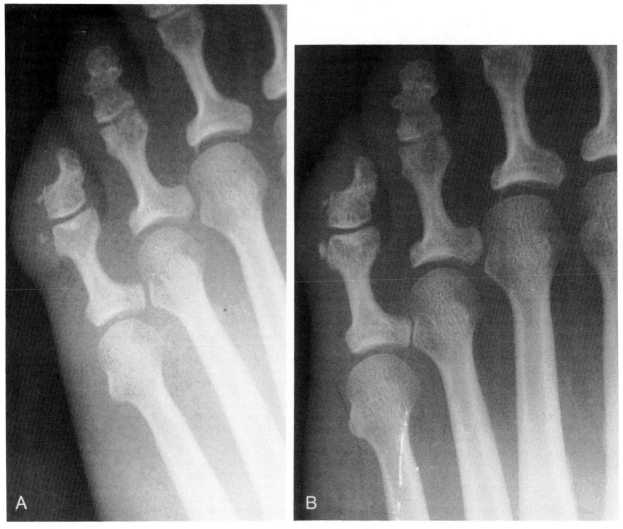

Figure 7.23.   Calcified bursitis. *A* shows early calcification of adventitious bursa on the dorsolateral aspect of the fifth digit. *B* shows further progression in the calcification of the bursa.

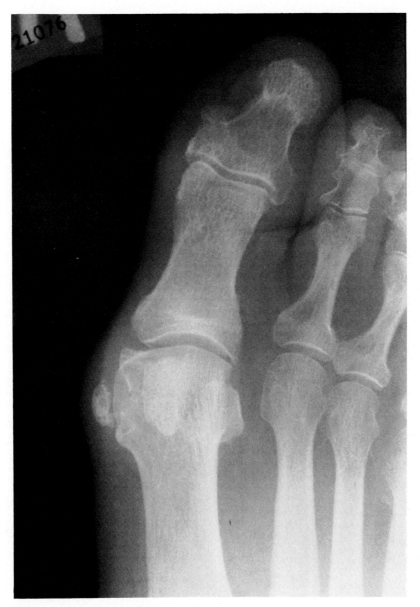

Figure 7.24.　Calcification of a bursa, medial to the first metatarsal head, associated with hallux-abducto-valgus and bunion deformity.

METASTATIC CALCIFICATION

Metastatic calcification implies a disturbance in the calcium or phosphorous metabolism leading to ectopic calcification in normal tissues. Examples are: hyperparathyroidism, secondary hyperparathyroidism, systemic lupus erythematosis, dermatomyositis, and scleroderma.[5,6]

Hyperparathyroidism

Hyperparathyroidism and secondary hyperparathyroidism can lead to profound alterations in calcium resorption and absorption leading to deposition in the soft tissues. There will be changes in the blood picture as well. Clinical manifestations include: cutaneous gangrene, peripheral vascular disease, and myositis. Radiographically, we will see subperiosteal bone resorption, a linear shadow of bone lying parallel to the cortex in the metatarsals, and calcium deposits within the media and intima of vessels (Figs. 7.24 and 7.25).[21]

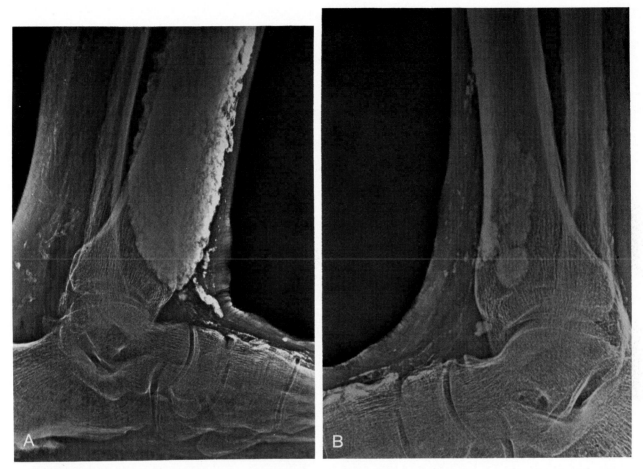

Figure 7.25. *A* and *B*, calcinosis due to secondary hyperparathyroidism causing extensive deposits of calcium in the soft tissues of the lower leg and blood vessels of the lower leg.

Systemic Lupus Erythematosus (SLE)

There are basically three patterns of soft tissue calcification that can occur in SLE. These include the diffuse linear pattern, the streaky pattern, and the nodular calcific pattern, as well as combinations of the three above. In this disease, we can see periarticular calcifications, calcifications of arteries, and, focal plaque-like calcific deposits in the soft tissues. Some of the soft tissue calcification can be precipitated by recurrent tissue ulcerations (Figs. 7.26 to 7.28).[22]

Scleroderma

Patients with long-standing scleroderma will frequently show atrophy of the skin and subcutaneous tissues. Radiographically, in these areas, we can see many calcific deposits, especially in the subcutaneous tissues of the digits. These calcifications also occur in pressure areas. They can be seen in the muscles and viscera as well. Radiographically, they tend to be punctate or conglomerates of small punctate bodies with sharply defined borders (Fig. 7.29).

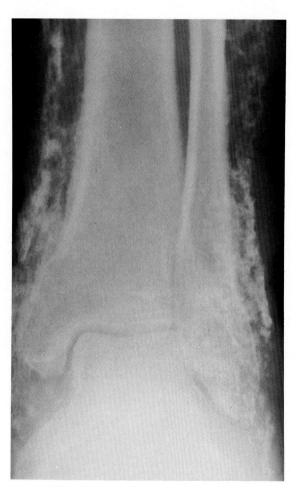

Figure 7.26. Systemic lupus erythematosus causing a streaky pattern of calcification in the lower leg.

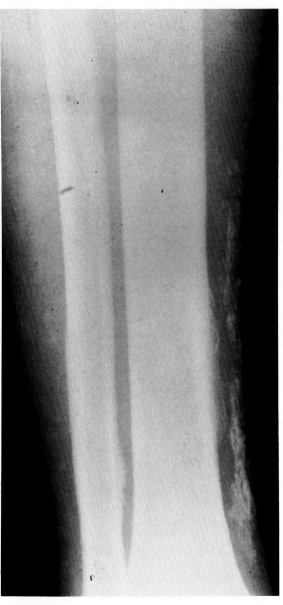

Figure 7.27. Systemic lupus erythematosus causing a streaky pattern of calcification in the lower leg.

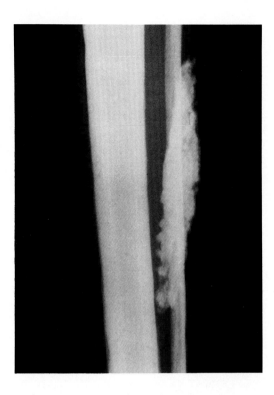

Figure 7.28.   SLE causing a diffuse linear pattern of calcification in the lower leg.

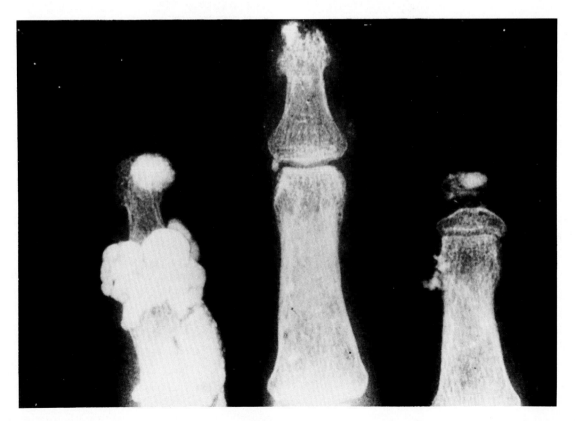

Figure 7.29.   Scleroderma. This patient was diagnosed as having CRST syndrome consisting of calcinosis, Raynaud's phenomenon, sclerodactyly, and telangiectasia. This syndrome causes punctate calcification near the tips of the digits and a resorption of portion of the distal phalanges. Radiograph compliments of Dr. Harvey Lemont.

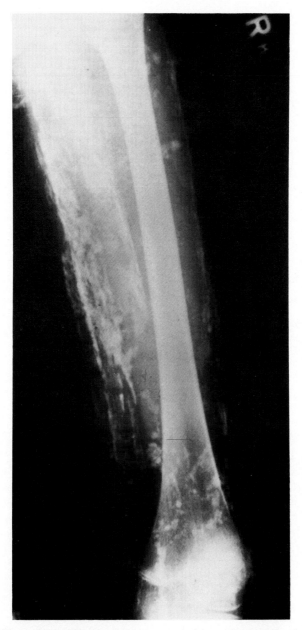

Figure 7.30. Dermatomyositis causing diffuse subcutaneous and muscular calcifications. Note the extensive soft tissue atrophy of the lower leg.

Dermatomyositis

Dermatomyositis can cause diffuse subcutaneous and muscular calcifications which may assume any configuration, but tend to be thinner, more finely linear, or net-like and less sharply defined than those of scleroderma (Fig. 7.30).

SOFT TISSUE OSSIFICATION

Traumatic Myositis Ossificans

Of all the myositis ossificans seen, approximately two-thirds are secondary to trauma. A lesion will become apparent 1–2 weeks after trauma as a subcutaneous mass. Within 4–6 weeks it will become calcified. Histologic examination shows three layers or zones: an inner zone of undifferentiated fibrous tissue, a middle zone containing osteoid elements, and a peripheral zone of well-organized bone and fibrous capsule. The bone becomes well organized and mature with a trabecular pattern and a thin cortex that is well defined. This is in direct opposition to extraosseous osteogenic sarcoma (Figs. 7.31 and 7.32).

Myositis ossificans progressiva occurs as soft tissue masses in early childhood. The ossification

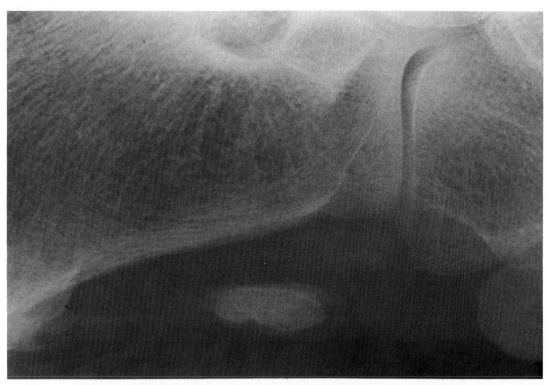

Figure 7.31.   Posttraumatic myositis ossificans in the intrinsic musculature of the sole. Note the trabeculations in the calcific area.

begins as an exostosis at tendon insertions. Later it invades muscles and deep connective tissues, and in the latter stages fusions of joints can occur. These affected people frequently have skeletal changes consisting of shortening of the great and little toes. The first metatarsal and proximal phalanx may be hypoplastic or the great toe may have only one phalanx.[4, 5, 11, 23]

THE PERIOSTEUM

Elevation of the periosteum from the cortex followed by new bone formation is a fundamental response of bone to a disease process.[12] The terms periosteal new bone, and reactive bone formation, usually imply a pathologic process, but at times, only represent acceleration of normal subperiosteal bone growth. Whereas osteogenic and chondrogenic tumors alone are able to produce tumor-

ous new bone, many neoplasms, as well as infections, trauma, and other diseases, can stimulate reactive new bone. It is of paramount importance to differentiate one from the other.[13] It is also important to the diagnosis to know if inflammation is present or absent.

The cambium layer of periosteum retains its osteogenic properties, and if not destroyed, will form new bone. Reactive new bone usually is well organized and appears as a thickened cortex. Tumorous new bone is disorganized, appearing as areas of ivory-like density, or as multiple dense flecks of bone. The former is produced by osteogenic tissue, the latter by chondrogenic tissue.[13] Periosteal reactions are common occurrences in most bone lesions, and the pattern of the elevation is really of greater significance than the presence of the elevation. There are three basic forms of periosteal reactions.

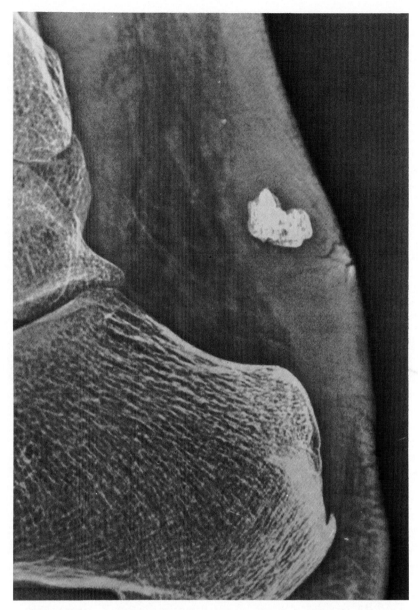

Figure 7.32.   Pellegrini-stieda disease or calcification within a tendon.

SOLID PERIOSTEAL REACTIONS

The solid periosteal reactions may be defined as a single layer of new bone greater than 1 mm in thickness. They are of uniform density, and when seen, can be considered the hallmark of a benign process.[13] Although persistent, they remain relatively unchanged for weeks, and are not useful as a diagnostic indicator. The uniformity of its roentgen density changes very little, even as they increase in size. It is the uniformity and solidarity that are important, not the thickness or density (Fig. 7.33).

The thickness and density seem related to the aggressiveness of the irritant. Solid periosteal new bone formation may be caused by eosinophilic granuloma, fractures, osteomyelitis, hemorrhage, hypertrophic pulmonary osteoarthropathy, osteoid osteoma, vascular diseases, and the storage diseases.[13]

INTERRUPTED PERIOSTEAL REACTIONS

Interrupted periosteal reactions are non-uniform and pleomorphic. They are indicators of intermittent or cyclic processes, and seem to lack stability, changing constantly. Included are parallel, onion skin or lamenated, and perpendicular or sunburst reactions. Interrupted periosteal reactions are caused by periosteal elevations, such as in osteomyelitis, hemorrhages, and tumors.

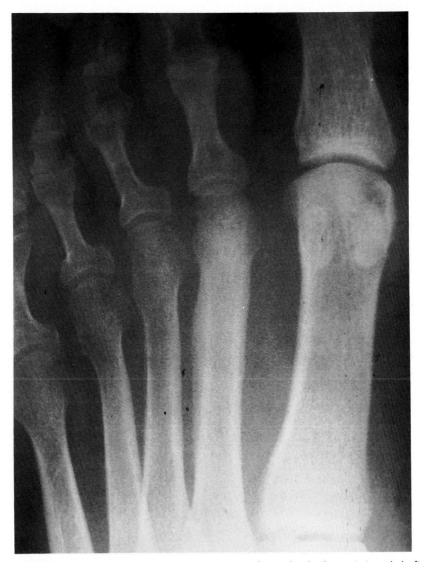

Figure 7.33. Solid pattern of periosteal new bone formation in the metatarsal shafts.

Lamenated periosteal reactions, due to intermittent growth, occur in active conditions, such as acute osteomyelitis and malignant tumors. During the slow growth, the periosteum has time to form a layer of bone analagous to the involucrum of infection.[13]

"Sunburst," or perpendicular reactions, are the result of new bone growing at right angles to the shaft of the host bone, and frequently are caused by a malignant tumor, which elevates the periosteum.[13]

AMORPHOUS REACTIONS

Amorphous calcific densities are often found in malignant tumors, in addition to lamellations, and perpendicular striations. These densities lie between the periosteal new bone, and its parent cortical bone, and may represent extension of bone tumor rather than a periosteal response to the tumor.[13]

While the "sunburst" pattern is often considered characteristic of primary bone sarcoma, occasionally, such a pattern is found in association with metastatic bone tumors as well.[14]

BENIGN CONDITIONS CHARACTERIZED BY GENERALIZED PERIOSTEAL ELEVATIONS

Pulmonary Hypertrophic Osteoarthropathy

Pulmonary hypertrophic osteoarthropathy is composed of a triad of periosteal new bone, clubbing of the toes and fingers, and synovitis. It is associated with a wide variety of pulmonary and plural conditions. In adults, it is most commonly caused by carcinoma of the lung, while in children, fibrocystic disease or pulmonary metastasis may cause this reaction. The x-ray manifestations of pulmonary hypertrophic osteoarthropathy may be present long before the lung disease becomes apparent. A neurogenic mechanism produces the changes that are seen radiographically, and it has been found that the osteoarthropathy regresses after removal of the primary lung lesion.[5]

In pulmonary osteoarthropathy, the tubular bones show wavy, cortical thickening caused by new bone apposition, which is most apparent along the shaft. The epiphyses are usually not involved. The osteoperiostotic deposit is at first sharply demarcated from the original cortex, but as it thickens, it eventually merges with the cortex.

Radiographically, clubbing of the digits at the terminal tufts is noted. Thin, undulating periosteal reactions are located primarily on the concave aspect of long bones.[13] It is seen frequently in the metatarsal shafts. The periosteal pattern may vary from a simple solid elevation of the periosteum with a radiolucent area between the periosteum and cortex to an onion skin appearance caused by regular bursts of periosteal new bone, to simply a solid, wavy contour to the thickened cortex.

Thyroid Acropachy

Thyroid acropachy is a rare complication of hyperthyroid disease in which there is exophthalmos, asymptomatic swelling of the feet and hands, clubbing of the digits, pretibial myxedema, and periosteal new bone formation. This generally gives the bones a fusiform contour with asymmetrical involvement. It is particularly prevalent in the metatarsal bones and phalanges.[5]

Pachydermoperiostosis

Pachydermoperiostosis, or chronic idiopathic hypertrophic osteoarthropathy with pachydermia and osteolysis, is characterized by thickening of the skin of the face, forehead, forearms, and legs; clubbing of the digits; and there are painful edematous joints; osteolysis; and hyperhidrosis. Nontender periosteal new bone formation and resultant cortical thickening occurs. X-rays will show irregular periosteal new bone formation, which tends to blend with the cortex. It will be symmetrical, and the bone ends may on rare occasions be involved. Osteolysis with clubbing of the digits helps to differentiate this condition.[15]

Caffey's Syndrome or Infantile Cortical Hyperostosis

Caffey's syndrome is a familial condition in which there are soft tissue swellings, periosteal new bone formation and hyperirritability, or colic. The areas of soft tissue swelling are usually tender and precede the periosteal changes on x-ray. Swelling is frequently found over the anterior tibial region and gives a convex profile to the leg.

In the earliest phase, the cortex is narrow with blurring of the outer edge of the bone. This develops into fine linear densities adjacent to the cortex, which within several days become more distinct, and gives a pencil-streak appearance. The pencil-streak widens, increases in density, and appears separated from the older cortex by a radiolucent zone. The new subperioteal bone later becomes incorporated into the old cortex; the end result being a spindle-shaped long bone with massive cortical thickening and widening of the bone.

A new generally known fact is that roentgenologically visible new bone in infants frequently is normal. An area of periosteal new bone in a child is not necessarily diagnostic of Caffey's syndrome. Many conditions give rise to periosteal new bone in children, such as trauma, osteomyelitis, congenital syphillis, rickets, scurvy, hypervitaminosis-A, infantile cortical hyperostosis, leukemia, and neuroblastoma.[16]

Hypervitaminosis-A

In hypervitaminosis-A tender masses are seen over the long bones with periosteal new bone formation beneath them. Diaphyseal involvement usually is present in the form of smooth to wavy undulating cortical thickening.[5]

Codman's Triangle

When the periosteum of a bone is locally elevated in a triangular shape, a periosteal cuff called Codman's triangle is seen. The significance of the triangular Codman's cuff merits particular attention. It was long considered a manifestation of malignant bone disease, but it is now generally accepted that it may be the result of anything that lifts the periosteum either benign or malignant (Fig. 12.1).[14]

Pseudoperiostitis

During periods of increased osteoclastic activity, reflecting rapid demineralization, occasionally a picture occurs which simulates periostitis. This change must be recognized as a reflection of osteoporosis, so that misdiagnosis as an inflammatory disease does not occur.

Exaggerated osteoclastic activity in which there is a rapid disillusion of calcium may occur and appears radiographically as separation of a margin of cortical bone, which is similar to the cortical tunneling described in hyperparathyroidism. Since this condition mimics periostitis, it is called pseudoperiostitis. It appears as a linear radiodense shadow paralleling the contour of the diaphysis, appearing as though the cortex has been split.

Usually this condition occurs along with mottled decalcification of the medullary space. Loss of mineral from the long bones can result in cortical tunneling simulating periosteal new bone. Pseudoperiostitis has been known to occur in the intense inflammation that sometimes occurs in rheumatoid arthritis, and may be exaggerated by disuse or treatment with steroids.[17]

ABNORMALITIES IN BONY MINERALIZATION

Evaluation of bony mineralization can be very difficult and must be approached in a manner similar to evaluation of the soft tissues: "Is there too much or too little, and is the change generalized or limited?"[6] It must be remembered that the appearance of bones can be altered simply by technical factors, and there is no baseline by which to judge changes from the norm.

The three major metabolic diseases resulting in a generalized defuse loss of bone density are: osteoporosis, osteomalacia, and hyperparathyroidism. Osteoporosis may be defined as an increased porosity of bone, and refers to a condition caused by diminution of bone mass. The bone substance is of normal quality. In osteomalacia, there is abnormal bone with excess uncalcified osteoid. This is similar to demineralization, which is defined as loss of calcium salts from the bone. Hyperparathyroidism results in increased resorption of bone by osteoclasts. This is accompanied by proliferation of fibrous connective tissues.[3,6]

Osteoporosis

Osteoporosis is a skeletal condition, generalized or localized, in which the quantity of bone per unit volume is decreased in amount but is normal in composition.[5]

When the bone formation rate falls below the bone resorption rate, diminution of bone mass

develops. Decreased bone mass leads to increased skeletal fragility, and can result in fractures.

Close evaluation of the cortical bone on film can be used to access the changes in the amount of bone. As bones become osteoporotic, the cortex begins to thin and the trabeculae within the medullary canal begin to disappear. While trabecule can disappear from overexposure of an x-ray, the cortex usually does not thin from overexposure. In an osteoporotic bone, the central shaft will appear grayish from loss of trabeculae and the cortex will usually stand out in sharp contrast. This can be deceiving, giving one the false idea that the cortex is hypertrophied. On close examination, it will be determined that the cortex has become thinner and stands out only because of the contrast with the ground glass appearance of the medullary canal from the loss of trabeculation. "In the normal, the cortex encroaches on the medullary portion of the bone."[6] The bones in osteoporosis will become brittle, but will not bend, in contrast to hyperparathyroidism and osteomalacia.

Local osteoporosis reveals a patchy or moth-eaten appearance which usually indicates a rapid calcium loss. Most commonly, it results from disuse atrophy. This may be associated with treatment for a fracture, plaster immobilization, muscular paralysis, or denervation. It will appear as a spotty loss of density with mottled irregular rarefraction and endosteal resorption. This can, of course, in later stages progress to a generalized osteoporosis, in which there is a typical ground-glass appearance (Figs. 7.34 and 7.35).

Sudek's Atrophy

Patchy demineralization of all the bones of the foot is a sign of Sudek's atrophy. Sudek's atrophy is a reflex neurovascular dystrophy which occurs after a minimal or trivial trauma. Clinically there is intense pain and edema and a limitation of motion. The skin can become glossy and smooth. The temperature is increased, and there is an extreme porosis of the bone. The clinical manifestations and residual dysfunctions that are noted are far beyond what one would expect as a result of the minimal trauma that has occurred. Although the symptoms may subside, normal bone density usually never reoccurs (Fig. 7.36).

In inflammatory conditions, such as rheumatoid and psoriatic arthritis and osteomyelitis, either a generalized or localized osteoporosis can occur, depending upon the severity of the condi-

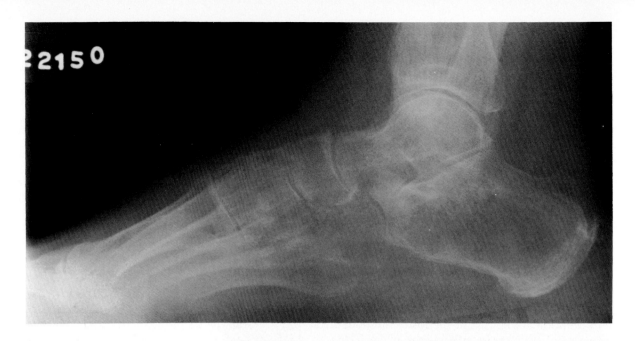

Figure 7.34. *Above*, osteoporosis secondary to old age.

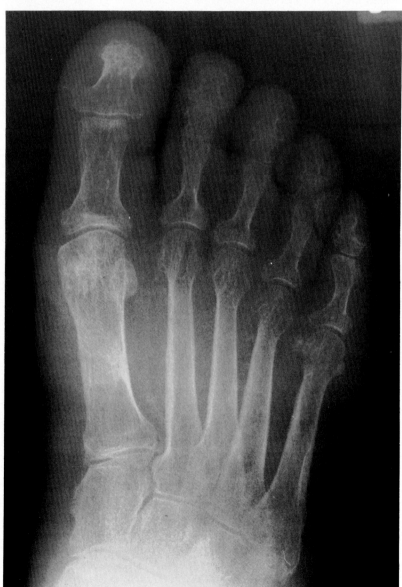

Figure 7.35. Severe osteoporosis secondary to long-term immobilization.

tion. If the inflammatory process involves the joint capsule, the ends of the bones enclosed by the capsule will often become demineralized, while the shaft is spared. This is referred to as juxta-articular demineralization.[6]

Osteomalacia

Osteomalacia results from insufficient mineral within the matrix of bone. There is an accumulation of increased amounts of uncalcified osteoid. Among its causes are inadequate absorption of calcium, as in steatorrhea, excessive loss of calcium, vitamin D deficiency, and hypophosphatemia. In osteomalacia, there is a loss of bone density due to the lack of mineralization. The bony trabecular pattern is coarsened and there is a decrease in the total number of trabeculae. This gives a lace-like appearance to the cancellous bone. In addition, subperiosteal bone resorption may occur (a pathonomic sign of hyperparathyroidism). Thinning and lack of definition of the cortex and the bony trabeculae will not be as well defined as it was in the osteoporosis.[5]

Endosteal New Bone

Just as the periosteum can form new bone, so too can endosteal new bone form. This widens the cortical frame from the inside rather than from the outside. The medullary cavity is reduced while the cortex thickens, and the overall outer bony diameter remains constant.

Osteopetrosis is the most striking example of endosteal new bone formation. The distinction between cortex and medulla is lost. There appears to be "bone within a bone."[18]

Terminal phalangeal sclerosis may occur in osteopetrosis as well as in rheumatoid arthritis, progressive systemic sclerosis, dermatomyositis, disseminated lupus erythematosus, and in psoriatic arthritis.

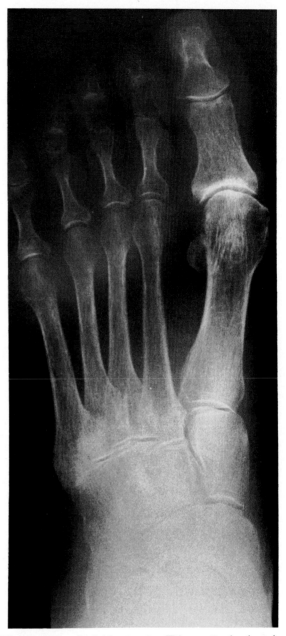

Figure 7.36. Sudek's atrophy. This spotty demineralization occurred approximately 3 months following an ankle sprain.

REFERENCES

1. KROLL, H. G., AND THURSTON, D. E.: Soft tissue injuries. J. Kansas Med. Soc., **80:** 267, 1979.
2. LEMONT, H., AND LIEBER, G. A.: The posterior triangle of the ankle. J.A.P.A., **72:** 363, 1982.
3. TABER, C. W.: *Taber's Cyclopedic Medical Dictionary*, 9th Ed, F. A. Davis, Philadelphia, 1968.
4. LICHTENSTEIN, L.: *Diseases of Bone and Joints*, 2nd Ed, C. V. Mosby, St. Louis, 1975.
5. GREENFIELD, G. B.: *Radiology of Bone Disease*, 3rd Ed, J. B. Lippincott, Philadelphia, 1980.
6. RESNICK, D., AND NIWAYAMA, G.: *Diagnosis of Bone and Joint Disorder*, W. B. Saunders, Philadelphia, 1981, vol. 3.
7. FAIRBAIRN, J. F., JURGENS, J. L., AND SPITTEL, A., JR.: *Peripheral Vascular Disease*, 4th Ed, W. B. Saunders, Philadelphia, 1972.
8. JUERGENS, J., ET AL.: *Peripheral Vascular Disease*, 5th Ed, W. B. Saunders, Philadelphia, 1980.
9. HACIHANEFIOGLU, U.: Tumoral calcinosis. J. Bone Jt. Surg., **60-A:** 1131, 1980.
10. PAUL, L. J., AND JUHL, J. H.: *Essentials of Roentgen Interpretation*, 4th Ed, Harper & Row, Philadelphia, 1981.
11. MCCARTY, D. J.: *Arthritis and Allied Conditions*, 9th Ed, Lea & Febiger, Philadelphia, 1979.
12. VOLBERG, F. M., WHALEN, J. R., ET AL.: Lamellated periosteal reactions. Am. J. Roentgenol., **128:** 85, 1977.
13. EDEIKEN, J., HODES, P. J., AND CAPLAN, L. H.: New bone

production and periosteal reaction. Am. J. Roentgenol. **97:** 708, 1966.

14. LEHRER, H. Z., MAXFIELD, W. S., AND NICE, C. M.: The periosteal sunburst pattern in metastatic bone tumors. Diagn. Radiol., **108:** 154, 1970.

15. GRUYER, P. B., BRUNTON, F. J., AND WREN, M. W.: Pachydermoperiostosis with acro-osteolysis. J. Bone Jt. Surg., **60-B:** 219, 1978.

16. DITKOWSKY, S. P., GOLDMAN, A., ET AL.: Normal periosteal reactions and associated soft-tissue findings. Clin. Pediatr. **9:** 515, 1970.

17. FORRESTER, D. M., AND KIRKPATRICK, J.: Periostitis and pseudoperiostitis. Diagn. Radiol. **118:** 597, 1976.

18. DEQUEKER, J.: Periosteal and endosteal surface remodeling in pathologic conditions. Invest. Radiol., **6:** 260, 1971.

19. FROST, H. M.: Bone dynamics in metabolic bone disease. J. Bone Jt. Surg., **48-A:** 1191, 1966.

20. PIRKEY, E. L., AND HURT, J.: Roentgen evaluation of the soft tissues in orthopedics. Am. J. Roentgenol., **82:** 271, 1959.

21. PETERSON, R.: Small vessel calcification and its relationship to secondary hyperparathyroidism in the renal homotransplant patient. Diagn. Radiol., **126:** 627, 1978.

22. BUDIN, J. A., AND FELDMAN, F.: Soft tissue calcifications in systemic lupus erythematosus. Am. J. Roentgenol. **124:** 358, 1975.

23. STAPLE, T. W., NELSON, G. L., AND EVENS, R. G.: Miscellaneous soft tissue lesions of the extremities. Semin. Roentgenol. **3:** 117, 1973.

24. NAIDICH, T. P., AND SIEGELMAN, S. S.: Paraarticular soft tissue changes in systemic diseases. Semin. Roentgenol., **3:** 101, 1973.

25. GOODMAN, N.: The significance of terminal phalangeal osteosclerosis. Radiology, **89:** 709, 1967.

26. YAGHMAE, I., AND MIRBAD, P.: Tumoral calcinosis. Am. J. Roentgenol., **3:** 573, 1971.

27. GAMBLE, F. O., AND YALE, I.: *Clinical Foot Roentgenology*, 2nd Ed, Krieger, Hungtington, NY, 1975.

CHAPTER 8

Osteochondritis

ISCHEMIC NECROSIS

Osteonecrosis indicates that ischemic death of the cellular constituents of bone and marrow has occurred."[1] Historically, this was first thought to be related to sepsis in the osseus segments. However, continued studies led to the use of the term "aseptic necrosis." Subsequent observations indicated that the necrotic areas of bone were not only aseptic, but were also avascular. This led to the terms "ischemic necrosis," "avascular necrosis," and "bone infarction." Today, the terms aseptic and avascular necrosis are generally applied to areas of epiphyseal or subarticular involvement, whereas bone infarct is usually reserved for metaphyseal and diaphyseal areas of involvement.[1]

Ischemic necrosis of bone results from a significant reduction in or obliteration of blood supply to the affected area.[1] The various bone cells, including osteocytes, osteoclasts, and osteoblasts, usually undergo anoxic death in 12 to 48 hours after blood supply is cut off. The infarct that has thus developed is three-dimensional and can be divided into a number of zones: 1) a central zone of cell death; 2) an area of ischemic injury, most severe near the zone of cell death, and lessening as it moves peripherally; 3) an area of active hyperemia; and 4) the zone of normal unaffected tissue. Once ischemic necrosis has begun, the cellular damage provokes an initial inflammatory response, which typically is characterized by vasodilatation, transudation of fluid and fibrin, and local infiltration of inflammatory cells. This response can be considered the first stage in repair of the necrotic area.[1]

Because the osteonecrotic segment is without circulation, repair can only begin at the outer peripheral zone and must work inward toward the dead zone.

While extensive circulation is available in the cortex and intermedullary cavity, the epiphyseal ends of long bones have limited circulation because much of their surface is covered by articular cartilage, which does not have its own circulation. In the growing bone, arterial access to the epiphysis is even more tenuous because the epiphysis is separated from the metaphysis by the growth plate or physis. Since in all likelihood there is a single dominant artery supplying a developing epiphysis, compromise of this artery is a probable mechanism for Legg Calvé-Perthes' disease, Köehler's disease, and Freiberg's disease. Accordingly, ischemic necrosis of cortical bone is relatively rare, due to the extensive blood supply.[1]

A series of responses then occurs in an attempt toward revival, rehabilitation, removal, and reconstruction of the affected portion of bone.

The first phase of osteonecrosis in the initial response is cell death. This phase leads to necrosis of hematopoietic elements, osteocytic cellular constituents, and the marrow fat cells.[1] There are no recognizable radiographic changes in the architecture of the bone in this stage.

The next phase is dependent upon the inflammatory response of the body within the viable tissue surrounding the necrotic area. During this phase, two distinct zones will become apparent radiographically. The generalized active hyperemia results in osteoporosis in adjacent viable bone tissue. This leaves the necrotic area as a radiodense-appearing wedge of bone. This dense appearance is relative to the less dense appearance of the osteoporotic viable tissue. During the next phase of repair, a reactive margin forms about the osteonecrotic zone.[1] The process continues with remodeling and repair along the entire reactive interface between the viable and necrotic zones. At this stage there is no evidence of articular buckling.

During the next phase, the supporting bony architecture becomes sufficiently weakened by the continued resorption of trabecular bone on the reactive interface that the stress of weight-bearing results in fracture, and buckling of the articular cartilage with eventual collapse. Fragmentation and compaction of subchondral bony fragments leads to the development of a subchondral lucent area along the fracture line, the crescent sign. Thus, in this phase, the articular flattening and collapse can be visualized radiographically.[1,2]

Radiologic Progression of Epiphyseal Ischemic Necrosis

Initially, dense areas in the epiphyseal end of the long bone will appear. These areas may take the form of a band-like opacity or may follow the epiphyseal line. The relative opacity is due more to the resorption of calcific density from the viable tissue, leaving the necrotic tissue appearing more radiopaque. It is followed by widening of the epiphyseal plate and a so-called "snow-cap" appearance.

The next radiographic stage is that of structural failure, which appears as a fracture line in the subcortical areas. At times this may precede the bony sclerosis previously mentioned. The articular surface then collapses with fragmentation and compaction, looking like a step-off in the bone. The "step formation" occurs at the junction of the normal with the necrotic bone. There is sequestration or necrosis of this portion of the bone substance. A fibrous band surrounds the lesions and mottled cystic areas are usually present. Advanced destructive and absorptive changes continue, and periosteal new bone formation about the fracture site is a prominent feature of this stage radiographically.

These changes may then be summarized as fragmentation, compression, and resorption of dead bone followed by proliferation, revascularization, and production of new bone with remodeling as the final stage. In early cases, the subchondral fracture line or crescent sign may be demonstrated radiographically by applying traction to the distal portion of the extremity. The vacuum thusly created will accentuate the fracture line.

Following the fracture process, flattening of the head of this long bone will occur in the vast majority of the cases.

Reossification usually occurs with reconstruction and remodeling to either a spherical or mushroom shape with flattening and widening of the head and broadening of the neck. In the late stages of the disease, there will be considerable deformity of the joint with degenerative arthritic destruction and osteophytic proliferation present.[1,2]

Legg-Perthes' Disease

Legg-Perthes' disease (Legg Calvé-Perthes' disease or osteochrondosis of the femoral head) is a condition of ischemic necrosis of the femoral capital ossification center. It occurs between the ages of 4 to 8 and involves males, predominently. Radiographic changes in Legg-Perthes' disease have been extensively studied and are usually used as a model for ischemic necrosis in other long bones of the body. They follow, rather closely, the previously described radiographic changes for ischemic necrosis and its repair.[1-3]

Osgood-Schlatter's Disease

Osgood-Schlatter's disease, or osteochrondosis of the tibial tuberosity, is thought to result chiefly from trauma to the tibial tuberosity. Usually it results in pain and soft tissue edema. Because of the extreme variation in shape and configuration of the apophysis of the tibial tuberosity, radiographs are not an aid in diagnosing this condition (Fig. 8.1).[2]

FREIBERG'S INFRACTION

In 1914, Freiberg described a series of patients with metatarsalgia in whom the metatarsal head appeared to be crushed or collapsed, terming the condition an infraction of bone.[1] Infraction is defined as an incomplete fracture of a bone in which the parts do not become displaced.[4] While the second metatarsal head predominates as that which is affected most often (68% of the cases), the third (27% of the cases), the fourth (approximately 4%), and the fifth (1%) are also affected. In rare instances, the first metatarsal head may possibly be affected as well. The changes are usually unilateral and usually only one lesion is found in a foot.

The infraction seems to occur on the metatarsal bone subjected to the greatest weight. In many instances, the longest metatarsal is the one affected, and in other cases, the lesion seems to be caused by an insufficient support by an adjacent metatarsal bone. They seem to occur in structurally weak feet with short or hypermobile first metatarsals. This seems to account for the high predominance of lesions in the second and third metatarsals. Frequently, unusual activity was observed prior to the actual infraction. The lesions occur more frequently in females and usually occur in adolescents between the ages of 13 and 18 years of age. The epiphysis of the second metatarsal is most vulnerable to injury because of its relative length and firm fixation, the second

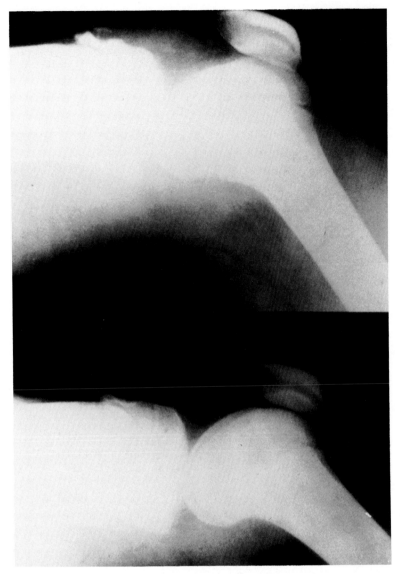

Figure 8.1. Osgood-Schlatter's disease. This patient had long-standing pain of the tibial tuberosity and a diagnosis of Osgood-Schlatter's disease was made.

metatarsal being the most firmly fixed. The high incidence of the disorder in women could conceivably be related to the wearing of high-heel shoes, which creates increased stress on the second metatarsal.

Clinical manifestations consist of local pain, tenderness, and swelling, with limitation of motion of the corresponding metatarsophalangeal joint.

A Freiberg's infraction seems to progress through stages similar to those already described under osteonecrosis. A subchondral bone fracture is the initial lesion, and the osteonecrosis is caused by the absence of vascularity in the fracture fragment. Through a series of surgical interventions,

it has been determined that usually the central and dorsal part of the metatarsal head seem to be detached by the stress fracture in the metatarsal. At first it is attached by a plantar hinge, but finally separates completely from the metatarsal head, and becomes a loose body. It eventually becomes compressed in a cavity, the lateral margins of which eventually give way as it collapses (Fig. 8.2 to 8.6).

Roentgenographic abnormalities include, at first, mild flattening with increased radiodensity of the metatarsal head. Occasionally, a crescent sign can be observed and cystic-lucent lesions of the metatarsal head are predominent. As the disease progresses, the metatarsal head tends to widen. Flattening of the metatarsal head progresses with sclerosis occurring, and periostitis with increased cortical thickening of the adjacent metaphysis and diaphysis of the bone occur. The final result usually is premature closure of the growth plate, deformity and enlargement of the metatarsal head, and secondary degenerative arthritic changes, including enlargement and flattening of the base of the proximal phalanx and osteophyte proliferation about the metatarsal head.[1,2,5-7]

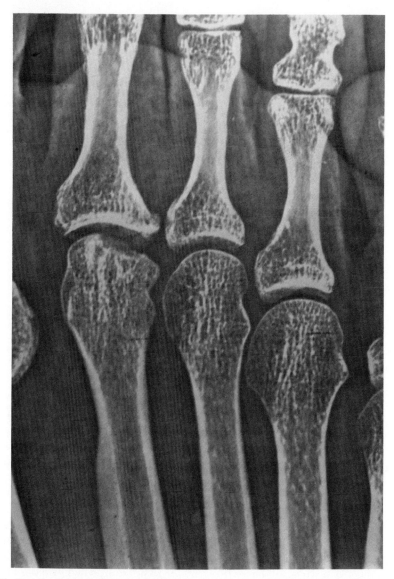

Figure 8.2.   Early Freiberg's disease. Structural failure has occurred, a portion of the metatarsal head imploding. A portion of the bony sclerosis or snowcap is evident.

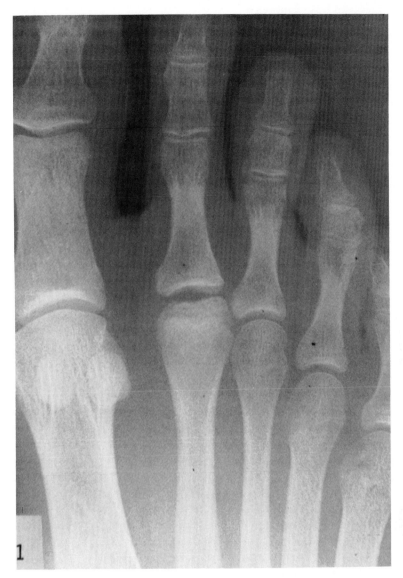

Figure 8.3. Freiberg's disease of the second metatarsal in a 14-year-old female. The second metatarsal, excessively long, and probably bearing an excessive amount of weight, developed Freiberg's disease.

KÖEHLER'S DISEASE

In 1908, Köehler first described an abnormal radiographic appearance of the tarsal navicular bone. Since that time, much debate about the cause of this appearance has occurred. Köehler's description characterized this as a self-limiting condition of the tarsal navicular characterized by flattening, sclerosis, and fragmentation. However, these same signs are not uncommon in the absence of symptoms, and it has been proposed that these radiographic features may represent a normal variation in the process of ossification of the navicular. Köehler's disease is relatively rare, and it can be almost impossible to distinguish the radiographic abnormalities from those occurring as a normal variation of growth.

The diagnosis of Köehler's disease is made in a child presenting with a limp and local pain and tenderness over the navicular bone. If affects boys 4 to 6 times more commonly than girls, usually between the ages of 3 and 7 years, which seems to coincide with the timing of the ossification of the navicular. Unilateral involvement is evident in 75–80% of the cases.

There are two distinct radiographic patterns described in the literature. The more common pattern reveals the navicular to be flattened, as if squashed, with patchy areas of increased bone density and loss of the normal trabecular pattern.

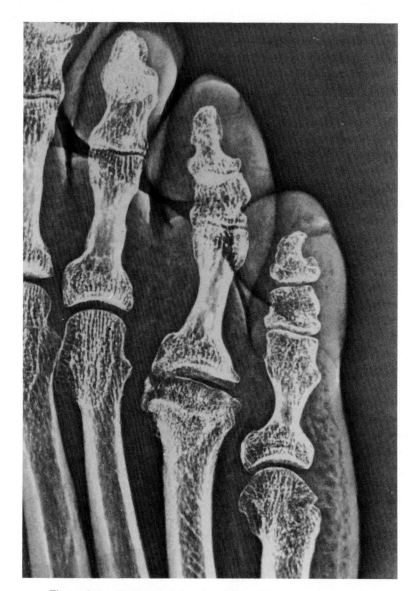

Figure 8.4. Freiberg's infraction (of the 4th metatarsal head).

This is referred to as the "discoid navicular." The second type shows the navicular to be of normal shape, but uniformly increased in density when compared with the surrounding bones (Figs. 8.7 and 8.8).

There is evidence that Köehler's disease may have a mechanical basis. During pronation, the talus is displaced plantarly, medially, and distally, thus concentrating considerable force on the navicular during normal ambulation. It has been determined that in cases of osteochondritis of the navicular, the talus projects further distally than in the normal, by an average of from 16–35%. It has further been shown that the space allowed for the navicular is less in feet with Köehler's disease than in normal feet. The conclusion drawn from these findings is that distal displacement of the talus and the decrease in the navicular space are either anatomical variations or sequellae of pronation that predispose to the disease and facilitate its development. They also tend to lead to compression of the bony nucleus at a critical phase of growth, which could very well result in altered ossification. Though Köehler's disease has long been considered an avascular necrosis of bone, the only confirmatory factor to this conclusion is the fact that radionuclide examination tends to reveal diminished uptake in Köehler's disease.

It is the self-limiting and reversable nature of

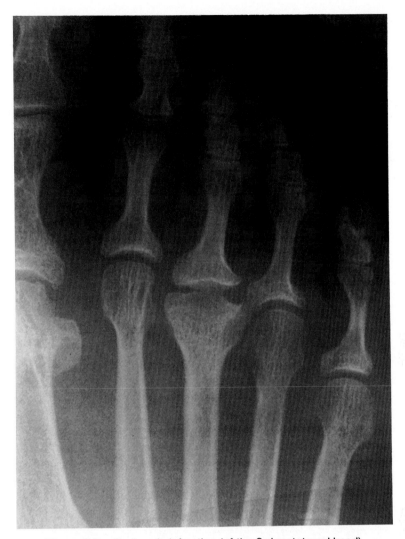

Figure 8.5. Freiberg's infraction (of the 3rd metatarsal head).

the process that has lead to speculation that this "disease" is simply a variation in the sequence of tarsal ossification, rather than actually a disease.[1,2,8,9]

SEVER'S DISEASE

Sever's disease, or ischemic necrosis of the apophysis of the calcaneus, may not truly exist as a disease entity. The normal ossification center varies widely in appearance between the ages of 8 to 13 years of age. The apophysis usually has a greater density than the body of the calcaneus.

Radiographs of children with symptoms and normal children show similar changes in the calcaneal apophysis, including fragmentation and sclerosis.

The symptoms usually include pain and tenderness to palpation in the area of the apophysis of the calcaneus. The disease usually affects 8- to 13-year-old males. There is speculation that the symptoms may be due to trauma in the area of the apophysis, or that it may be due to an abnormal pull, from a shortened Achilles tendon, upon the superior portion of the calcaneal apophysis into which this tendon inserts (Fig. 8.9).[1,2]

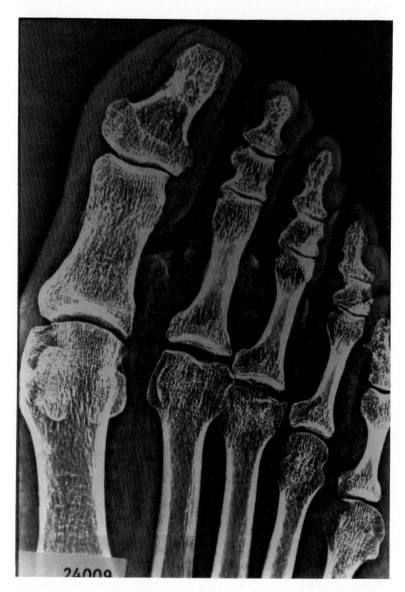

Figure 8.6.   Freiberg's infraction (of the 2nd and 3rd metatarsal heads).

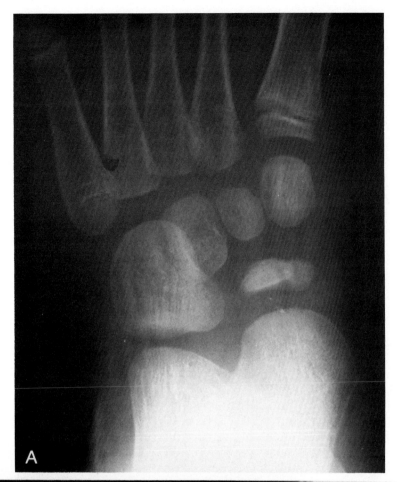

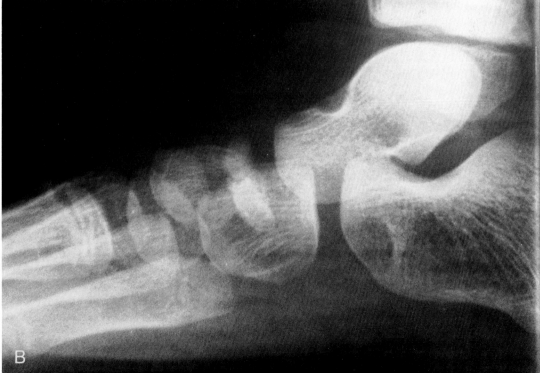

Figure 8.7. *A* and *B*, a normal navicular, while ossifying, may be somewhat irregular, and may possibly begin as two ossification centers.

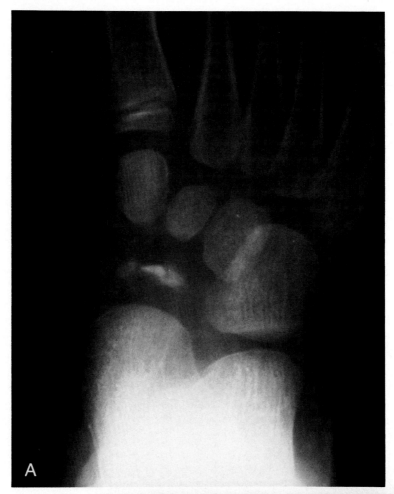

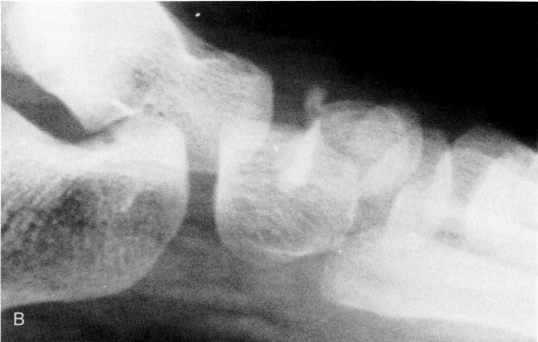

Figure 8.8. *A* and *B*, Köhler's disease. Note the discoid navicular and the more irregular and retarded ossification of the navicular with sclerosis. The contralateral foot is seen in Figure 8.7.

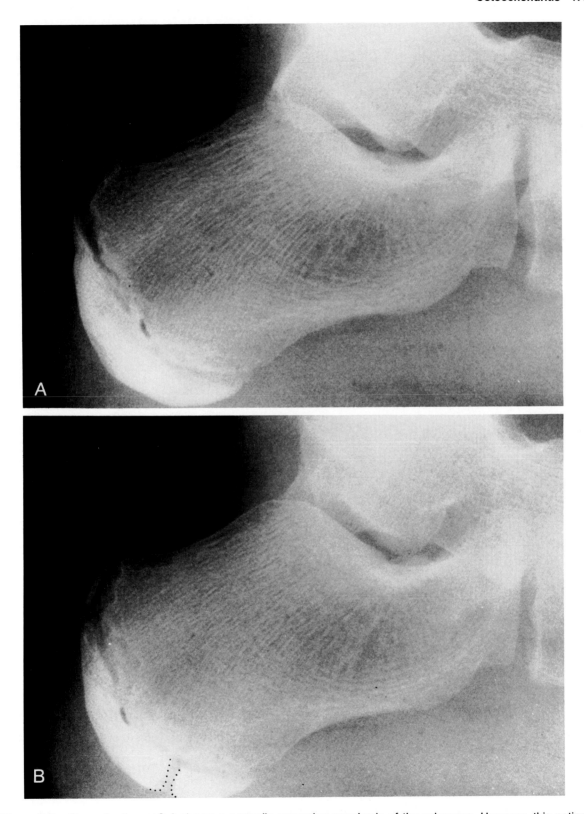

Figure 8.9. Severe's disease? *A* shows a normally appearing apophysis of the calcaneus. However, this patient had symptoms that were diagnosed as Severe's disease. The calcaneus in *B* was fragmented, but the patient had no symptoms. The diagnosis of Severe's disease cannot be made radiographically.

OSTEOCHRONDRITIS DISSECANS

Osteochrondritis dissecans or segmental is-chemic necrosis is most commonly seen in males. A small segment of bone with its articular cartilage detaches from the body of the bone, and lies either in the depression of the joint surface or floats free as a joint mouse. It may be more dense than the surrounding bone and is frequently demarcated by a crescentic radiolucent zone. Adolescents are chiefly affected. This may represent either a post-traumatic sequelum or a true case of aseptic necrosis (Fig. 8.10).[2]

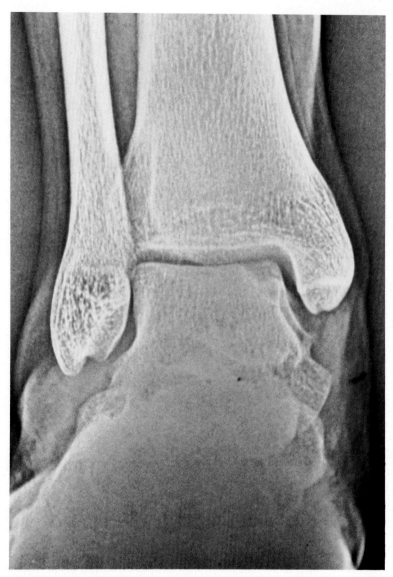

Figure 8.10.   Osteochondritis dissecans. The lateral portion of the dome of the talus has broken loose and is lying in the posterior portion of the ankle joint.

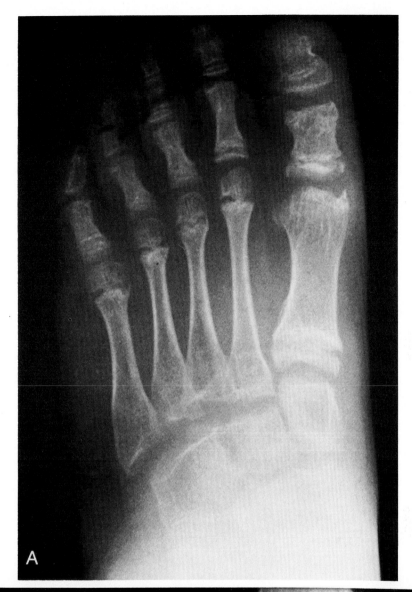

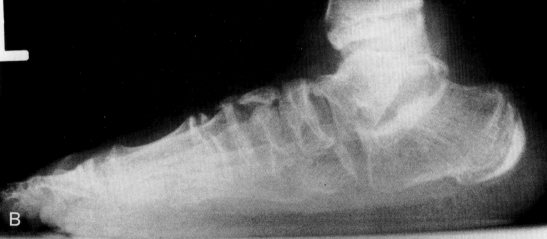

Figure 8.11.   *A* and *B*, Multiple epiphyseal dysplasia. Fairbank's disease is characterized by an irregular mottled ossification of multiple epiphyseal plates. Note the short stubby phalanges of the first toe.

MULTIPLE EPIPHYSEAL DYSPLASIA

Multiple epiphyseal dysplasia, or Fairbank's disease, is characterized by an irregular mottled ossification of multiple epiphyses. Maturation of these epiphysis is delayed. These findings are usually bilateral and symmetrical and occur between the ages of 5 and 14. There are some reported cases in which there is a familial tendency. The chief complaints are pain and stiffness of the hips and extremities. Involvement of the primary ossification centers of the tarsals and carpals is common. Short, stubby digits and metatarsals are sometimes present, but the feet seem less frequently involved than the hands (Fig. 8.11).[2]

REFERENCES

1. RESNICK, D., ET AL.: *Diagnosis of Bone and Joint Disorders*, W. B. Saunders, Philadelphia, 1981, vol. 3.
2. GREENFIELD, G. B.: *Radiology of Bone Disease*, 3rd Ed, Lippincott, Philadelphia, 1980.
3. CATTERALL, A.: *Perthes' disease.* Br. Med. J., **11:** 1145, 1977.
4. *Taber's Cyclopedic Medical Dictionary*, 9th Ed, F. A. Davis, Philadelphia, 1962.
5. SMILLIE, I. S.: Freiberg infraction (Köehler's second disease). J. Bone Jt. Surg., **39-B:** 580, 1957.
6. GAUTHIER, G., AND ELBAZ, R.: Freiberg's infraction: A subchondral bone fatigue fracture. A new surgical treatment. Clin. Orthopaed. Relat. Res. **142:** 93, 1979.
7. BRADDOCK, G. T. F.: Experimental epiphysial injury and Freiberg's disease. J. Bone Jt. Surg., **41-B:** 154, 1959.
8. SCAGLIETTI, O., STRINGA, G., AND MIZZARE, M.: Plus-variant of the astrogalus and subnormal scophoid space. Two important findings in Köehler's scophoid necrosis. Clin. Orthopaed. **32:** 499, 1962.
9. MCCAULEY, G. K., AND KALIN, P. C.: Osteochondritis of the tarsal navicular. Radiology, **123:** 705, 1977.

CHAPTER 9

Infections of Bone and Neurotrophic Foot

OSTEOMYELITIS

Osteomyelitis, or an infection of bone, is a very debilitating disease that can occur anywhere in the body, but especially in the lower extremity. The bone infection may be due to bacteria, viral infections, or mycotic infections, but usually is due to bacteria. The most commonly involved organism is *Staphylococcus aureus*. In osteomyelitis, the usual clinical picture reveals infectious edema, soft tissue changes, subperiosteal alterations, active bone destruction, areas of dead bone, and areas of new bone production. Osteomyelitis must be distinguished from inflammatory disorders, Arthritis, Paget's disease, neurofibromatosis, multiple myeloma, malignant disease, endocrine disorders, and metabolic disorders. All of these conditions may cause changes that can be confused with osteomyelitis.

There are two basic types of osteomyelitis: hematogenous and direct extension. The hematogenous route of infection is a more indirect route, and is the more difficult of the two to diagnose. Bacteria traveling through the blood stream will become lodged in a bone, and eventually cause an infection in the bone without any outward signs of infection for quite some time. The direct extension route seems by far the more common method of spread of osteomyelitis in the lower extremity. Usually the spread is from a skin ulceration which continues to deepen down to the bone, finally involving the osseous tissue.

It must be emphasized that bone itself responds very slowly to inflammation and to infection. Hematogenous osteomyelitis, for example, will show no radiographic changes for about 10–14 days, and medullary changes are seldom detectable, except in the most advanced stages of the disease. Furthermore, the osteomyelitis may be well controlled clinically, while the radiographs give the appearance of unchecked deterioration.[1]

The cardinal radiographic signs of osteomyelitis are as follows.

Radiolucency

Radiolucency is nearly always present in one form or another.[1] This constitutes an area that is regular or irregular and of decreased density. It is usually accompanied by a loss of trabeculations, leaving a ground, glass-like darkened region (Figs. 9.1 and 9.2).

Sclerosis

Sclerosis is evidence of an area of more advanced stage of bone repair or the reverse, dead bone.[1]

Sequestration

A sequestrum is a piece of dead bone. The process of producing a sequestrum occurs when purulent exudation eliminates the blood supply to a portion of bone. It may become separated from the bone proper and can be seen on x-ray (Fig. 9.1).

Involucrum

Involucrum is an area of new bone production. With the accumulation of pus beneath the periosteum, the periosteum becomes elevated and new bone is laid down on its inner surface. It appears as a region of increased density immediately adjacent to an area of active osteomyelitis (Fig. 9.1).[1]

Cloaca

A cloaca is an area of decreased density at the bone-periosteal interface, and represents numerous openings for discharge of pus and debris. The region was previously taken up by the bone which formerly constitutes a sequestrum (Fig. 9.1).

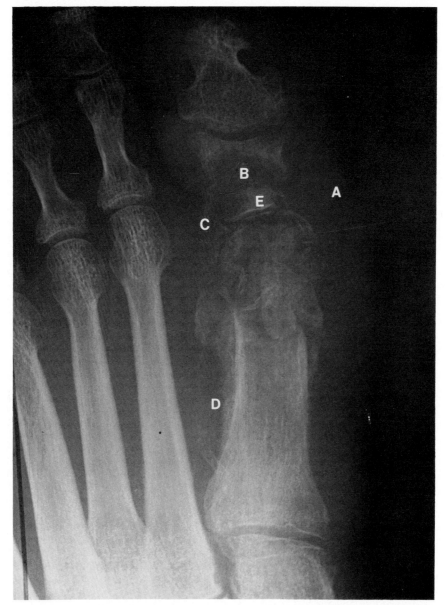

Figure 9.1. Acute osteomyelitis and septic arthritis. This radiograph shows the typical cardinal signs of osteomyelitis. There is hazy edema in the soft tissues about the area *A*, bone destruction (*B*), cloaca (*C*), involucrum (*D*), and sequestrum (*E*).

Subperiosteal Calcification

Subperiosteal calcification is a common finding in which the underlying osteomyelitis initiates an elevation of the covering periosteum with calcification of the intervening space.[1]

HEMATOGENOUS OSTEOMYELITIS

Acute hematogenous osteomyelitis usually affects infants and children. These is a latent period of 10–14 days between the onset of symptoms and evidence of osseous x-ray change. The symptoms are pain, edema, and limitation of movement which occurs about 1 week prior to the x-ray changes. Soft tissue change occurs within a few days.[2]

Hematogenously spread osteomyelitis is "seeded" into bone via the bloodstream and most often involves the medullary region which is rich in cancellous bone.[1] This soft bone offers little resistance to the rapid extension of the infection.

The invading bacteria settles in terminal capil-

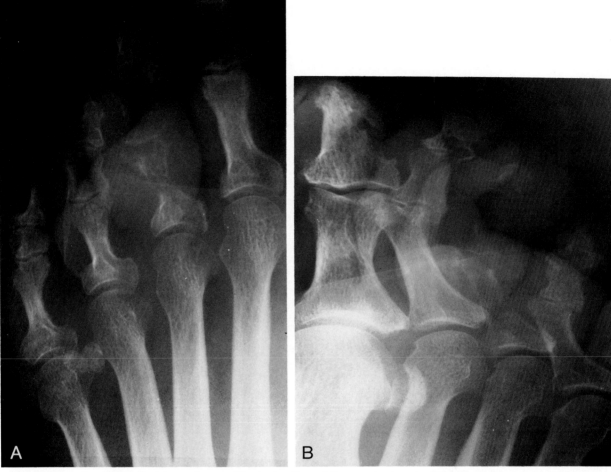

Figure 9.2. A and B, extensive osteomyelitic destruction of the proximal and middle phalanges of the third digit. There are numerous sequestra and cloacae. Small areas of new bone proliferation can be seen about the head of the proximal phalanx.

lary loops of the metaphysis and epiphysis of bone and causes multiple abscesses leading to bone destruction. This initial focus is followed by one of several events, including: penetration of articular cartilage into the joint space; or extension to part or all of the medullary canal. Metaphyseal involvement with destruction of cancellous bone may later extend to the cortex at the end of the shaft; or most commonly, the disease, if unrestrained, will extend through the Haversian system to the cortex and into the subperiosteal space. When this occurs, the periosteum is stripped from the cortex and elevated, appearing as a thin strip of increased density paralleling the shaft of the bone. This happens because the bacteria spread throughout the subperiosteal space and periosteum is forced to balloon out.[2] Reactive periostitis initiates production of new bone or involucrum. Subperiosteal calcification is not to be interpreted

as a thickening of the periosteum itself. The development of involucrum tends to proceed irregularly, leaving necrotic or devitalized defects at intervals.[1]

The cortex has two main blood sources: nutrient vessels and periosteal vessels. The nutrient vessels become occluded from arterial emboli, and the periosteal vessels will rupture as the periosteum is elevated, due to pressure from the buildup of bacterial and necrotic material.[2] The cortical bone will then become necrotic due to the lack of blood supply. The ballooned periosteum retains its osteogenic properties and thereby forms new bone at the elevated sites. There will be destruction, dead bone, and new bone developing superficially all in the same general area. Inflammation and increased circulation lead to demineralization in the uninvolved or unaffected bone in the general region of the osteomyelitis. Pus exudes from

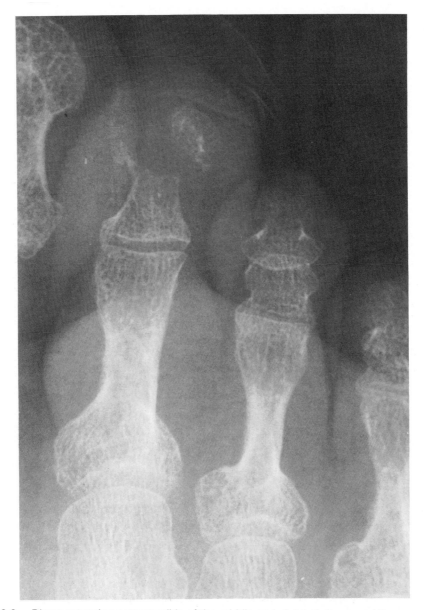

Figure 9.3. Direct extension osteomyelitis of the middle and distal phalanges of the second digit.

the cloaca in the cortex. When healing occurs, the involucrum remodels and gradually assumes a more normal contour.

Radiographically, osteomyelitis will present the following scenario: initially there will be no osseous findings. Deep soft tissue edema will be noted adjacent to the involved area of the bone, and there will be obliteration of soft tissue planes. In children, the earliest x-ray sign will usually be bone destruction in the metaphyseal area. These destructive changes may also be present in the epiphyseal ossification center and may extend down the shaft of the bone. Periosteal new bone formation then occurs as a solid or cloaking pat-

tern forming the involucrum about the involved area. Regional osteoporosis will occur as a response to the inflammation in the area. The roentgen criteria for sequestrum are: separation of a piece of bone from the main mass of bone and chaulky white appearance to the separated osseous fragment (Figs. 9.1 to 9.5).

There is a greater tendency toward involvement of a joint in adults than in children. The most common form of osteomyelitis in an adult is direct extension osteomyelitis in which there is an ulcer that extends down to the bone. Frequently, a corn or callus will cover the ulcer, and will cloud the diagnosis somewhat.

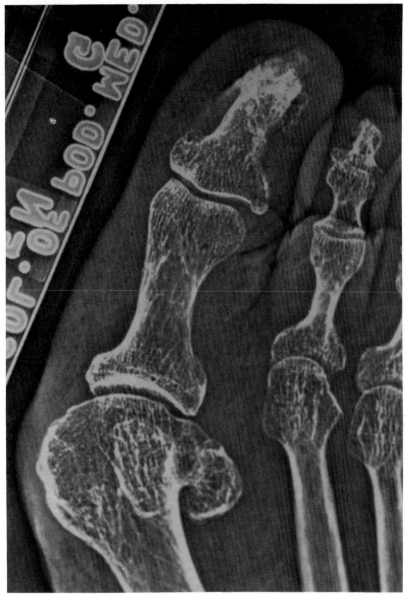

Figure 9.4. Early osteomyelitis of the tuft of the distal phalanx of the hallux showing early involucrum and bone destruction.

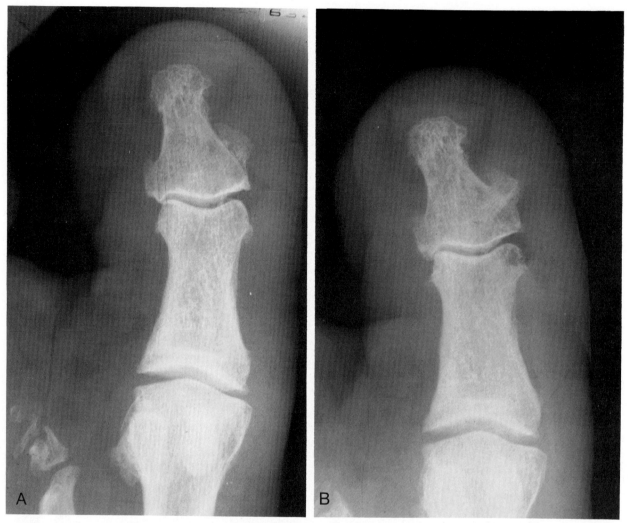

Figure 9.5.   *A,* infectious edema can be observed about the entire great toe and a skin defect can be seen under the medial aspect of the interphalangeal joint. The second digit was sacrificed 3 years earlier to acute osteomyelitis. *B,* two and one-half months later, the area of radiolucency has become more profound and there is absence of trabeculation at the medial, distal aspect of the first proximal phalanx. *C,* eleven weeks later, active osteomyelitis is seen along with a concomitant increase in the soft tissue defect. The osteomyelitis now involves the head of the proximal phalanx and the base of the distal phalanx. The ulceration had completely perforated the toe from plantar through to the dorsum. *D,* three weeks later following hospitalization and extensive systemic and local therapy, bone destruction has ceased and the skin defect is healing. *E,* one week later, the skin defect can still be observed, the bony portions of the proximal phalanx are beginning to coalesce. Involucrum is seen along the shaft of the proximal phalanx. A negative culture has been present for at least three weeks at this point. The entire proximal interphalangeal joint went on to self-arthodese.

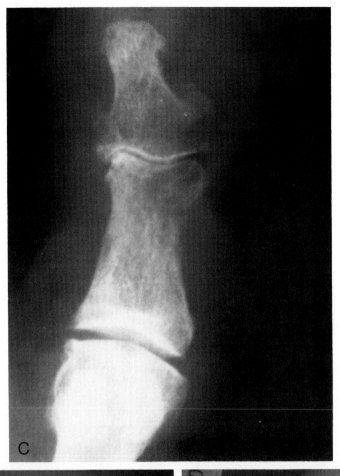

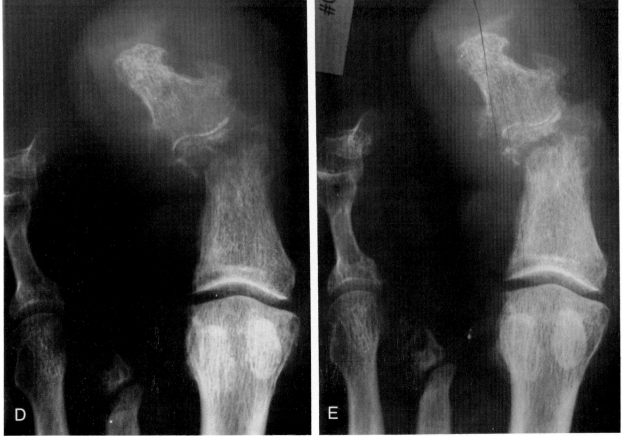

Figure 9.5. (*C* to *E*)

CHRONIC OSTEOMYELITIS

Adult osteomyelitis shows a greater tendency toward chronicity. The patient is no longer obviously ill, but has a local infection of low grade with persistent drainage from one or more sinuses and recurrent episodes of pain, rubor, and calor.[3] Radiographically, it appears as a thickened, irregular sclerotic bone containing several radiolucent areas with elevated periosteum. It must be stressed that osteomyelitis rarely, if ever, is cured. Generally, the patient has it for life, no matter which antibiotics are used. The ostemyelitis can only be controlled to a degree. Low-grade infection persists and undergoes periods of exacerbation and remission. In this instance, periosteal reactivity may produce a layered ebernation in the cortical areas. The ultimate sequelae may involve gross structural changes. Limb shortening may result from destruction of the epiphyseal plate during an acute phase of the disease in the child. Chronic hyperemia associated with osteomyelitis which does not destroy the epiphyseal plate actually accelerates limb growth, maturation, and precocious closure of the epiphysis which is frequently observed radiographically (Fig. 9.6).

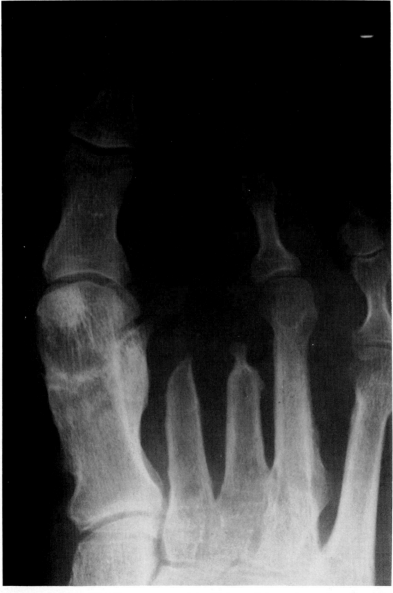

Figure 9.6. Chronic osteomyelitis. The first metatarsal is thickened, irregular, sclerotic, and contains radiolucent areas throughout its shaft.

BRODIE'S ABSCESS

Brodie's abscess is a chronic abscess that never went through an acute stage. It is a form of localized osteomyelitis within a long bone that develops several years after an initial trauma. It is really a slow infection with no indication of inflammation. The abscess has a thin wall of fibrous tissue and sclerotic bone with a center filled with pus.[3]

Radiographically, the abscess gives the appearance of a cyst-like rarefaction in the bone. It can be very slowly expansive and will have increased density surrounding the radiolucent area. It can be a painful lesion and can be surrounded by marked sclerosis. Eventually, it can break through a cortex and become an active osteomyelitis. Brodie's abscess is differentiated from the bone cyst using the following criteria:

1) It occurs in the metaphyseal area.
2) It is usually smaller than a cyst.
3) There is evidence of infection, clinically. A cyst usually shows no inflammation.
4) It cortical shell is more dense than a cyst (Figs. 9.7 and 9.8).[2]

SYPHILITIC OSTEOMYELITIS

Luetic osteomyelitis can be present in both congenital and acquired tertiary syphilis. It pre-

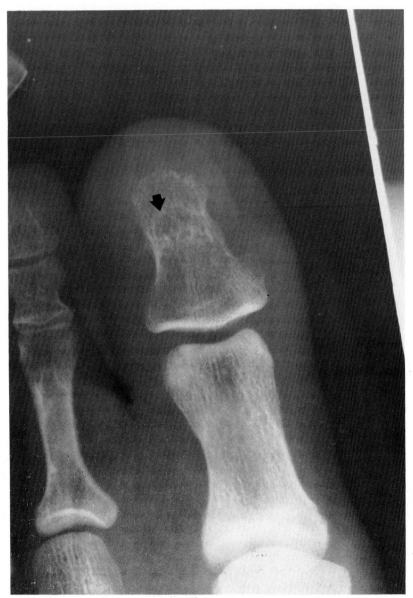

Figure 9.7. Brodie's abscess. One of the more common areas of the foot for a Brodie's abscess is the distal phalanx of the hallux, usually in the vicinity of the posterior nailfold.

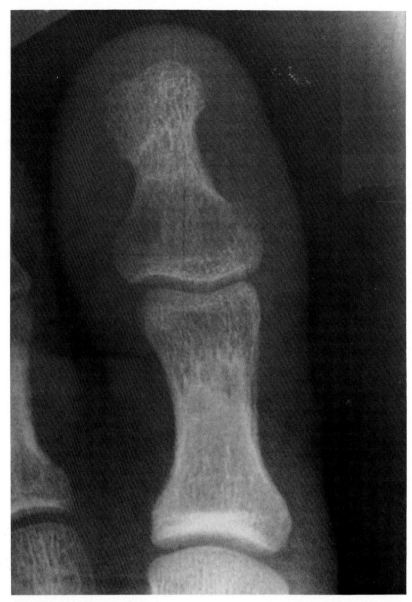

Figure 9.8. Brodie's abscess. Lateral portion of base, distal phalanx of hallux. This abscess caused a chronic inflammation of the posterior nailfold.

sents as a bone-producing disease. The femur and tibia are affected late in childhood, but the feet are rarely affected. In advanced cases of the disease, it presents nearly a pathognomonic radiographic finding of "saber shin."[1] In the first 6 months, the epiphysis may be involved. A serology is usually taken to establish the diagnosis. Osseous lesions develop in approximately 50% of the patients having congenital syphilis.

This disease can occur at any age in either sex and is a multiple process involving one or several bones. It is primarily proliferative, usually occur-

ring in the shaft of long bones. This disease usually involves the periosteum and subperiosteal calcification, and new bone formations are typical on x-ray.[1] Demineralization does not occur as there is little inflammation. A "lace-like" subperiosteal calcification is an outstanding x-ray criterion for luetic osteomyelitis. Bony outlines are characteristically curved, wavy, and irregular. Osseous tissues may be laid down in parallel laminae or as an irregular lacework. Osteolytic activity results in areas of cortical destruction called gummatus destruction.[1] Neurotrophic changes frequently occur in the syphilitic patient.

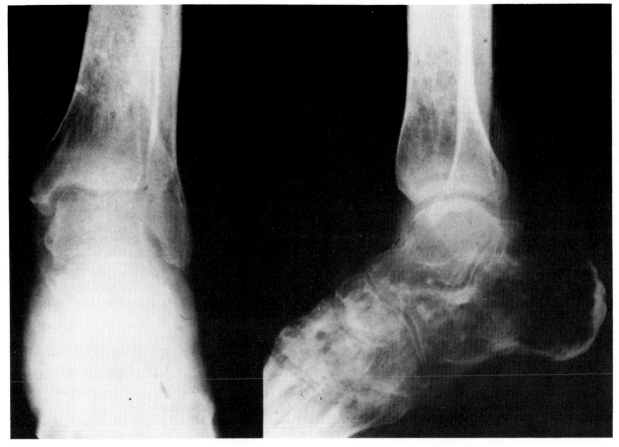

Figure 9.9. Tuberculous of bone. Note the severe osteolytic activity causing severe osteoporosis with little to no sclerosis and involucrum.

TUBERCULOSIS OF BONE

The origin of tuberculous osteomyelitis is always hematogenous and is usually, but not always, secondary to pulmonary involvement. It is most common in children, adolescents, and young adults less than 30 years old. Symptoms are usually absent. The radiographic appearance of tuberculous osteomyelitis is often the antithesis of syphilitic osteomyelitis.[1] Cancellous bone and the epiphyseal areas are usually invaded by the tuberculosis. In youngsters, fusiform swelling of the digits will be present. Epiphyseal tuberculosis is common and it usually presents as a single lesion. The involved bone will end up being quite small because of the affected growth centers. Neighboring uneffective bones are demineralized. The radiographic appearance is that of single or multiple disseminated areas of rarefaction of bone. This osteolytic activity occurs without any proliferation of new bone. One of the more common areas of involvement is the body of the calcaneus. The radiographic appearance of the phalanges is particularly significant to the podiatric physician. The fusiform shape of these digits has been termed "tuberculosis dactylitis." As the tubercular infection progresses, the shaft is seen radiographically to become both dilated and rarefied, and the external circumference of the bones of the fingers and toes will have an increased diameter. It is basically similar to pyogenic osteomyelitis except that the osteoporosis is earlier and greater. The sclerosis and periosteal new bone are less (Fig. 9.9).[3]

GARRE'S NON-SUPPURATIVE OSTEITIS

In 1983, Garrè described a form of chronic osteomyelitis. It was sclerosing osteitis, usually in the shaft of long bones. The major symptom is pain and it is due to organisms of low virulence. The condition is non-suppurative and is limited to a single bone. Radiographically, one sees cortical thickening, which produces an irregular fusiform thickening of the bone, with sclerotic changes in the spongiosa and increased density of the cortex.[2,3] Periosteal proliferation is absent in this very rare condition. The sclerosis may obliterate the normal trabecular patterns of cancellous bone.

LEPROSY

Hansen's disease may affect bone and cause severe soft tissue contracture. Active destruction of bone with loss of bone substance may occur. There may be complete absence of phalanges and entire digits. Neutrophic changes are common in this condition.

FUNGAL INFECTIONS OF BONE

In tropical and sub-tropical regions, including the southern United States, mycetoma may occur. In this condition the foot may be swollen to twice its normal size. The roentgenologic findings include:
1) Marked increase in soft-tissue density.
2) Sinus tracts may become visible.
3) Secondary bacterial infection may occur with active destruction and the usual osteomyelitic pattern.
4) Large spotted areas of decreased density will be present.

Coccidioidal granuloma of bone will be seen in the desert areas of Southwestern United States. It will present with soft-tissue swelling, linear calcifications, and loss of bone substance with marked thickening of long bones.

Ainhum is a spontaneous amputation of a digit. The severity of pain that is present in this patient will be in proportion to the extent of the constricting band and overlying hyperkeratosis. This is a non-inflammatory condition, characterized by dry gangrene in fibrous bands which envelops an entire toe. Radiographically there will be a bulbous soft tissue swelling at the end of the toe (Fig. 9.10).

The constrictive band of fibrous tissue can be visualized radiographically. There will be a narrowed transverse diameter of bone beneath the constrictive bands. In the late stages, necrosis of bone may be recognized.

THE DIABETIC FOOT

The diabetic foot presents the podiatrist with a number of interesting disease manifestations that represent a dilemma in diagnosis. Understanding the etiology of these conditions helps considerably

in arriving at a diagnosis. Osteomyelitis, diabetic osteopathy, and Charcot foot must be considered and differentiated. Excluding the osteomyelitic foot, which has already been covered, the remaining two disease conditions have been described as neuropathic, neuroarthropathic, osteoarthropathic, osteopathic, neurogenic, and atrophic. This vast array of descriptive names is due only to the fact that the etiology is so poorly understood. We will first differentiate between these two conditions by classifying them as either atrophic or hypertrophic.

That disease that has in the past been called diabetic osteopathy consists of an alternation between bone absorption, erosion, and disappearance, alternated with osteosclerosis, periosteal proliferation, fragmentation of bone, and sequestration. It is now clear that we have been mixing two different disease entities that have a similar etiology.

ATROPHIC ARTHROPATHY

The term atrophic arthropathy will be used to denote that bone condition which exhibits on x-ray, osteoporosis, atrophy, destruction, disappearance of bone substance, and sometimes dislocation. To qualify for this condition, the joint must be free of osteophytes, sclerosis, eburnation, and fragmentation. That is, it must lack the criteria commonly attributed to the hypertrophic variety of Charcot foot. This condition results in bones that may be called pointed, or may be said to exhibit penciling, or a sucked-candy deformity. These changes are commonly observed in sensory neuropathic osteopathy, a bone disease associated with sensory nerve disturbances of variable etiology, which usually involve the metatarsal and metacarpal bones and the phalanges of the extremities.

There are a number of other conditions that cause similar changes, including: frostbite, trench foot, burns, rheumatoid arthritis, psoriatic arthritis, Raynaud's disease, progressive systemic sclerosis, and surgical amputation.

Most investigators believe that the pathological process leading to this deformity is a gradual concentric absorption of the phalanges and/or metatarsals, and that the narrowing process commences at the distal end, extending gradually toward the base, and terminating in a pointed deformity.

The epiphyseal ends gradually vanish while the shafts taper with pencil-point narrowing. Bones tend to become sclerotic, thereby simulating an

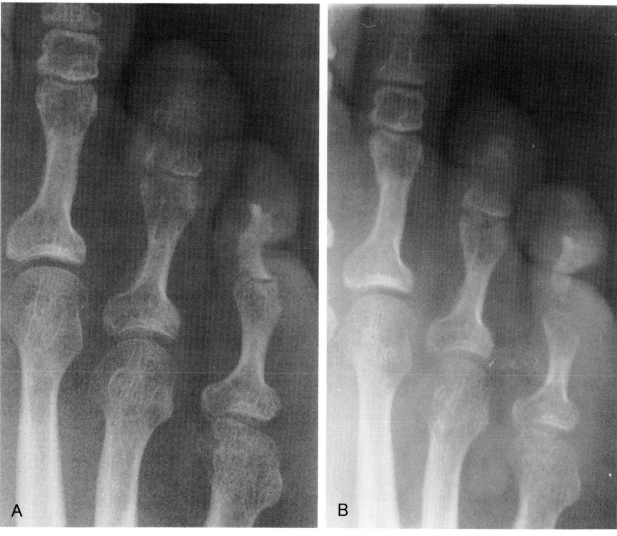

Figure 9.10. *A,* ainhum. A spontaneous amputation of the fifth digit at the level of the distal phalanx is occuring. *B,* one year later the constricting band has increased and the distal end of the toe has become bulbous.

osteomyelitis. At times the bases of the proximal phalanges broaden and form a cup-shape. Varieties of resulting deformities are known as intrusion, mortar-in-pestle, pencil-in-cup, and balancing pagoda. There usually is a dorsiflexion of toes, and a talipes cavus occurs. This is in contrast to the valgus deformity in the hypertrophic type.

In the description of the pathogenesis, one fact remains blaringly obvious, and that is that adequate blood supply is a prerequisite for the occurrence of the osteolysis that has been just described. Diabetic neuropathy constitutes an increasingly frequent basis for Charcot joint disease, and now outranks syphilitic tabes dorsalis in this respect.

The etiology in this condition is now thought to be that of a peripheral neuropathy. The spinal nerve is affected, as opposed to cord lesions. Remember that this contains sympathetic as well as sensory and motor fibers. These sympathetic fibers normally carry vasoconstrictive impulses. When the function of the postganglionic peripheral nerve is damaged, two events will take place: 1) loss of protective pain sensation will lead to mechanical over-use of the joint, and 2) loss of vasoconstrictive impulses will lead to hyperemia. Only when both events combine does the atrophic variety of Charcot foot occur.

One is inclined, therefore, to judge the ultimate effect of peripheral diabetic neuropathy upon a given joint according to whether or not an "autosympathectomy" has occurred. When this autosympathectomy occurs, we will see a complete

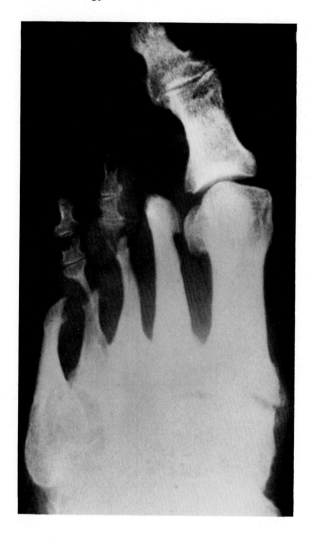

Figure 9.11. Atrophic arthropathy. Note the pencil-pointing of the third, fourth, and fifth metatarsals, and the dissolution and tapering of the proximal phalanges of the third and fourth digits in this diabetic. X-ray compliments of Dr. Harvey Lemont.

resorption of the metatarsal heads, and severe tapering of the shafts with pencil-point narrowing. The bone that remains tends to become sclerotic. Loss of bone and remodeling of the bases of the proximal phalanges result in a variety of deformities of the metatarsophalangeal joints. In time the proximal phalanges may be completely absorbed. Osteoporosis is present and destruction may lead to dislocation. No osteophytes, sclerosis, fragmentation, or soft tissue debris is present.

The tapering of the distal aspect of the metatarsal results in a mortar and pestle or pencil-in-a-cup deformity. Generally, there will be a pointing of the convex member of the joint and a hollowing or broadening of the convex member of the joint. Joint effusion usually precedes the destructive changes. Simply locating these findings on an x-ray does not give a diagnosis of diabetes.

Any disease that affects the spinal nerve such as trauma, alcoholism, and diabetes, which presumably affect postganglionic nerve segments,

carrying sympathetic vasoconstrictive as well as sensory and motor fibers, can cause this to occur.

Inflammatory arthritis, such as psoriatic arthritis, may cause a pencil-in-a-cup deformity, but the pathological process is quite different. Only the end-product appears similar.

Neuroarthropathy may also be related to a neurally initiated vascular reflex leading to increased osteoclastic bone resorption in an area supplied by a particular vascular bed (Figs. 9.11 to 9.13).

HYPERTROPHIC OSTEOARTHROPATHY

The atrophic form of osteoarthropathy must be distinguished from the neurotrophic arthropathy of the hypertrophic variety. This form of Charcot joint is an extreme progression of degenerative osteoarthritis. Following a loss of proprioceptive and pain sensation, with normal sympathetic innervation, the normal protective reactions are not invoked. Relaxation of supporting structures

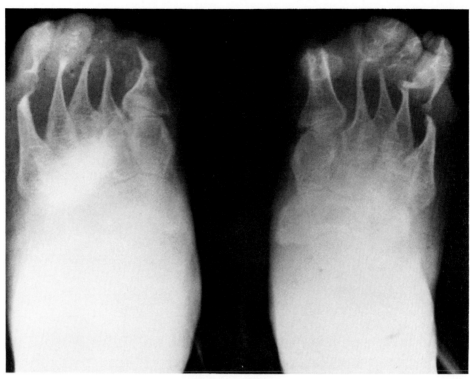

Figure 9.12.   Bilateral atrophic arthropathy. There are no fractures or new bone proliferation, only dissolution and osteoporosis. X-ray compliments of Dr. Harvey Lemont.

eventually leads to joint instability. The neurotrophic joint may paradoxically be painful due to the capsular distention and soft tissue trauma. Productive changes have been linked with central spinal cord lesions, such as trauma, tumor, congenital malformation, and diseases which commonly spare the sympathetic nervous system.

Peripheral neuropathy usually is diagnosed on the basis of decreased pin-prick sensation and decreased joint position sense. All affected joints usually are painless on passive or active motion. The hypertrophic arthropathy is usually associated with a lesion in the posterior tracts or the central portion of the gray matter of the spinal cord. These lesions exempt the sympathetic system by virtue of their anatomic location.

Mention of a Charcot joint has invariably conjured up a classical, clinical roentgenographic complex, involving swelling, hypermobility, malalignment, and osteosclerosis without pain in a peripheral joint.

Charcot joints are normally assumed to start with spontaneous fractures which, when combined with ligamentous laxity, lead to progressive destruction of the joint. The frequent spontaneous fractures in patients with neuropathic disorders have led some authors to believe that intrinsic

bone disease may be present. There is little evidence to substantiate this theory, however.

When joint surfaces become incongruous due to ligamentous laxity, bone destruction becomes imminent, and eventually becomes more severe with fracture and fragmentation, resulting in bone spicules in the synovium and soft tissues. At this stage of the disease, a zone of subchondral osteoporosis is frequently present. It most likely represents fracture in the subchondral bone because it usually is subsequently replaced by sclerotic bone when the lesion is healed.

The involved bones and joints usually go through three stages; the destructive stage; the stage of healing, and stage of coalescence.

The x-rays of this disease entity will show varying degrees and combinations of destructive and hypertrophic changes. There is a loss of articular cartilage, fragmentation, and absorption of subchondral bone with proliferation of new bone at the joint margins. Pathologic fractures are common and usually involve the articular surface. There may be considerable destruction of epiphyseal substance accompanied by bone fragmentation. These changes in general are similar to nonneuropathic degenerative joint disease. However, it is the exaggerated degree of the changes that leads to the diagnosis of Charcot joint. They are much more florid and more profound. It is osteoarthrosis with a "vengance." The osteophytes attain a size out of all proportion to joint space narrowing, forming huge, haphazard, widely based hypertrophic shelfs of bone. The foot in this stage may be described as a bag of loose bones or loose sand. Additional productive changes in the form of intense ill-defined sclerosis obliterating normal trabecular arthitecture are usually found (Figs. 9.14 to 9.20).[4-15]

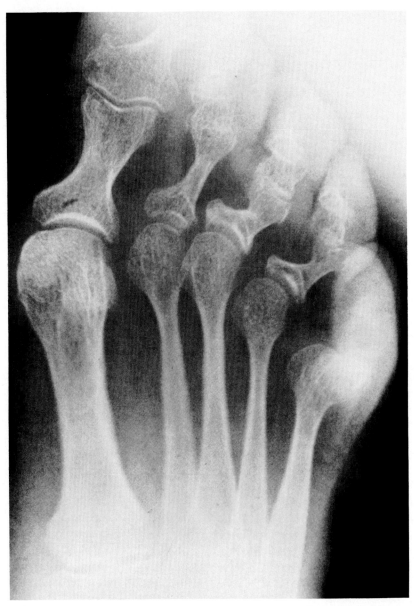

Figure 9.13. Early osteolysis in atrophic arthropathy. Note the early tapering of the second, third, and fourth metatarsals and the partial dissolution of the base of the proximal phalanges.

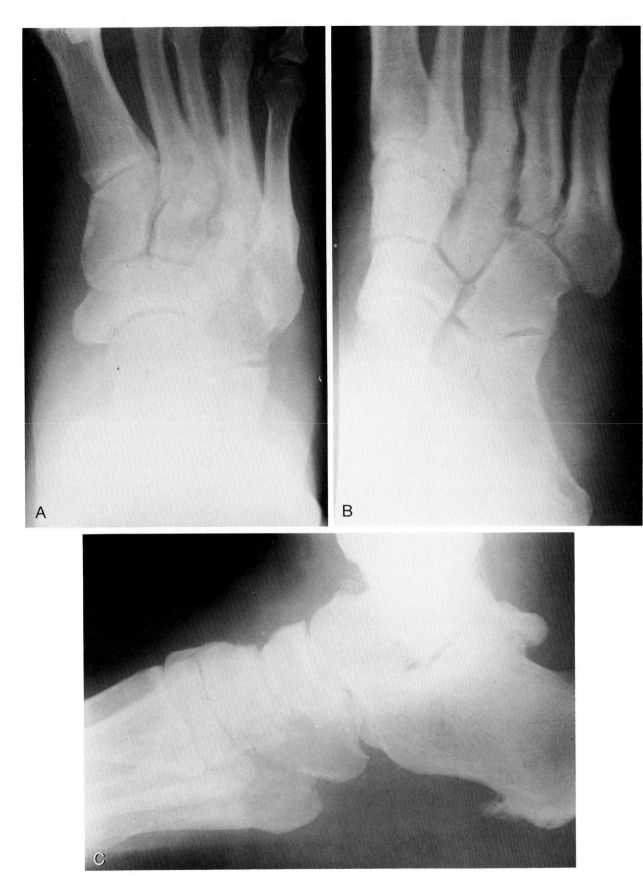

Figure 9.14. *A* to *C*, hypertrophic osteoarthropathy. This 40-year-old male injured his foot 3 months prior to these radiographs. The injury caused the neurotrophic process to begin. Note the periosteal proliferation along the shafts of the metatarsals and the severe sclerosis in the tarsal area.

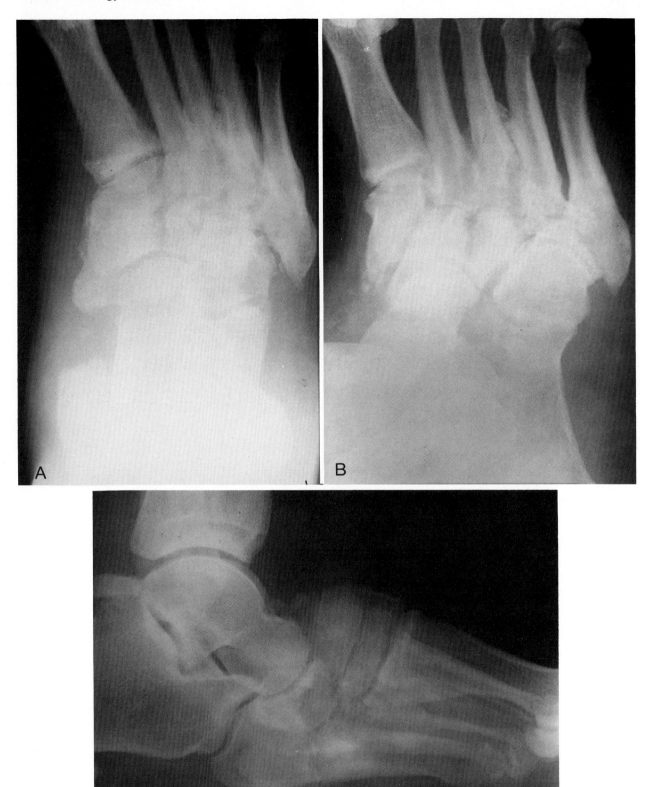

Figure 9.15.   Same patient as in Figure 9.14 three months later. Multiple fractures and dislocations have occurred throughout the tarsal area. Exuberant bone callus is present throughout the area. The navicular has crumbled and is sitting on top of the talus. The patient experienced no pain, only severe edema. On motion, the foot felt like a bag of loose sand.

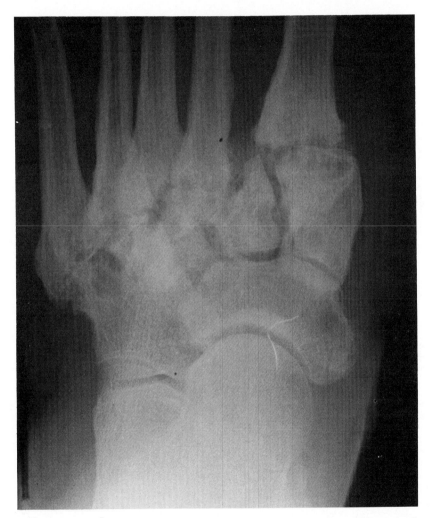

Figure 9.16. Hypertrophic arthropathy. Lisfranc's joint seems to be the commonest area for hypertrophic arthropathy to begin.

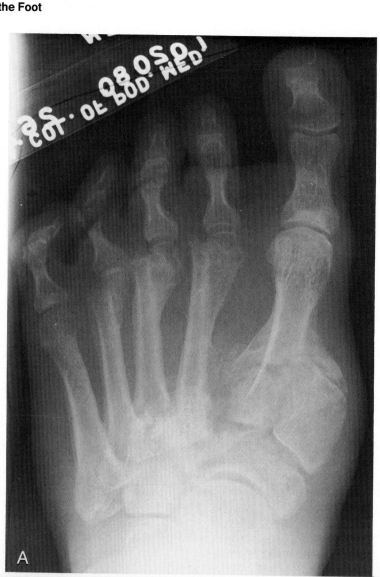

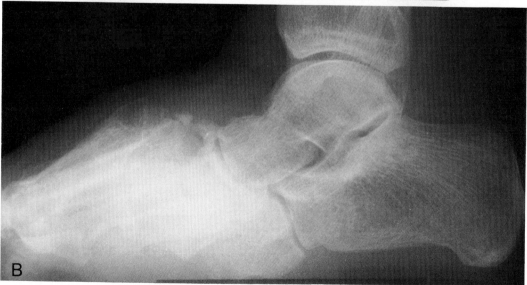

Figure 9.17. *A* and *B*, hypertrophic arthropathy. This 24-year-old female suffered a spinal injury one year prior to this film. The contralateral foot was completely unaffected.

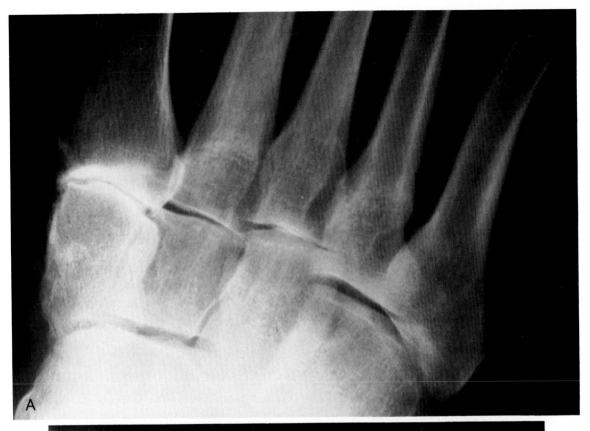

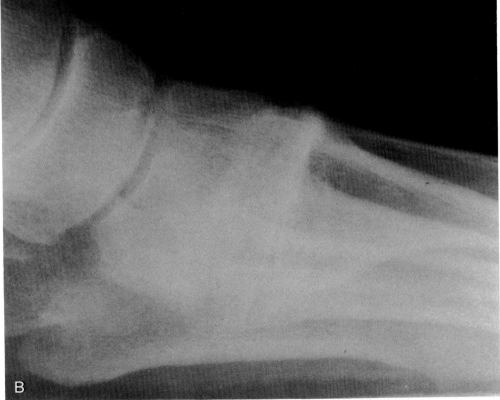

Figure 9.18. *A* and *B*, early hypertrophic arthropathy. Painless, severe, degenerative arthritis that seems out of proportion and exhibits a great deal of sclerosis is the hallmark of hypertrophic arthropathy.

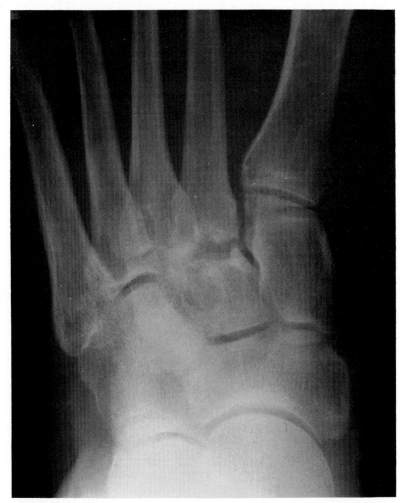

Figure 9.19.   Early hypertrophic arthropathy in the area of Lisfranc's joint.

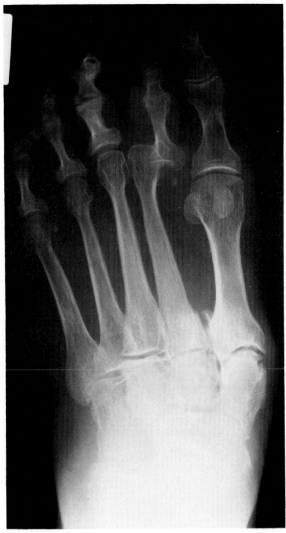

Figure 9.20.   Hypertrophic arthropathy in the area of Lisfranc's joint. Note that the foot appears severely pronated. This is typical of hypertrophic arthropathy.

REFERENCES

1. KEHR, L. E., ZULLI, L. P., AND McCARTHY, D. J.: Radiographic factors in osteomyelitis. J.A.P.A., **67**: 716, 1977.
2. GREENFIELD, G. B.: The joints. *Radiology of Bone Disease*, 3rd Ed, J. B. Lippincott, Philadelphia, 1980, p. 787.
3. SHANDS, A. R., AND RANEY, R. B.: *Handbook of Orthopaedic Surgery*, 7th Ed, C. V. Mosby, St. Louis, 1967.
4. KRAFT, E., SPYROPOULOS, E., AND FINBY, N.: Neurogenic disorders in diabetes mellitus. Am. J. Roentgenol., **124**: 17, 1975.
5. GONDOS, B.: The pointed tubular bone. Diag. Radiol., **105**: 541, 1972.
6. CLOUSE, M. E., GRAMM, H. F., LEGGS, M., AND FLOOD, T.: Diabetic osteoarthropathy. Am. J. Roentgenol., **121**: 22, 1974.
7. MUGGIA, F. M.: Neuropathic fracture. J.A.M.A., **191**: 160, 1965.
8. NEWMAN, J. H.: Spontaneous dislocation in diabetic neuropathy. J. Bone Jt. Surg., **61B**: 484, 1979.
9. EL-KHOURY, G. Y., AND KATHOL, M. H., Neuropathic fractures in patients with diabetes mellitus. Diag. Radiol., **134**: 313, 1980.
10. FELDMAN, F., JOHNSON, A. M., AND WALTER, J. F.: Acute axial neuroarthropathy. Diag. Radiol., **111**: 1, 1974.
11. RESNICK, D., AND NIWAYAMA, G.: *Diagnosis of Bone and Joint Disorders*, W. B. Saunders, Philadelphia, 1981, vol. 3, p. 2436.
12. McCARTHY, D. J., AND RODMAN, G. P.: Neuropathic joint disease (Charcot joints). *Arthritis and Allied Conditions*, 9th Ed, Lea & Febiger, Philadelphia, 1979, pp. 897–902.
13. SCHWARTS, G. S., BERENYI, M. R., AND SIEGEL, M. W.: Atrophic arthropathy and diabetic neuritis. Am. J. Roentgenol., **106**: 523, 1969.
14. WEISSMAN, S. D., AND WEISS, A.: Diabetic neurotrophic osteoarthropathy: A case report. J.A.P.A., **70**: 196, 1980.
15. FORRESTER, D. M., AND MAGRE, G.: Migrating bone shards in dissecting Charcot joints. Am. J. Roentgenol. **103**, 1133, 1978.
16. ANTES, E. H.: Charcot joints in diabetes mellitus. J.A.M.A., **156**, 602, 1954.
17. SHEPPE, WM.: Neuropathic (Charcot) joints occurring in diabetes mellitus. Diabetes, **8**: 192, 1959.

CHAPTER 10

Joint Disease and Arthritis

An x-ray examination is essential in the diagnosis and evaluation of the arthritities. Most arthritities are first suspected by the clinician, and x-ray evaluation of these entities along with laboratory testing is important for confirmation of the clinical diagnosis and in staging of the disease process. Several arthritities are often diagnosed first by the podiatrist on x-ray evaluation, including pseudogout, ankylosing spondylitis, early rheumatoid arthritis, degenerative joint disease, and tuberculosis of bone.[1]

The joint responds to insult in only a limited number of ways that become apparent on x-ray.[1] The soft tissues surrounding the joint, the articulating bones, and alignment of the joint space may all be involved by the arthritic process. On roentgenographic examination, the soft tissues must be examined for edema, masses, calcifications, and atrophy (see Chapter 8). The articulating bones must be examined for demineralization, erosions, osteophytes, periosteal reaction, cysts, and sclerosis.[1]

An examination of the joint space is of prime importance. In the inflammatory and the crystal-induced arthritities, it is common to see an increase in joint space in the early and acute stages, due to a soft tissue effusion. This effusion of fluid causes the joint capsule to balloon out and causes a greater separation between the articulating bones. This must be distinguished from an increase in the mass of the cartilage, which would show an increased joint space, as in acromegaly. The joint space should be examined for loose bodies, and increased density, possibly resulting from the presence of crystalline matter or purulent matter, or intraarticular fractures. The joint also

must be checked for abnormalities in alignment. This will occur in hallux-abducto-valgus, contractures of the digits, subluxation, deviations, and dislocations.

EROSIONS

In the inflammatory arthritities, lysosomal enzymes from hypertrophied synovium attacks the paraarticular bone near the attachment of the joint capsule, where the hyaline cartilage ends and the synovium begins. The enzyme-laden synovium eats away bone and cartilage, causing irregularities called erosions. It is important to examine the erosions closely as they can aid in determining which of the many arthritities you are dealing with.

In rheumatoid arthritis, the erosions are poorly outlined, often irregular, and without sclerotic margins. The joint space narrowing of rheumatoid arthritis is typically uniform. The erosions are fuzzily marginated (Fig. 10.1).

The early erosions of psoriatic arthritis may resemble those of rheumatoid arthritis. However, with progression of the disease, they become somewhat irregular, and become rimmed by sclerotic margins. They frequently are associated with a fluffy periostitis, which seems fairly characteristic (Fig. 10.2).[1–3]

The erosions of gouty arthritis are well outlined with definite sclerotic margins. As the tophus erodes the bone, it seems to stimulate a periosteal reaction, which extends partially over the tophus, producing an overhanging C-shaped edge of bone. This is called the martel sign, and is fairly characteristic of gouty arthritis (Fig. 10.3).

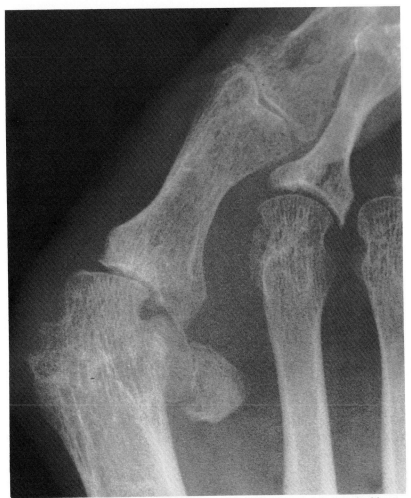

Figure 10.1. The erosions of rheumatoid arthritis are poorly outlined, irregular, and without sclerotic margins.

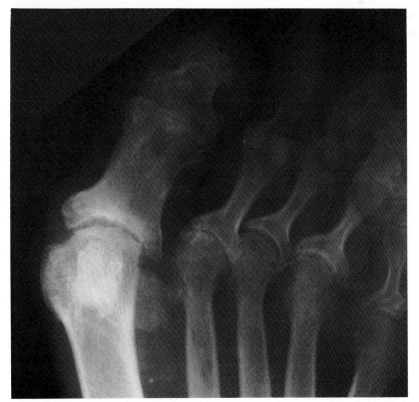

Figure 10.2. The erosions of psoriatic arthritis are similar to those of rheumatoid arthritis, but usually are rimmed with a sclerotic margin.

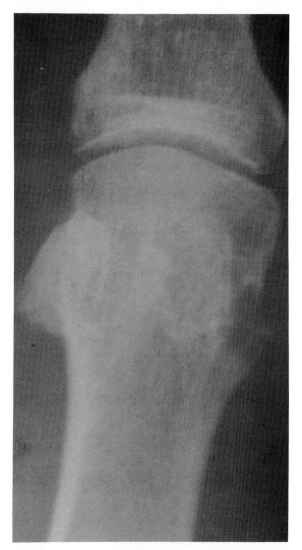

Figure 10.3. The erosions of gouty arthritis are well outlined with sclerotic margins and frequently have an overhanging edge of bone, the martel sign.

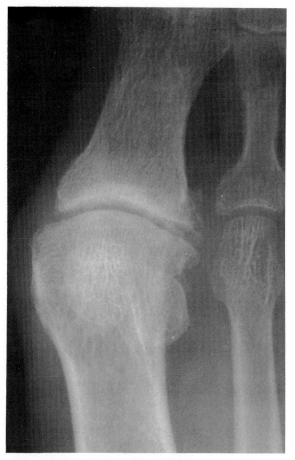

Figure 10.4. Osteophytes. Osteophytes represent new bone that is formed as the result of degenerative arthritis. Osteophytes are seen on the lateral edge of this metatarsophalangeal joint exhibiting hallux limitus.

OSTEOPHYTES

Osteophytes represent new bone that is formed as a result of cartilage degeneration from any cause. They occur in degenerative or osteoarthritis, neurotrophic arthropathy, acromegaly, ochronosis, and following trauma (Fig. 10.4).

Resorption of bone can be seen in scleroderma, psoriatic arthritis, leprosy, occasionally in hyperparathyroidism, and in many other conditions.

A decrease of joint space usually implies destruction of the articular cartilage. It is important to determine whether the narrowing is symmetrical or asymmetrical, and whether it is unilateral or bilateral, involving single or multiple joints. In rheumatoid arthritis, the narrowing of the joint space is uniform, even, and frequently bilateral, whereas in osteoarthritis, the narrowing is uneven and non-uniform.[1]

RHEUMATOID ARTHRITIS

Rheumatoid arthritis is a systemic disease usually presenting a chronic progressive symmetrical inflammation of multiple joints. The metatarsophalangeal and metacarpophalangeal joints are among the commonest sites of involvement, the initial lesion being a proliferative synovitis.[2] It almost always involves either the hands and wrists or feet and ankles, frequently before any other joints are involved. Usually it is symmetrical, and among the earlier symptoms, causes fusiform swelling of the digits at the proximal interphalangeal joints. As a result of the inflammatory

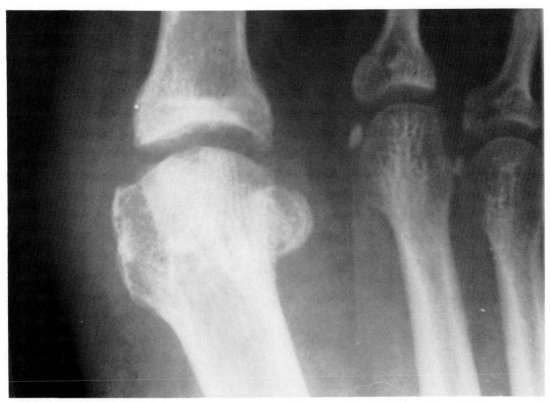

Figure 10.5. Early rheumatoid arthritis. The earliest sign of rheumatoid arthritis is a joint effusion as seen in the first metatarsophalangeal joint.

synovitis, there is a secondary demineralization that occurs in the juxtaarticular areas. This usually is first seen about the metatarsophalangeal or proximal interphalangeal joints. This occurrence leads to two of the earliest radiographic changes seen in rheumatoid arthritis: an increase in the joint space (Figs. 10.5 and 10.6), secondary to the edema present, and the juxtaarticular deossification (Fig. 10.7). As the disease progresses, a degeneration of cartilage occurs. Cartilage passes through several stages, initially losing its sheen and becoming soft and dull. Later it becomes gray and fibrillated, and still later becomes slightly pitted. Eventually, the underlying bone becomes exposed and an erosion has developed (Figs. 10.10 to 10.16).[2]

In contradistinction to most of the other arthritities, the erosions of rheumatoid arthritis usually lack sclerotic margins. Hammerman in 1969 stated that lysosomal enzymes released from proliferating rheumatoid synovium when in direct contact with cartilage may gain access to the cartilage matrix and degrade it. Cartilage is eventually destroyed and the matrix is replaced by pannus.[2] As the disease progresses, subluxation of the metatarsophalangeal joints occurs with fibular de-

viation, "swan-neck," and boutonniere deformities, along with a hallux-abducto-valgus deformity. The end-stage of rheumatoid arthritis is bony ankylosis.

Many factors are involved in the pathological processes that cause the deformity of the foot in rheumatoid arthritis. The joint pain causes a guarding and limitation of motion. This lack of motion eventually leads to weakness and atrophy of the muscles. Also contributing to the disuse atrophy is an interstitial polymyositis, which is found in a high percentage of rheumatoid arthritis patients. This causes miliary inflammatory foci in skeletal muscle (and interstitial myositis). Inflammatory cells will be found in the endomysial and perimysial connective tissue, usually around small blood vessels. The muscle fibers around these foci will be affected. The type II fibers are affected most often. These are the white fibers, which are involved in quick phasic activities.

There is also a possibility that a steroid myopathy contributes to the atrophy of the involved muscles. Muscles of the leg that are most commonly affected are the tibialis anterior and tibialis posterior. This leads to weakness in the primary inverters of the foot, and allows the peroneus

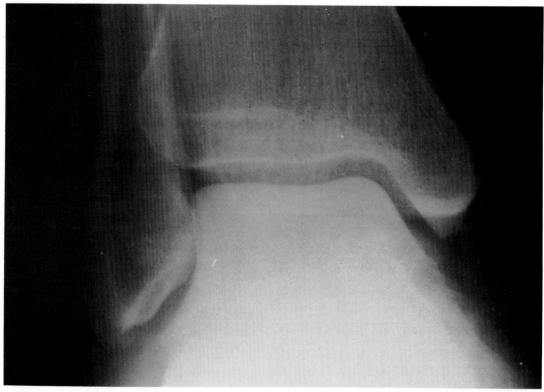

Figure 10.6. Joint effusion of early rheumatoid arthritis. The normal ankle joint space should be up to 3 mm in width.

longus and brevis, soleus, and the extensors of the toes to be strong enough to overpower the inverters and cause a severe pronation in the foot. A pronated foot requires intrinsic muscle activity more than a normal foot. This is necessary to stabilize the transverse tarsal joint and subtalar joints, but we know that the intrinsics become atrophic in rheumatoid arthritic patients, both in the hand and in the foot. This, in combination with the overpowering of the inverters of the foot, leads to a severe pronation of the foot. As the pronation develops the gait becomes abducted and the patient toes off on the medial side of the first metatarsophalangeal joint. The adductor hallucis becomes somewhat decreased in strength, but the abductor loses most of its strength, so it is overcome by the weakened adductor hallucis. With a valgus rotation of the hallux, the abductor, if it is able to act, becomes a flexor. With a valgus rotation, the insertion of the adductor hallucis moves to the lateral plantar side of the great toe. The flexor hallucis brevis becomes displaced laterally as the metatarsal head drifts medially, giving an abductory pull. The sesamoids will essentially "wipe away" the crista on weight-bearing. The long axis of the first ray becomes shortened by the abnormal position of the great toe. This allows the extensor hallucis longus to become shortened

(Fig. 10.8) and, in this abnormal position, it exerts an abductory pull on the great toe, which tends to increase the deformity. This occurs similarly in the digits, so that the extensor digitorum longus also becomes an abductor of the lesser digits. The intrinsics lose their power because the distances between the origin and insertion of these tiny muscles shortens; therefore, the amount of pull they are able to exert decreases.

Claw Toes Development

At toe-off there is a passive extension of the metatarsophalangeal joints. In swing phase, the extensors normally contract to help the toes and foot to clear the ground. This leads to a dorsal subluxation of the metatarsophalangeal joints (Fig. 10.9). When the synovitis is active and edema is present, it tends to stretch the capsules of the metatarsophalangeal joints. The flexor tendons will become displaced into the intermetatarsal spaces and will tend to move dorsal to the center of rotation of the metatarsal head. They then become extensors. With disruption of the capsule, the fat pad will shift distally and will perpetuate the dorsal dislocation of the digits. The foot ends up with extension that is unopposed by flexion and gives a claw toe deformity. The fat pad shifting distally removes the normal padding that is usually found beneath the metatarsal heads and allows callous to be exacerbated beneath the metatarsal heads.[3-10]

HLA ANTIGENS

During the early years of skin-grafting and organ transplantation, studies of the rejection phenomenon led to the discovery of the histocompatibility "antigens." These antigens are found on the surface of cells throughout the body. The genes that control the expression of these antigens, are situated on chromosome #6 and were called histocompatibility genes. The antigens are most conveniently detected in the laboratory on peripheral blood leukocytes and as a consequence are called, human leukocyte associated antigens, or HLA antigens. Today there are over 50 distinct histocompatibility antigens that have been identified.

The HLA B-27 antigen has been associated with many of the inflammatory arthritities, including a 100% association with ankylosing spondylitis, 93% with Reiter's arthritis, 55% with psoriatic arthritis, and 12% with ankylosing hyperostosis.[11,18]

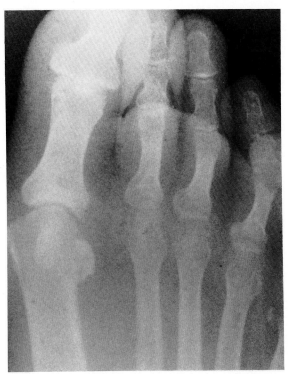

Figure 10.7. Rheumatoid arthritis. The earliest osseous sign of rheumatoid arthritis is juxtaarticular osteoporosis.

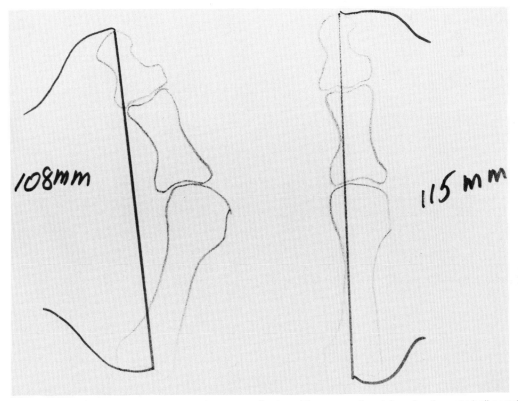

Figure 10.8. The extensor hallucis longus becomes short and increases the deforming force in hallux valgus.

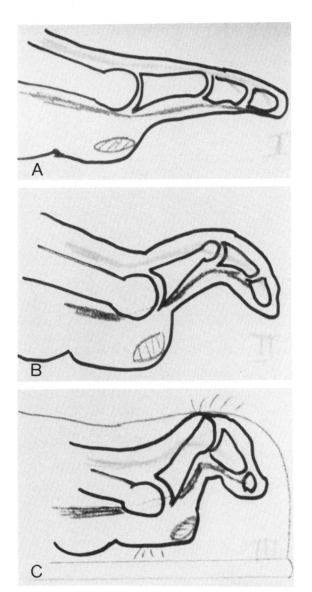

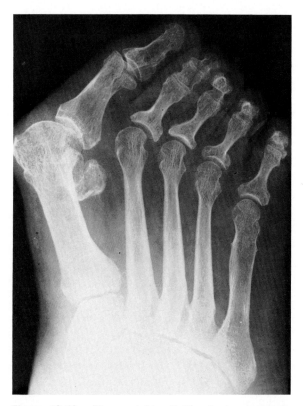

Figure 10.10. Rheumatoid arthritis. A classical radiograph of the rheumatoid foot with hallux-abducto-valgus, claw toes, fibular deviation of the lesser digits, and osteoporosis.

Figure 10.9. Claw toe development in rheumatoid arthritis. *A,* normal alignment of the long extensor and flexor tendons into a digit with a submetatarsal fat pad in place. *B,* following repeated bouts of synovitis, the metatarsophalangeal joint capsule becomes stretched, allowing the plantar fat pad to shift distally. The flexor tendons become displaced into the intermetatarsal space. *C,* they move dorsal to the center of rotation of the metatarsal head and become extensors of the digit.

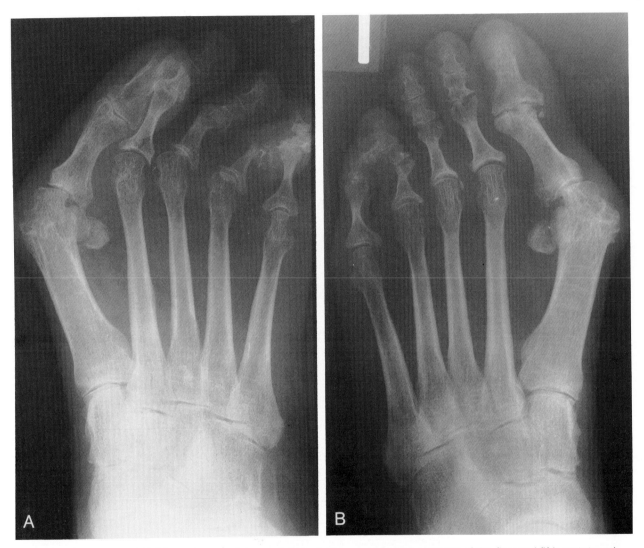

Figure 10.11.   *A* and *B*, bilateral case of rheumatoid feet. There are typical erosions of the first and fifth metatarsal heads without margins. Hallux-abducto-valgus and fibular deviation of lesser digits is typical.

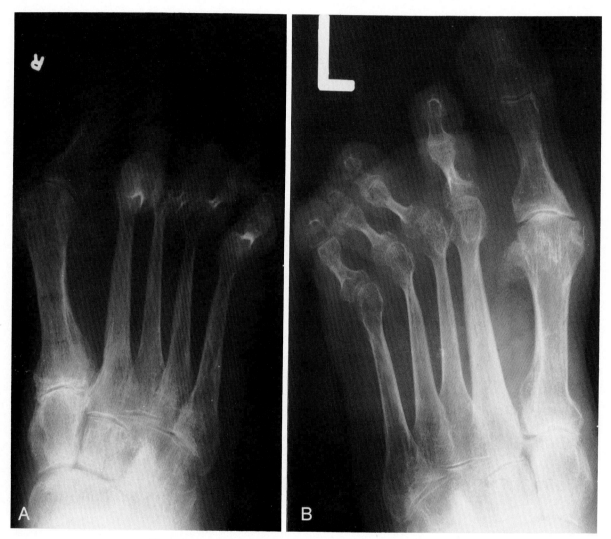

Figure 10.12.   *A* and *B*, rheumatoid arthritis bilaterally.

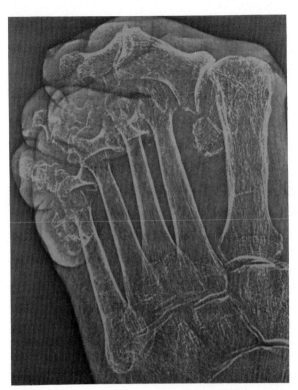

Figure 10.13. Severe rheumatoid of the foot. Note the severe osteoporosis present in this xeroradiograph.

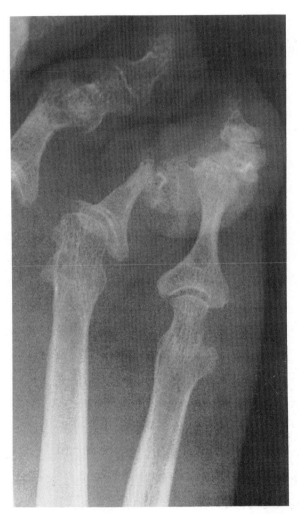

Figure 10.14. Rheumatoid forefoot. Fibular deviation with poorly marginated erosions of the metatarsal heads and phalanges.

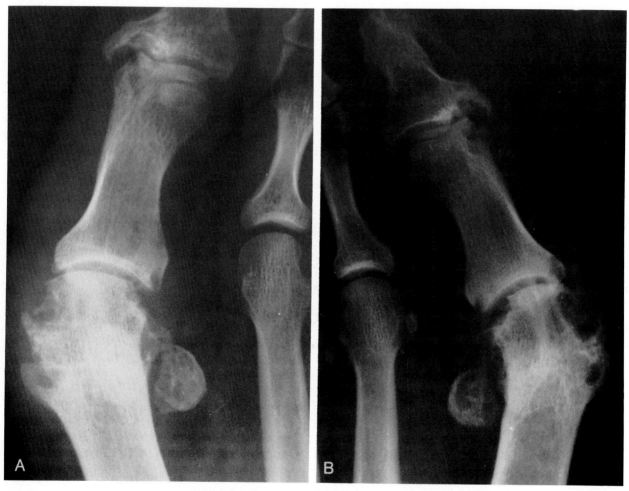

Figure 10.15.   *A* and *B*, severe erosive changes secondary to rheumatoid arthritis.

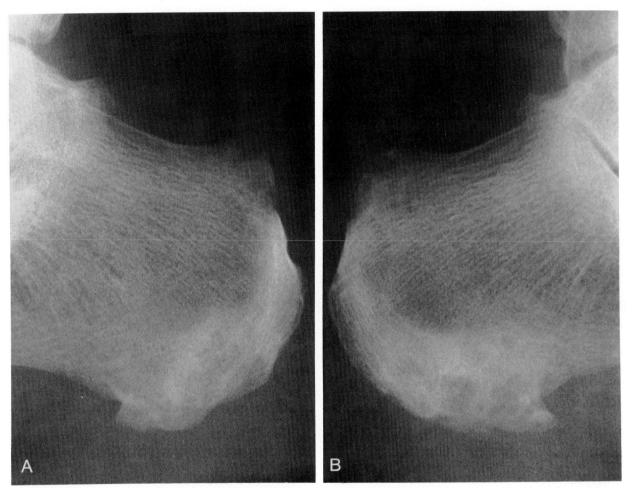

Figure 10.16. *A* and *B*, rheumatoid erosions of the calcaneus. The synovial lining of the preachilles bursa frequently causes erosions of the posterosuperior aspect of the calcaneus.

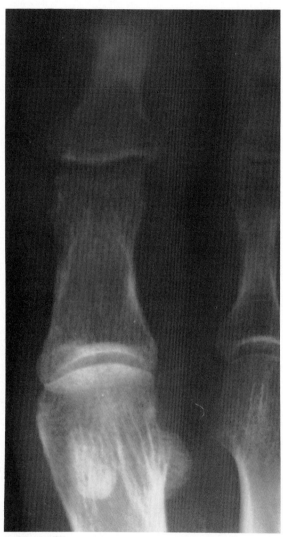

Figure 10.17. Psoriatic arthritis. This early erosion is typical of the commonest area to be affected by psoriatic arthritis in the foot, the interphalangeal joint of the hallux.

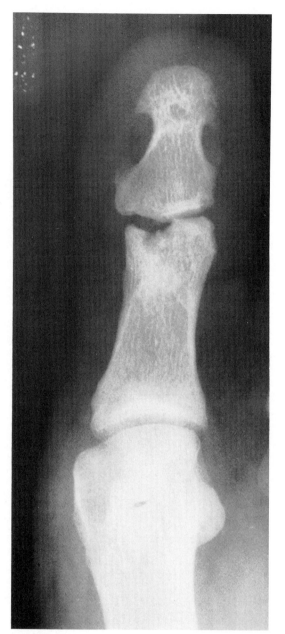

Figure 10.18. Psoriatic arthritis. The interphalangeal joint of the hallux is affected by an irregular erosion that is marginated by a sclerotic ring.

PSORIATIC ARTHRITIS

Psoriatic arthritis is an asymmetrical polyarthritis that is usually associated with psoriasis. It has a tendency for causing sausage-shaped swelling of the digits. Peripheral disease has been demonstrated in 91% of the patients having psoriatic arthritis, with the calcaneus being affected in 53% of those patients. The feet were demonstrated to have been involved in 81% of patients having

psoriatic arthritis.[11] The characteristics of psoriatic arthritis are as follows.

One or a few joints are involved at a time, usually in the digits. The most commonly affected joint in the foot is the proximal interphalangeal joint of the great toe. It affects the distal interphalangeal joints of the lesser digits most often, followed next by the proximal interphalangeal joints and the metatarsophalangeal joint involve-

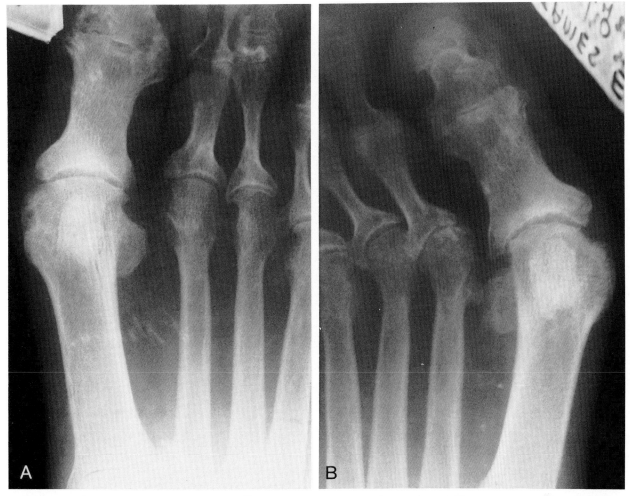

Figure 10.19. *A* and *B*, psoriatic arthritis. The interphalangeal joint of the hallux is affected and there are erosions in this area and about the metatarsophalangeal joint. Early "pencil-in-a-cup" deformities of the lesser metatarsophalangeal joints are occurring.

ment. Often all the distal interphalangeal joints are involved. Marginal erosion of subchondral bone in the phalanges is a very common sign. The periosteal reaction about these erosions is thick and fluffy and extends along the shafts of the metatarsals and phalanges. There usually is no deossification and no deviation of the affected joints. Swelling of the entire digit gives a sausage-like appearance. Frequently, there is resorption of the ungual tufts, which begins as small clefts in the distal tufts of the distal phalanges (Figs. 10.17 to 10.22).

The erosions of psoriatic arthritis are fairly distinct, are rimmed by sclerotic margins, and are usually associated with the thick fluffy periostitis. These marginal erosions of subchondral bone, when occurring on the metatarsal heads, cause whittling and eventually lead to a "pencil-in-cup

deformity." The metatarsal becomes pointed and the base of the proximal phalanx becomes widened and distorted, giving the cup shape. Bony ankylosis of the interphalangeal joints occurs in the end-stages of psoriatic arthritis. The bone destruction can at times be so severe that there can be telescoping of the digits, the so-called "main-en-lorgnette deformity." Complete resorption of joints can occur, the so-called arthritis mutilans. Calcaneal erosions are very frequent in psoriatic arthritis.[1, 10, 12]

REITER'S SYNDROME

Classically, Reiter's syndrome consists of four clinical features, including non-specific urethritis, arthritis, conjunctivitis, or iritis and mucocutaneous lesions (keratoderma blenorrhagicum).

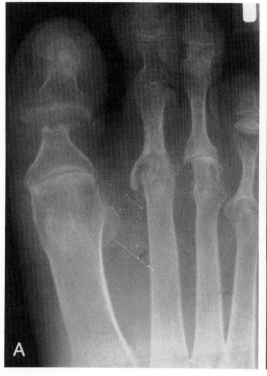
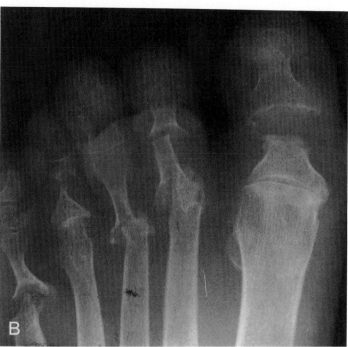

Figure 10.20. *A* and *B*, psoriatic arthritis. The head of the proximal phalanx of the hallux is completely resorbed. The "pencil-in-a-cup" deformities are typical of psoriatic arthritis. The lesser digits are sausage-shaped, exhibiting a "main-en-lorgnette" deformity.

Now the quadrad has been expanded to a sextad with the addition to mucosal ulcerations and balanitis circinata. It has also been known to involve the heart and the central nervous system. The diagnosis may be difficult because all of the clinical manifestations need not necessarily occur at the same time or even in close sequence to one another, and some of them may never occur. Only two of the classical symptoms are needed to make a diagnosis. It is because of this that the radiological features are of special significance. The feet show abnormalities in 84–93% of patients with Reiter's syndrome. The most common site of involvement is the foot and particularly the metatarsophalangeal joints and the heels.[11] The posterosuperior and posteroinferior aspects of the calcaneus are often selectively affected. Men are most commonly affected, and usually in the 20- to 30-year-old age bracket. Other joints in the feet may be involved, such as the proximal interphalangeal joints and the interphalangeal joints of the hallux. The ankles are also frequently in-

volved. Severe joint destruction is usually confined to the small joints of the foot, and, occasionally, of the hand. The bone erosions in the early stages appear as discrete marginal lesions, which are paraarticular, rather than subchondral. They appear at the chondro-osseus junction, the so-called "bare areas." Frequently, they will appear simply as a diffuse loss of cortical definition, in or adjacent to the joints, which may be blurred by coexistent periosteal bone formation. Arthritis mutilans seems to occur in only approximately 9% of the cases involved. Reiter's arthritis is usually unifocal or multifocal, but rarely is panarthritic in nature. While there may be small isolated areas of osteoporosis, regional osteoporosis is often absent or minimal despite severe joint destruction. Periosteal new bone formation is very fluffy and occurs particularly at bony prominances, such as about the calcaneus or at the malleoli. Sacroiliitis is very common. Following the initial edema, there is joint space narrowing and then destruction of the joints.[1, 10, 12, 13]

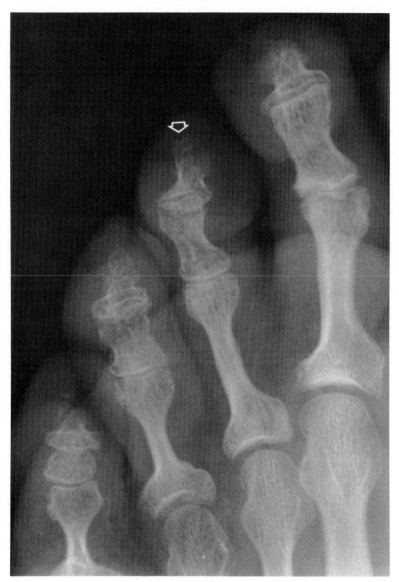

Figure 10.21.   Psoriatic clefts. Psoriatic arthritis frequently causes ''clefting'' at the tufts of the distal phalanges.

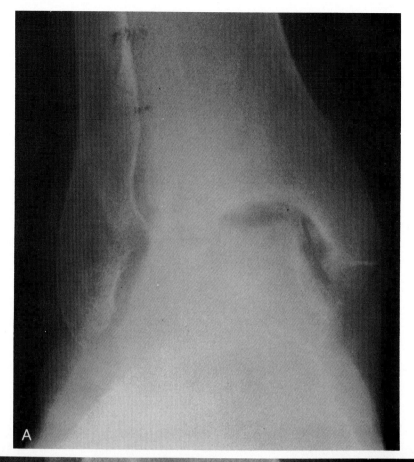

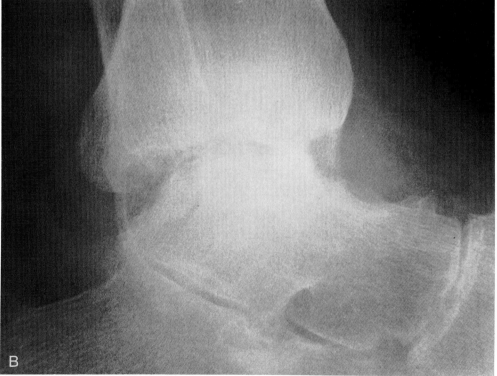

Figure 10.22. *A* and *B*, psoriatic arthritis of the ankle joint causing severe destruction.

Ankylosing Spondylitis

Ankylosing spondylitis is a chronic progressive arthritis characterized by involvement by the sacroiliac joint and the spinal joints. Ninety per cent of the patients are male, 100% of the patients have a positive HLA-B27 antigen, and foot abnormalities are present in approximately 18% of these patients. The usual age of onset is between the 2nd and 3rd decade with an insidious progression. It tends to affect the os calcis most often in the foot. The smaller joints are rarely affected. Erosions of the calcaneus occur along with a fluffy type of spur. The metatarsophalangeal joints can be affected in which paraarticular osteoporosis occurs, along with erosions, reactive sclerosis, and, as an end-result, bony ankylosis. The typical x-ray of the spine in these patients shows a "bamboo spine." It generally takes 3–6 months following the onset of symptoms for roentgen findings, suggestive of ankylosing spondylitis to be present. The radiologic changes of the os calcis can be divided into those involving the posterior aspect and those involving the plantar aspect.

Thickening of the Achilles tendon for several centimeters proximal to its insertion is one of the earlier findings of ankylosing spondylitis.[15] The swelling of the tendon and the concomitant edema tends to impinge on the pre-Achilles fat pad and bursa. Preerosive changes or cortical thinning without actual erosion occur anterior to the Achilles tendon and also tend to occur posterior to the insertion of the plantar fascia. Following these early changes, actual erosions can occur, they may be relatively small, but frequently can reach one centimeter in length. The characteristic appearance of the posterior type of erosion in ankylosing spondylitis is that of an "E," so that a central bone spicule is present. Although this appearance is characteristic, it is unfortunately not specific for ankylosing spondylitis. It may also be found in peripheral rheumatoid arthritis, as well as Reiter's syndrome. The plantar surface of the calcaneus may show erosive changes at the site where the cortical thinning occurs. They do not tend to be as deep here as they were at the posterior aspect, and do not have a central spicule. Osteoporosis is usually generalized throughout the entire calcaneus and adjacent tarsal bones (Figs. 10.23 to 10.25).

The formation of the plantar spur at the sight of insertion of the plantar fascia is important in the disease process. Early on in the disease, there is a minute speck of calcium deposit at the site which may require a magnifying glass to visualize. With a lapse of several months or even up to one year, the area of calcification increases, and a woolly-like appearance of new bone formation is noted which can extended distally and may become a solid amorphous mass. The inferior margin is straight and does not curve anterosuperiorally as in a degenerative type spur. Periosteal new bone formation at the posterosuperior aspect of the calcaneus may give rise to a squaring-off or puffed-out appearance, like a Haglund's deformity. In the late stages, a complete fusion of an entire tarsus may occur.

In the rare cases when the forefoot is affected, erosions may occur at the medial aspect of the metatarsal heads, as in rheumatoid disease. These erosions may also involve the interphalangeal joints, but are less marked. There will be narrowing of the joint space that is usually uniform and complete obliteration and fusion may finally occur. Periosteal new bone formation may occur along the shafts of the metatarsal bones and the phalanges. This periosteal new bone formation may also occur at the site of tendonitis.[12, 14, 16]

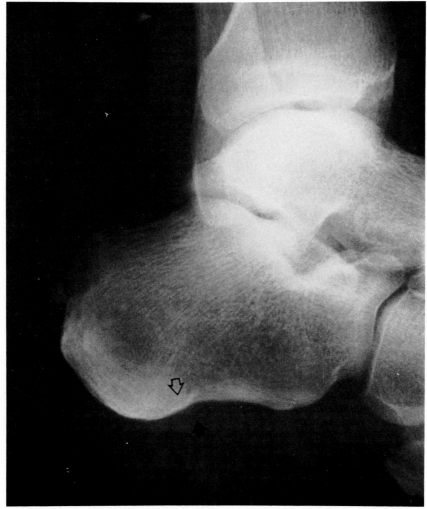

Figure 10.23.   Anklyosing spondylitis. Anklyosing spondylitis frequently causes erosions of the posterosuperior aspect of the calcaneus. An early sign of the disease is a minute speck of calcium at the attachment of the plantar fascia to the calcaneus.

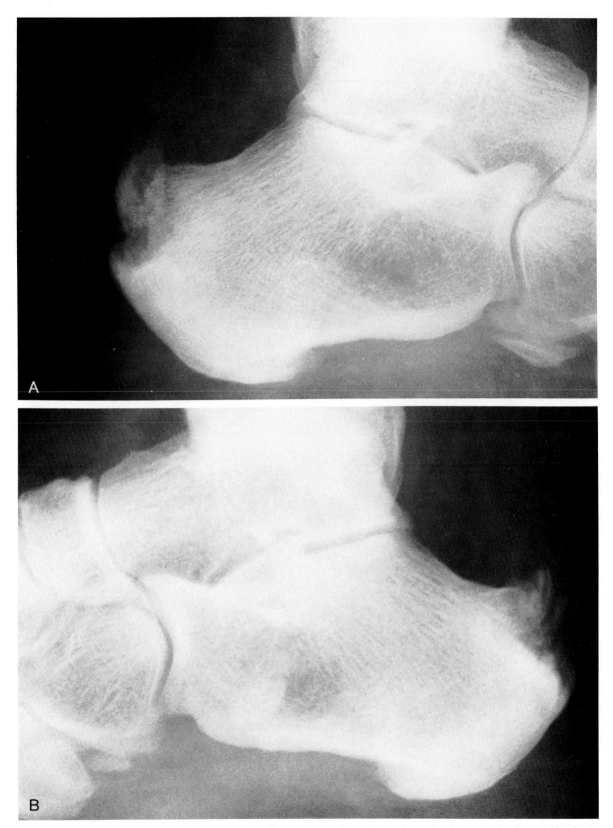

Figure 10.24.   *A* and *B*, anklyosing spondylitis. Severe posterior calcaneal erosion is present, along with plantar calcaneal spur formation. This patient exhibited thickening of the tendoachilles bilaterally.

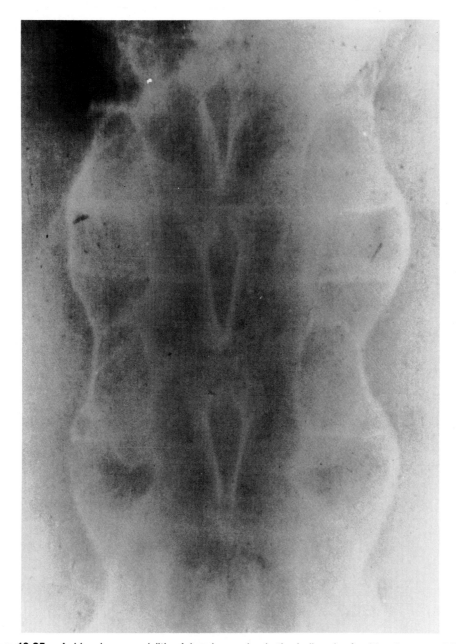

Figure 10.25. Anklyosing spondylitis. A bamboo spine is the hallmark of anklyosing spondylitis.

Degenerative Arthritis (Osteoarthritis)

Osteoarthritis, or as many authorities now call it, osteoarthrosis, is a progressive, non-inflammatory disorder of movable joints that is characterized by deterioration of the articular cartilage and by new bone formation. These osteophytes usually are proliferated at the joint margins and in the subchondral regions. Degenerative arthritis is the most common form of arthritis. X-ray changes include a non-uniform joint space narrowing, subchondral sclerosis or ebuneration, osteophyte proliferation, subarticular cysts with sclerotic margins, and pseudocysts. There usually is a lack of periarticular osteoporosis since there usually is not a major inflammatory phase. In severe cases, loose bodies, called joint mice, may become detached and float free within the joint space. Seldom does bony ankylosis occur (Figs. 10.26 and 10.27).

The bone cysts of osteoarthritis are frequently situated in areas of greatest bone sclerosis and greatest loss of joint space. There will be a concentric arrangement of healthy trabeculae around an enlarged marrow space that is filled frequently with ordinary adipose tissue. The cysts are usually multiple and are surrounded by a zone of dense bone. Some are multilocular. The smaller cysts always lie in the bone immediately adjacent to the joint space. There is usually one place where the cysts come close to the joint cavity, and in many cases, it is possible to demonstrate an opening between the two, usually in the form of a linear fissure. The cartilage over the cyst is never normal. The cysts that communicate with the joint space may burrow extensively under ebernated bone.

Bony protuberances at the dorsal margins of the distal phalangeal joints are known as Heberden's nodes, and at the proximal interphalangeal joints they are called Bouchard's nodes (Fig. 10.28).[17-21]

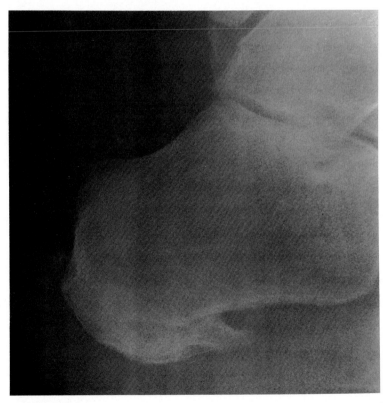

Figure 10.26. Degenerative arthritis. The plantar calcaneal spur is an osteophyte.

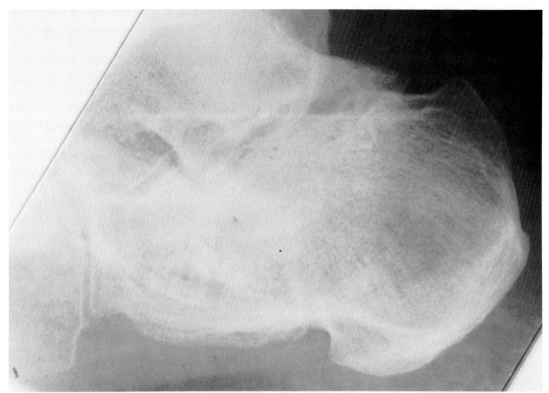

Figure 10.27.   Posttraumatic arthritis. The subtalar joint has developed severe arthritic changes following a traumatic episode, resulting in fracture of the calcaneus. Traumatic arthritis is a form of degenerative arthritis.

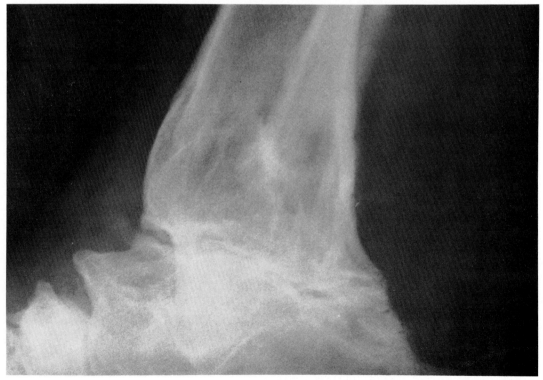

Figure 10.28.   Traumatic arthritis of the ankle joint.

GOUTY ARTHRITIS

Gouty arthritis is a condition of hyperuricemia, with urate crystal deposition in the soft tissues, and its resultant effects. The acute condition consists of marked edema and inflammation about a joint. The accumulation of uric acid in the system can be caused either by a catabolic state, in which a build-up of uric acid occurs, or by a failure in the excretory mechanisms to eliminate the normal uric acid in the body. In either case, uric acid crystals can be deposited in and around any joint in the body. There seems to be a preponderance for deposition in the foot, however, and the most commonly affected joint is the first metatarsophalangeal joint. The body seems to react rather strongly to the crystal deposition in the tissues, and there is an extreme infiltration of polymorphonuclear leukocytes in the tissues leading to a great deal of edema and pain. In an early case of gouty arthritis, the only x-ray finding will be that of an increase of soft tissue density and volume about the affected joint. These changes can be unilateral or bilateral; however, they are usually asymmetrical. Any joint in the body may be af-

fected. In long-standing cases of gouty arthritis, erosions of the bone may occur. The early erosions are shallow and are not rimmed by sclerotic margins. However, they quickly progress and are soon rimmed by sclerotic bone. In gouty arthritis there seems to be an attempt to heal over the bony erosion. This results in an overhanging edge of periosteal new bone that is C-shaped. This is called the martel sign (Figs. 10.29 to 10.35).

The crystal deposition within the joint eventually leads to an erosion of the articular cartilage, on both sides of the joint. While the early manifestations of this condition lead to joint widening, because of the extreme inflammatory response, the late changes include uneven joint narrowing. At this stage, the joint appears to be one that has been severely affected by degenerative arthritis. In rare cases of long-standing gouty arthritis, tophi may be deposited in the soft tissues anywhere in the body. They may clacify and can lead to further erosion of the bone. In the acute stages of gouty arthritis, there may be a localized deossification of the bone. However, this is usually not seen after the acute stage has subsided.[10, 22, 23]

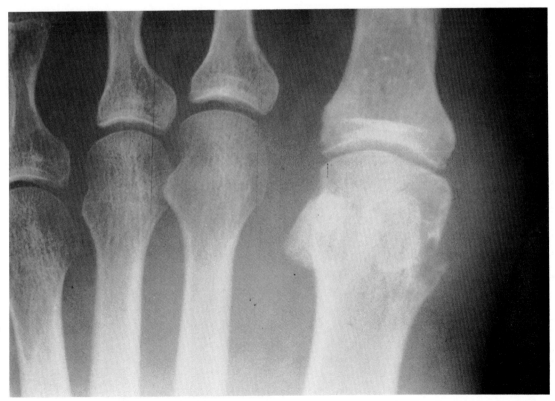

Figure 10.29.   Gouty arthritis. Erosion of the first metatarsal head that is rimmed with sclerotic bone and exhibits a martel sign.

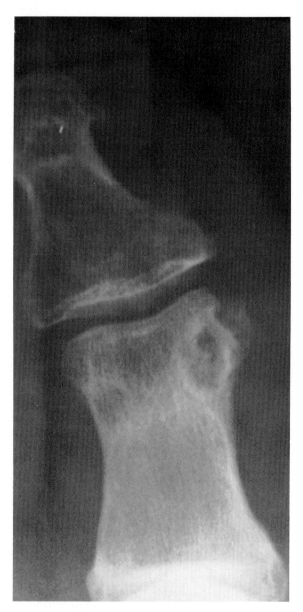

Figure 10.30.   Gouty arthritis.

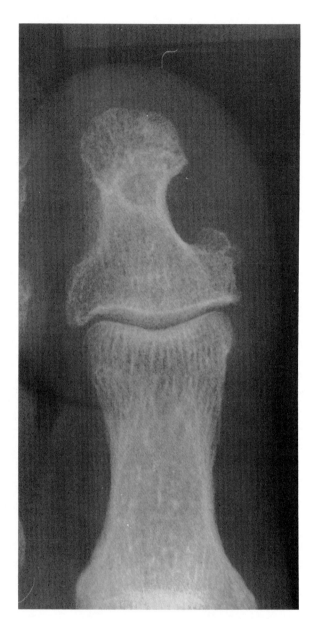

Figure 10.31.   Gouty arthritis.

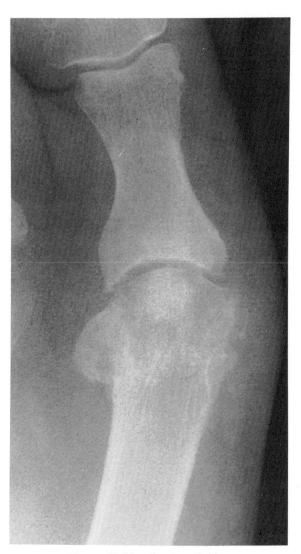

Figure 10.32. Gouty arthritis.

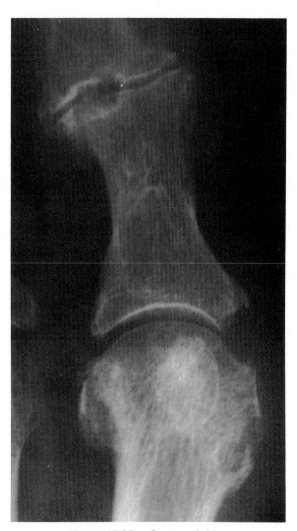

Figure 10.33. Gouty arthritis.

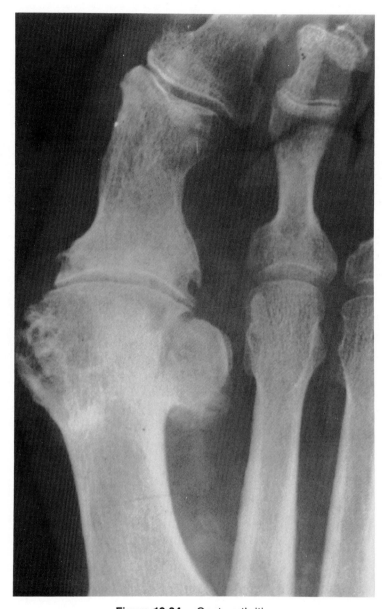

Figure 10.34.   Gouty arthritis.

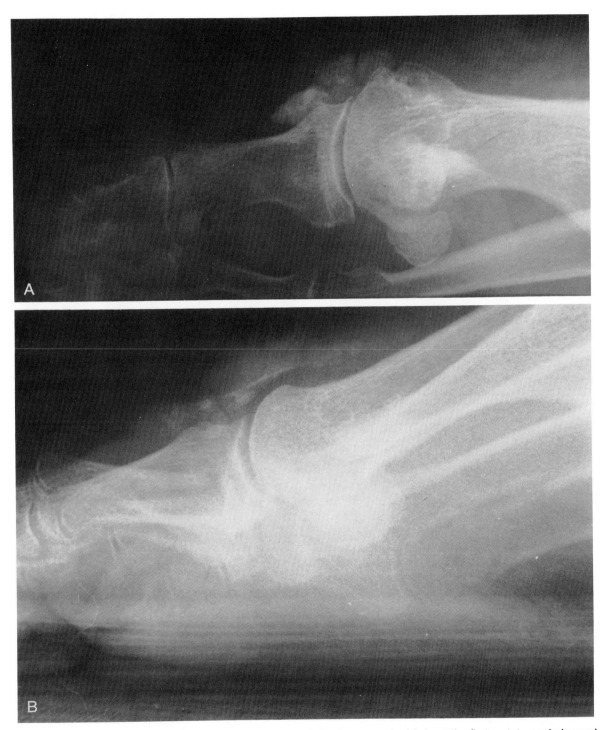

Figure 10.35.   *A* and *B*, tophaceous gouty arthritis. Note the radioopaque tophi about the first metatarsophalangeal joint.

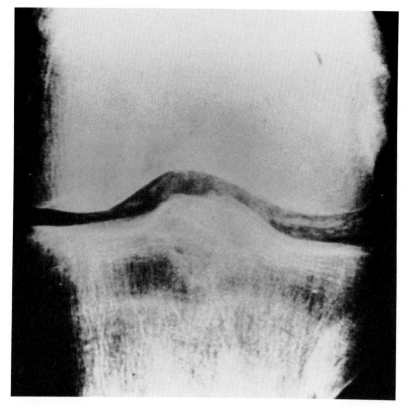

Figure 10.36. Pseudogout. Calcium pyrophosphate crystals are lining the hyaline cartilage of the knee joint forming a faint shadow within the joint.

PSEUDOGOUT

Pseudogout is an abnormality in which calcium pyrophosphate is deposited in the joints. The crystalline deposition causes a painful joint that responds very well to aspirin therapy. On x-ray, the calcium pyrophosphate crystals can be seen in larger joints, such as the knee and ankle. They form a very thin line, which lies parallel to the articular surface. This is because the crystals are deposited on and coat the cartilage of the involved joints (Fig. 10.36).

REFERENCES

1. KATZ, W. A.: *Rheumatic Disease, Diagnosis and Management*, JB Lippincott, Philadelphia, 1977.
2. MCMASTER, M.: The natural history of the rheumatoid metacarpo-phalangeal joint. J. Bone Jt. Surg., **54-B:** 687, 1972.
3. ADAMS, R.: *Diseases of Muscle, A Study in Pathology*, 3rd Ed, Harper & Row, New York, 1975, pp. 360–361.
4. DEFOREST, G. K., ET AL.: Rheumatoid arthritis: The diagnostic significance of focal cellular accumulations in skeletal muscles. Am. J. Med., **2:** 40, 1947.
5. SOHOLOFF, D., ET AL.: The diagnostic value of histologic lesions of striated muscle in rheumatoid arthritis. Am. J. Med. Sci., **219:** 174, 1950.
6. SOKOLOFF, L., ET AL.: Arthritis of striated muscles in rheumatoid arthritis. Am. J. Pathol., **27:** 157, 1951.
7. BLOOM, W., AND FAWCETT, D.: *A Textbook of Histology*, 10th Ed, W. B. Saunders, Philadelphia, 1975, pp. 334–345; 307–349.
8. BASMAJIAN, J. V.: *Muscles Alive. Their Functions Revealed by Electromyography*, 4th Ed, Williams & Wilkins, Baltimore, 1978.
9. STEINDLER, A.: *Disease and Deformities of the Spine and Thorax*, C. V. Mosby, St. Louis, 1929.
10. MCCARTHY, D. J.: *Arthritis and Allied Conditions*, 9th Ed, Lea & Febiger, Philadelphia, 1979, p. 584.
11. SCHUMACHER, T. M., ET AL.: HLA-B27, Associated arthropathies. Diagn. Radiol., **126:** 289, 1978.
12. RESNICK, D., FEINGOLD, M. L., ET AL.: Calcaneal abnormalities in articular disease. Diagn. Radiol., **125:** 355, 1977.
13. MARTEL, W., BRAUNSTEIN, E. M., ET AL.: Radiologic features of reiter disease. Diagn. Radiol. **132:** 1, 1979.
14. BERENS, D. L.: Roentgen features of ankylosing spondylitis. Clin. Orthop., **74:** 20, 1971.
15. BYWATERS, E. G. L.: Heel lesions of rheumatoid arthritis. Am. Rheumatol. Dis., **13:** 45, 1954.
16. FORESTER, J., JACQUELINE, F., ET AL.: *Ankylosing Spondylitis*, Charles C. Thomas, Springfield, 1956.
17. LANDELLS, J. W.: The bone cysts of osteoarthritis. J. Bone Jt. Surg., **35-B:** 643, 1953.
18. BRODSKY, A., ET AL.: HLA antigens and Heberden's nodes. Acta Rheumatol., **3:** 95, 1979.
19. MARKS, J. S., STEWART, I. M., AND HARDING, K.: Primary osteoarthrosis of the hip and Heberden's nodes. Ann. Rheum. Dis., **38:** 107, 1979.
20. HUSKISSON, E. C.: Osteoarthritis: Changing concepts in pathogenesis and treatment. Postgrad. Med., **65:** 97, 1979.
21. YAZICI, H., ET AL.: Primary osteoarthrosis of the knee or hips, J.A.M.A., **231:** 1256, 1975.
22. BLOCH, C., HERMANN, G., AND YU, T.: A radiologic reevaluation of gout: A study of 2,000 patients. Am. J. Roentgenol., **134:** 781, 1980.
23. GREENFIELD, G. B.: The joints. *Radiology of Bone Disease*, 3rd Ed, J. B. Lippincott, Philadelphia, 1980.

CHAPTER 11

Trauma

There is no other area of musculoskeletal disease in which x-rays play a more useful and important role than in the evaluation of trauma and foreign bodies (Figs. 11.2 and 11.3). It is important to remember when an extremity is injured and a fracture is found on radiograph, that the injury involves all layers of tissue, including the skin and subcutaneous tissues, tendons, periosteum, capsular tissues, nerves, and blood vessels in the area.

SOFT TISSUE INJURIES

A strain implies a stretching of the ligaments and soft tissues in the area, due to a mild form of trauma. A strain is inherently more mild than a sprain. The only radiological sign to be noted in a strain would be an increase in soft tissue density and volume in the involved area.

A sprain is a subcutaneous injury to the soft tissues of a joint. It involves the capsular ligaments, blood vessels, nerves, tendons, muscles, etc. It results from tearing of the soft tissues and involves edema, spasms, immobility, and pain. The most common sprain involving the lower extremity is an inversion sprain of the ankle. The inversion sprain can involve the three lateral ligaments of the ankle, as well as a possible tear of the joint capsule. In order to treat the patient properly, an accurate diagnosis of the extent of soft tissue injury must be made. The most commonly injured ligament is the anterior talofibular ligament, followed by the combination of anterior talofibular and calcaneofibular ligaments. The most severe soft tissue injuries involve all three ligaments of the ankle and can possibly even cause a diastasis of the ankle mortise. A number of special x-rays should be employed to aid in the diagnosis of these soft tissue injuries about the ankle. These studies include drawer sign x-rays, stress inversion x-rays, and arthrography.

DRAWER'S SIGN X-RAYS

It is frequently necessary to administer local anesthesia before taking these x-rays. The examiner should wear lead gloves and a lead apron to protect himself from excessive radiation. He should hold the involved leg with one hand on the anterior aspect of the leg and with the other hand should pull the foot in an anterior direction. A lateral non-weight-bearing view is taken in this position. This provides an excellent means for determining if a tear of the ankle capsule has occurred, as well as an injury to the anterior talofibular ligament. If the anterior talofibular ligament has been ruptured, the foot will ride forward distally, out of the ankle mortise, and it will be observed on this view. This view is not used very frequently, but perhaps should be used much more frequently.

STRESS INVERSION VIEWS

The involved ankle is usually given local anesthesia to prevent guarding and excessive pain to the patient during this examination. A non-weight-bearing mortise view is taken with the aid of an examiner (Fig. 11.1). The examiner will forcibly invert the foot during this exposure. Bilateral views must be taken of the stress inversion, as well as drawer sign x-rays. In the stress inversion films, we are interested in measuring the angle that is formed by the dorsal surface of the talar dome and the distal tibial plafont. The normal angle and stress inversion will be from 0° to ~5°. An increase to 5°–7° up to 15° indicates an injury to the anterior talofibular ligament. A 15°–25° angle indicates that the calcaneofibular ligament also has been ruptured. In the event that all three lateral ligaments are ruptured, the angle will be greater than 25°, and for all intensive purposes, the talus will be inverted out of the ankle mortise. This must be taken bilaterally and compared with the contralateral side. Frequent studies have shown that many people normally have greater than 5° of inversion available within the ankle joint. This is the reason for taking the comparison views. It is certainly possible that this increased inversion bilaterally could have been due to old ankle sprains on the contralateral side.[1]

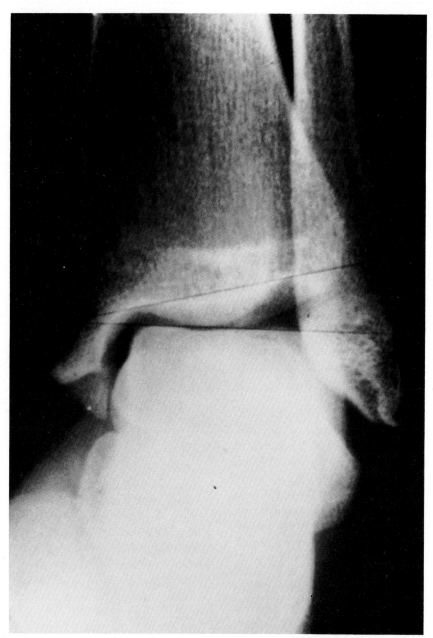

Figure 11.1.   Stress inversion views were taken following a sprain of this ankle and they revealed an abnormal amount of inversion of the talus within the ankle joint. On surgery it was found that a rupture of the anterior talofibular ligament had occurred.

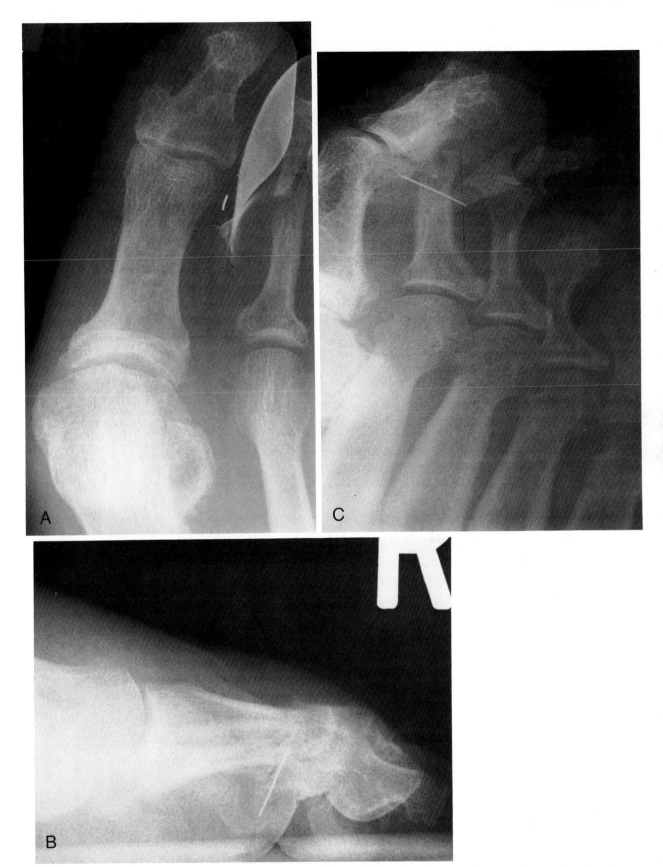

Figure 11.2.   Foreign body. Multiple views must be taken to determine the size, shape and exact location of a foreign body. Note the difference in appearance of this metallic foreign body in each different projection (*A* to *C*).

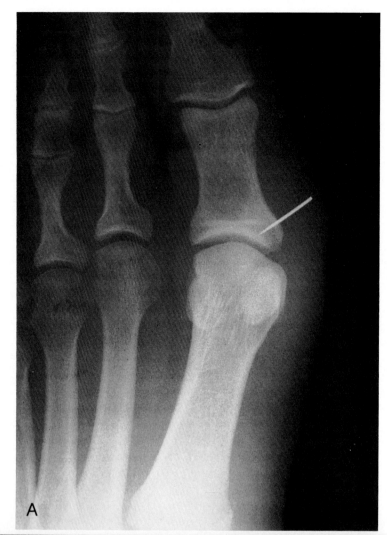

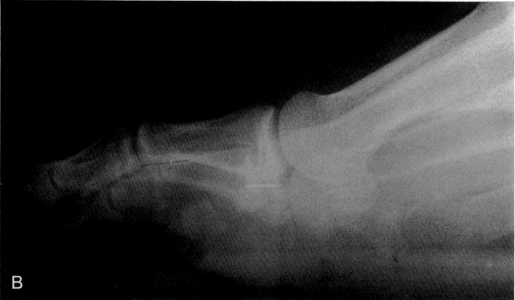

Figure 11.3.   Foreign body. Multiple views were taken to localize this metallic foreign body (*A* to *C*). At the time of surgery, sterile needles were inserted into the foot to help triangulate and find the exact location of the foreign body (*D* and *E*).

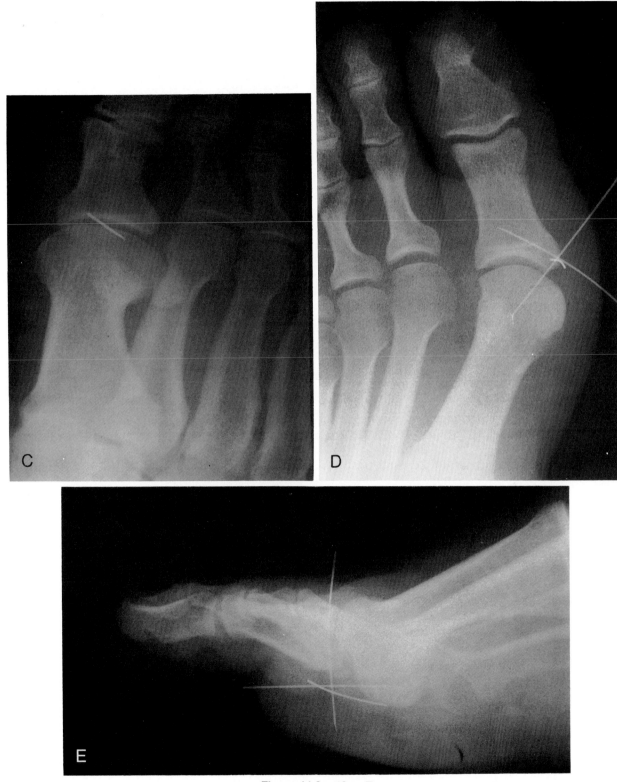

Figure 11.3.   (*C* to *E*)

ARTHROGRAPHY

A radioopaque dye is injected into the ankle joint and the ankle is then put through a range of motion followed by standard x-ray views. The object is to determine if a tear in the ankle joint capsule, ankle ligaments, or inferior tibiofibular ligaments has occurred. The anterior and posterior talofibular ligaments are contiguous with the ankle capsule. The calcaneofibular ligament may or may not be contiguous with the capsule, but is contiguous with the peroneal retinaculum. When there is a tear of any of these structures, the dye will leak out into the soft tissues, and may even extend up a tendon sheath. This occurs frequently with the peroneal tendons, and occasionally with the long flexor tendons in the posterior aspect of the ankle.

Arthrography is only useful within approximately 5 days of the injury. After this time the rupture will have fibrosed in or be plugged with a clot, and the dye will not leak. The major contraindication to arthrography is allergy to the injectible dye. It must be noted that people who are allergic to seafood frequently will be allergic to the iodine that is used in the dye. Anaphylaxis can result from this form of allergy (Fig. 11.4).

A diastasis involves a tear of the inferior tibiofibular syndesmosis, and represents a severe insult to the ankle. It is imperative that this be diagnosed and treated properly for the patient to function normally after the injury.[1,8]

DISLOCATION AND SUBLUXATIONS

A subluxation usually implies a chronic partial disruption of a joint, although it does not necessarily have to be chronic; acute subluxations can occur. A dislocation, on the other hand, means that a total disruption in the continuity of a joint has occurred. Usually the two previously articulating bones are no longer articulating with each other. While dislocations can at times be chronic or subacute, they are usually acute. It is rare to see an acute dislocation that does not also involve fractures. These fractures usually are from avulsions of the ligaments that support the joint structure (Figs. 11.5 to 11.11).

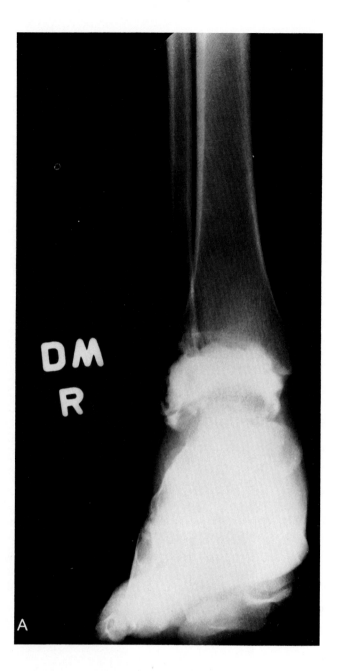

Figure 11.4. Arthrography of the ankle. *A,* an AP view of the ankle showing a normal distribution of dye about the ankle joint. *B,* a lateral view of the normal ankle showing the extent of the ankle joint on the anterior and posterior aspects, including folds or pouches in the posterior ankle capsule. *C,* a normal mortise projection showing dye extending into the inferior tibiofibular syndesmosis.

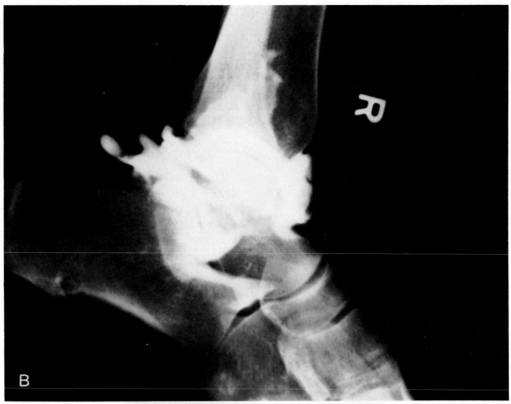

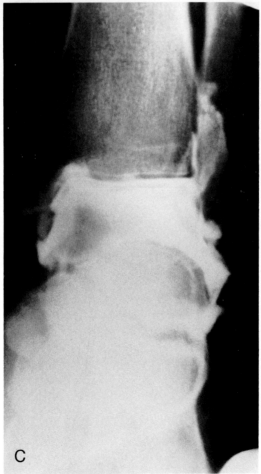

Figure 11.4.   (*B* and *C*)

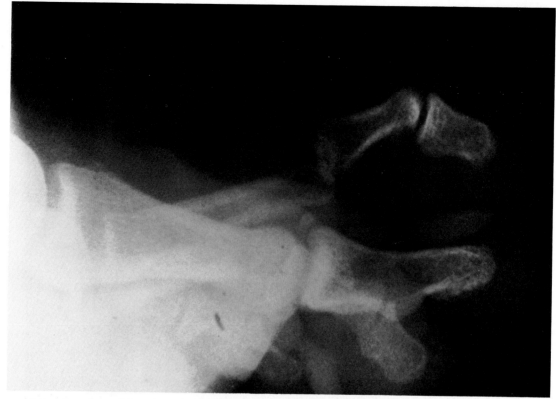

Figure 11.5. Complete dislocation of the proximal interphalangeal joint of the second digit. There usually are multiple avulsion fractures accompanying such dislocations.

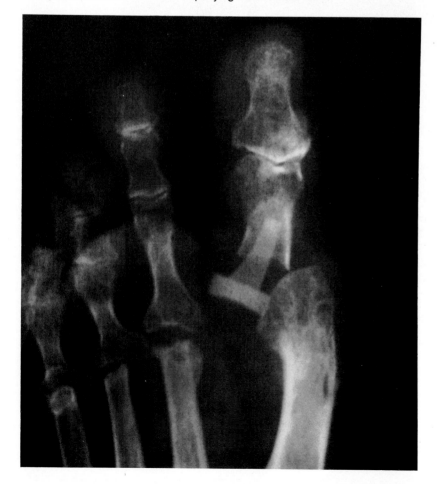

Figure 11.6. Dislocation of hemi-joint implant of the great toe following trauma. Radiograph compliments of Dr. Anthony Kidawa.

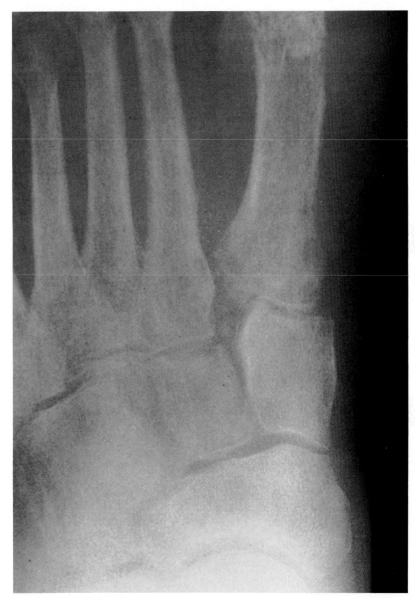

Figure 11.7.   Dislocation of the first metatarsocuneiform joint following trauma.

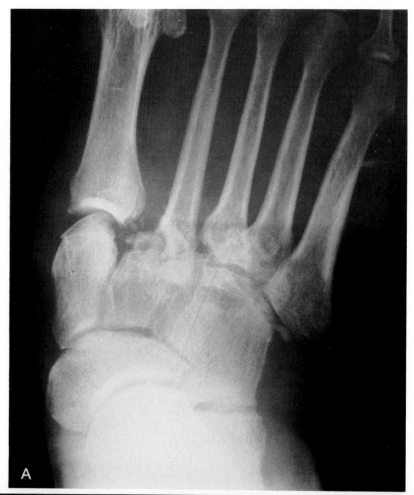

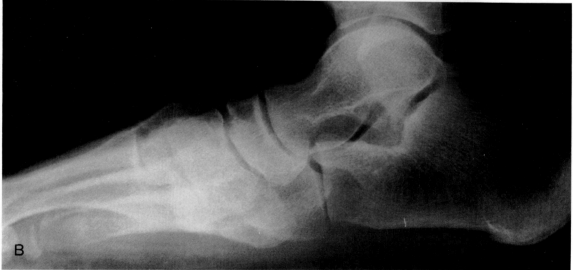

Figure 11.8. *A* and *B*, Lisfranc's dislocation. Note the multiple avulsion fractures accompanying the dislocation.

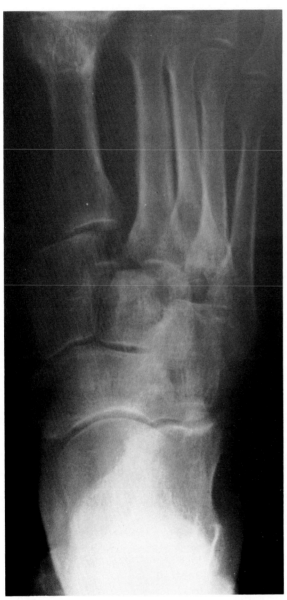

Figure 11.9. Lisfranc's dislocation. The tarsometatarsal joint is a common place for severe dislocation.

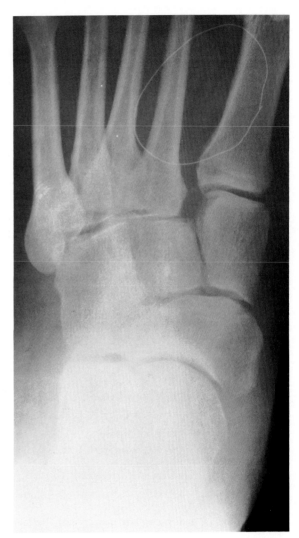

Figure 11.10. Dislocation of first metatarsocuneiform joint.

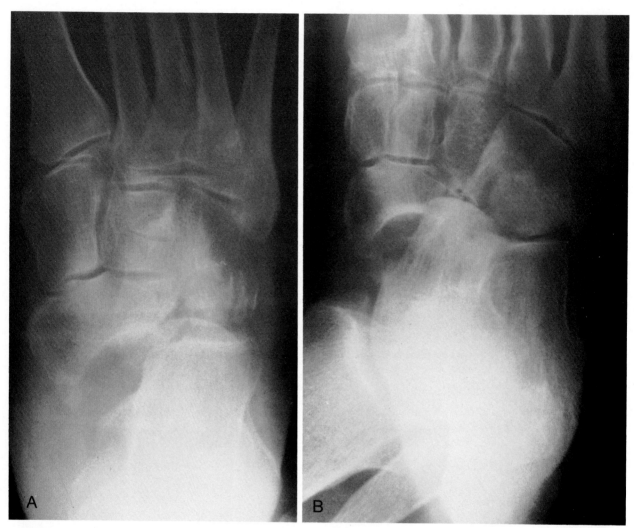

Figure 11.11.   *A* and *B*, peritalar dislocation. The talus has remained in the ankle mortise and the remainder of the foot has dislocated away from it. Severe dislocations of this type are medical emergencies. The circulatory and neurological status of the foot must be determined early and reestablished if impaired.

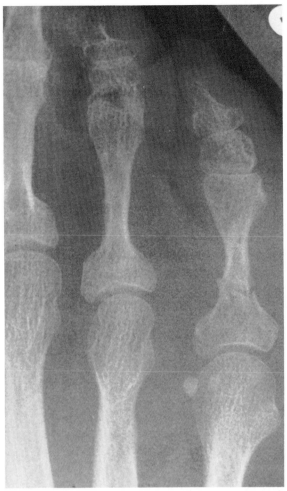

Figure 11.12. Transverse fracture, proximal phalanx, fifth digit.

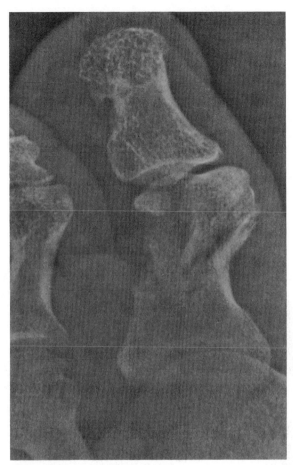

Figure 11.13. Severely comminuted displaced fracture of the proximal phalanx of the hallux.

FRACTURES

A fracture is a break or loss in the normal continuity of a bone. It involves periosteum, cortical bone, and cancellous bone. There are many types of fractures, depending on the bones involved and the etiology of the fracture. The most common fracture is secondary to either trauma or violence, and, as such, may be accompanied by general bodily manifestations such as shock. It must be remembered that there will always be internal bleeding when there is a fracture (Figs. 11.12 to 11.30).

Fractures must be differentiated from a number of other findings which may be incidental in the foot. These include the open epiphysis, accessory bones and anatomical variations, overlapping by soft tissue structures, bipartite sesamoids, and some epiphyseal lines that are variable in their presence, such as in the first metatarsal. Occasion-ally, an epiphysis is found in the neck of the first metatarsal, and can be mistaken for a fracture, following trauma. To differentiate any of the coincidental findings from a fracture, it is usually necessary to take bilateral x-rays, following trauma. The acute fracture line will appear uneven, jagged, and will be irregularly shaped. The space between the fracture fragment will be of varying widths, with the abutting surfaces showing signs of spiculization and irregularity. The bone margins will be angulated and the cortex will be broken. There will be a loss in the normal continuity of the bone. Old fractures, on the other hand, will be smooth, with rounded edges.

Avulsion Fracture

An avulsion fracture signifies a tearing away of a small fragment from the main body of bone. This usually occurs in areas where a known ana-

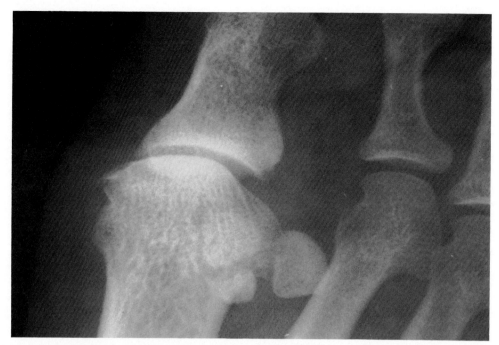

Figure 11.14.   Fracture tibial sesamoid. This must be distinguished from a bipartite sesamoid. Note the jagged edges at the fracture site.

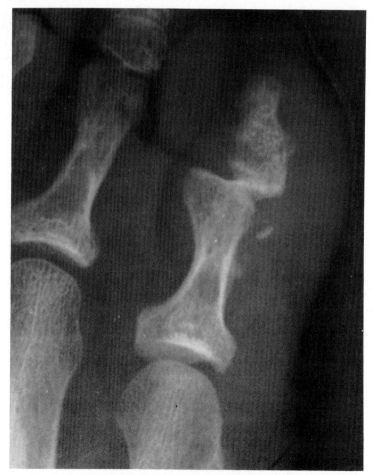

Figure 11.15.   Fracture dislocation of the fifth digit. A typical "bedroom" injury that occurs when stubbing a toe.

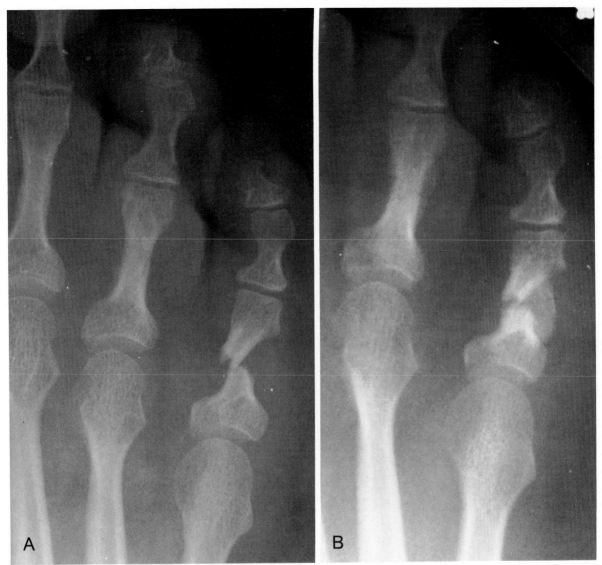

Figure 11.16. *A,* transverse fracture of the proximal phalanx, fifth digit, with lateral displacement of the capital fragment. *B,* 6 weeks following injury and immobilization, adequate bone callus is forming about the fracture site.

tomical structure attaches to a bone. These can include tendons and ligaments (Fig. 11.22).

Incomplete or Greenstick Fracture

An incomplete or green stick fracture is an incomplete fracture of a long bone which is usually seen in children. Like a green stick, the bone will not fracture completely. One cortex will fracture and the fracture will extend partially through the bone, but not through the second cortex. The second cortex will usually bend and become convex. There will usually be some splintering of bone when this occurs.

Compound Fracture

In a compound fracture, there will be an exter-

nal wound present which will usually lead to the break in the bone. This implies that the fracture has been contaminated.

Spiral Fracture

A spiral fracture is usually within a long bone, especially in a leg or a metatarsal and radiographically will appear as a spiral.

Fractures may also be named according to the direction in which the fracture runs, i.e., longitudinal, transverse (Fig. 11.16), or oblique.

Comminuted Fractures

This implies a fracture of the bone into more than two fragments. Possibly even a crushing type of injury (Fig. 11.13).

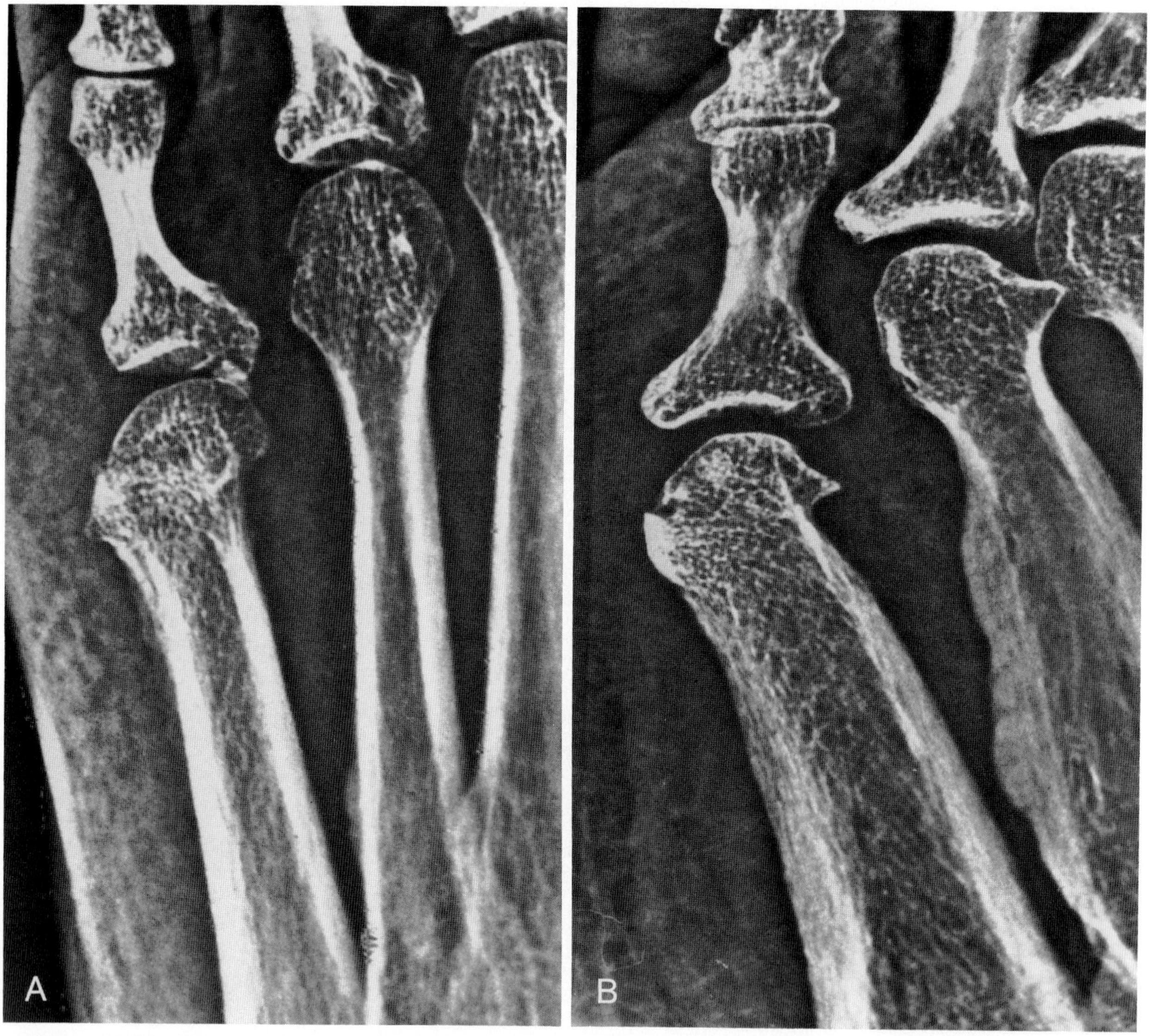

Figure 11.17. Impaction fracture, fifth metatarsal head. The fracture line running transversely through the center of the metatarsal head is very faint (*A* and *B*). Multiple views are needed to completely evaluate this fracture.

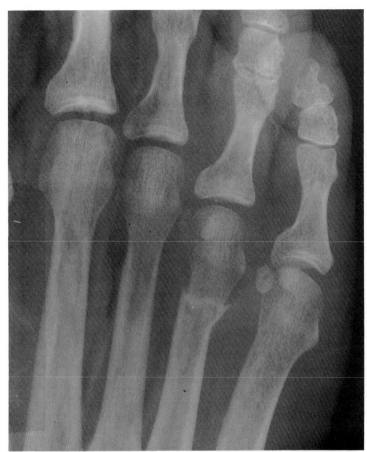

Figure 11.18. Impaction fracture, fourth metatarsal neck area. X-ray compliments of Dr. Morris Moss.

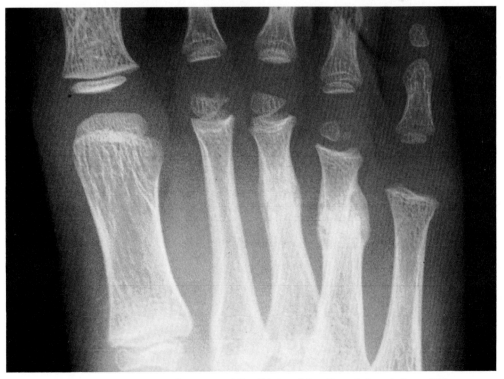

Figure 11.19. Healing fractures of the third and fourth metatarsals in a child.

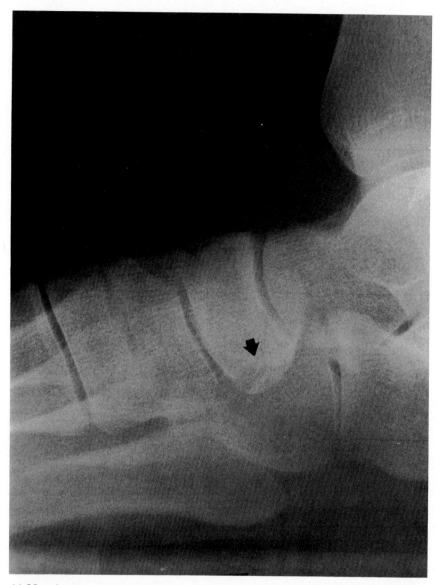

Figure 11.20.   A very unusual fracture of the navicular, observable only in the lateral projection.

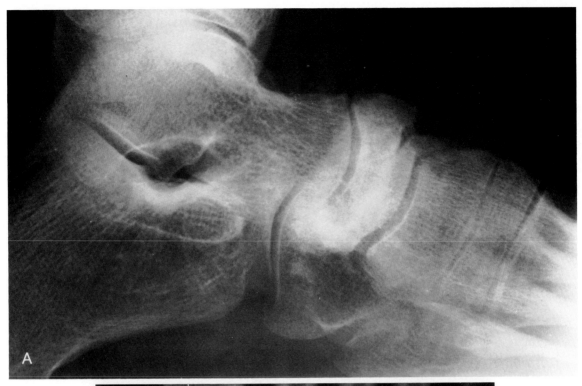

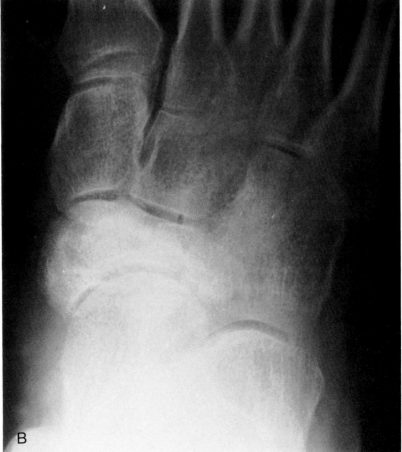

Figure 11.21. *A* and *B*, fracture of the navicular resulting from dropping a heavy weight on the foot.

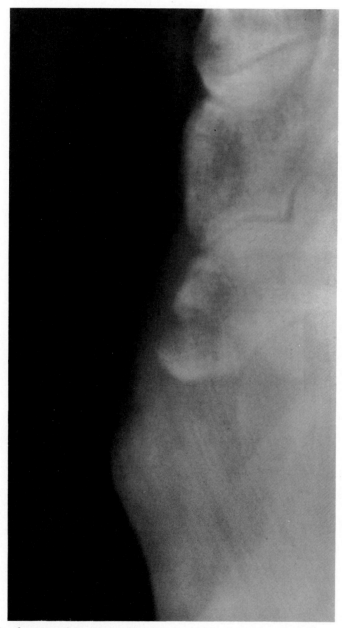

Figure 11.22.   Avulsion fracture of the tuberosity of the navicular from severe ankle sprain, seen on tomogram.

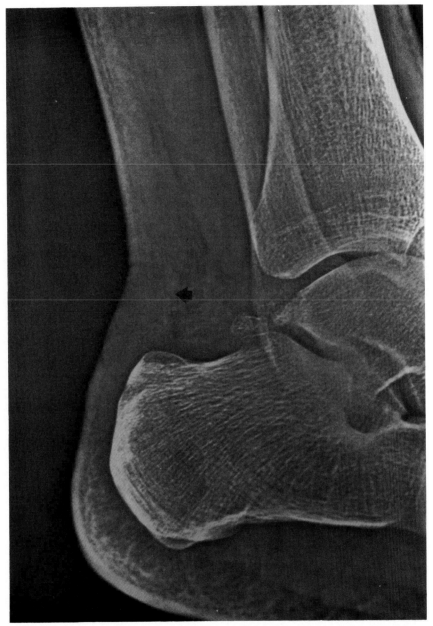

Figure 11.23.   Fracture of the posterior process of the talus and rupture of the tendoachilles (*arrow*) occurred while jumping during a basketball game.

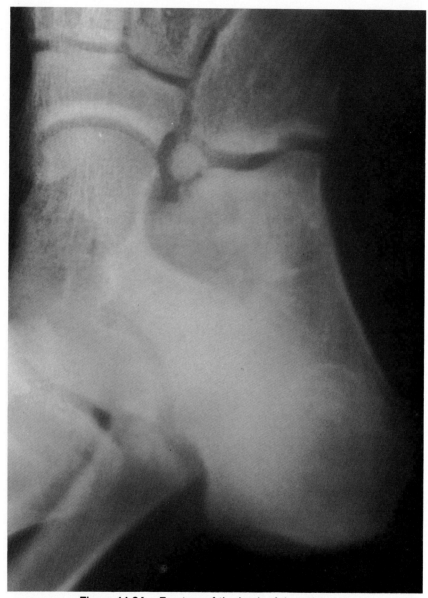

Figure 11.24.   Fracture of the beak of the calcaneus.

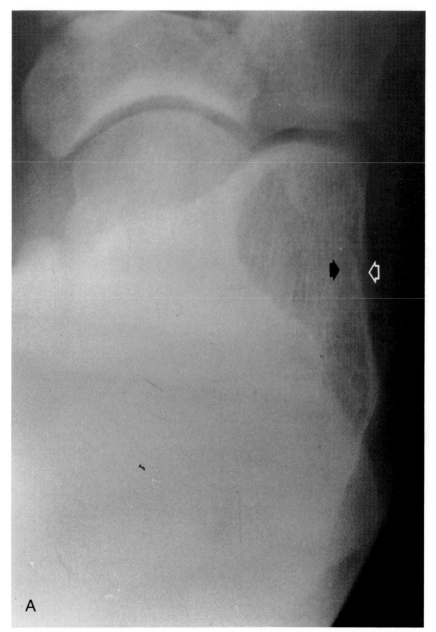

Figure 11.25.   This fracture of the calcaneus is barely noticeable on the dorsoplantar projection (*A*) (see *arrow*), but shows up quite well on the axial calcaneal (*B*) and oblique (*C*) projections.

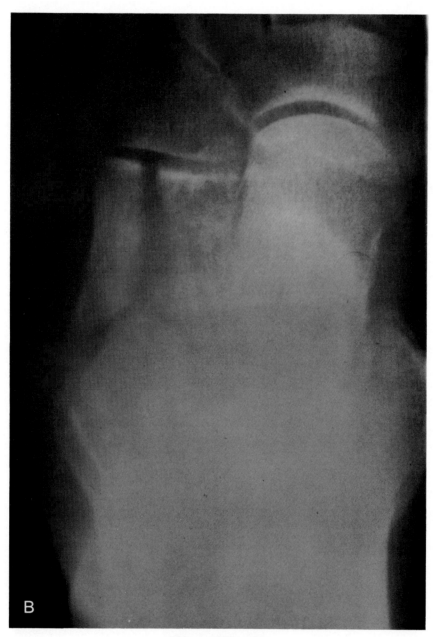

Figure 11.25. (*B*)

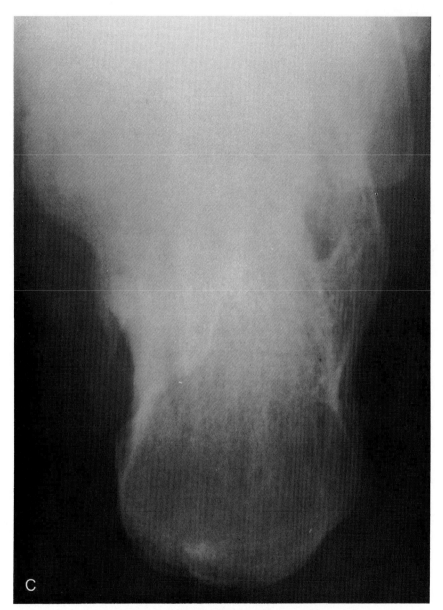

Figure 11.25.   (*C*)

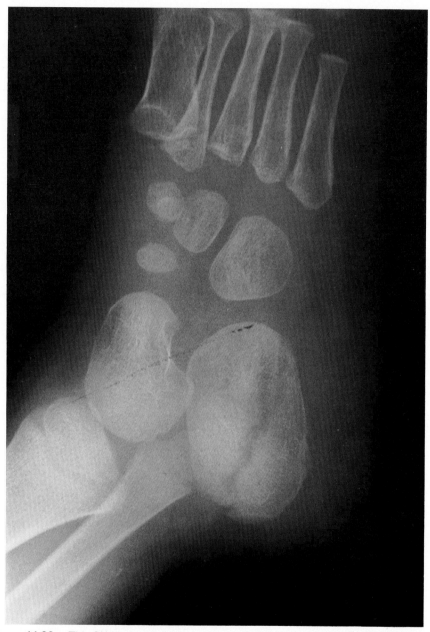

Figure 11.26.   This 2½-year-old child knocked a radiator over, fracturing his calcaneus.

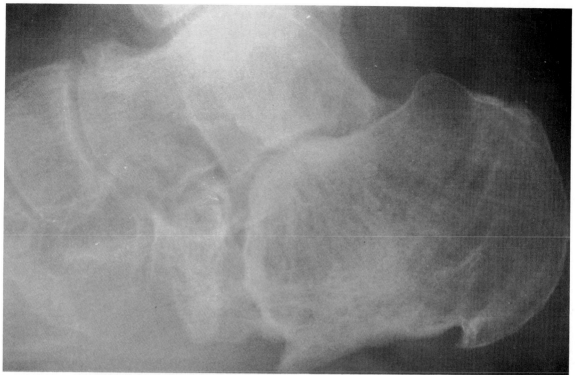

Figure 11.27. Non-healed fracture of the calcaneus. There is an extra bony segment between the body of the calcaneus and the cuboid.

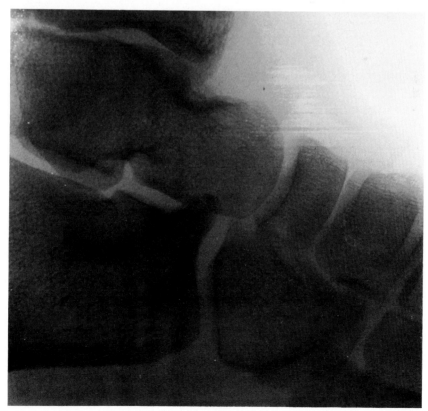

Figure 11.28. Polaroid radiograph revealing a fracture of the beak of the calcaneus. This child remembered no trauma.

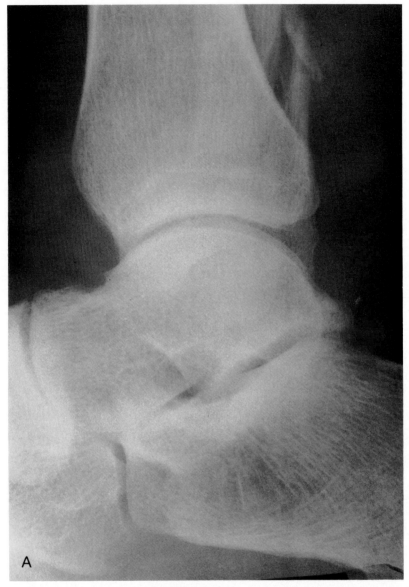

Figure 11.29. *A* and *B*, severely comminuted fracture of the fibula is associated with a diastasis of the ankle. The joint space on the lateral aspect of the ankle is widened.

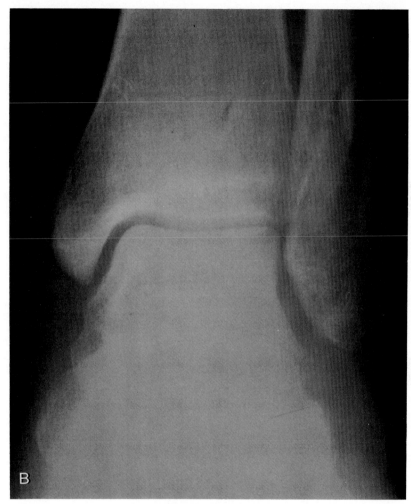

Figure 11.29. (*B*)

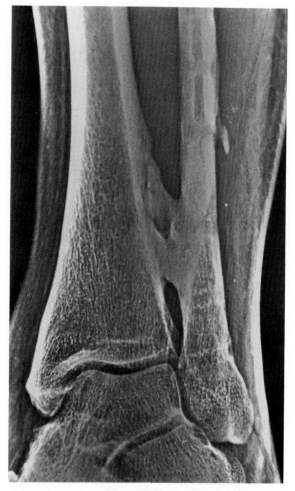

Figure 11.30. Healed fracture of the ankle. There are tracks running through the fibula from the screws used to reduce the deformity. Bony bridging has occurred between the tibia and fibula.

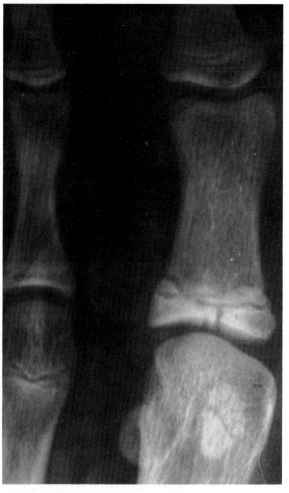

Figure 11.31. A type III Salter-Harris fracture. Proximal phalanx.

Epiphyseal Fracture

An epiphyseal fracture is a fracture involving the epiphysis of a bone. There are five types of epiphyseal fractures based on the Salter-Harris classifications.

1) Type I is a fracture that runs completely through the cartilaginous plate with no fracture of the actual osseous structure.
2) Type II is a Salter-Harris fracture that extends partially through the plate and also breaks off a portion of the diaphysis of the bone.
3) Type III is a Salter-Harris fracture that runs partially through the plate and then extends distally into the joint.
4) Type IV is a Salter-Harris fracture that starts proximal to the epiphysis and runs through the epiphysis and into the joint.
5) Type V is a Salter-Harris fracture that implies a crushing injury to the epiphysis.

Injuries to children before the age of 1 year old may be considered as a Type I Salter-Harris fracture (Figs. 11.31 and 11.32).[2]

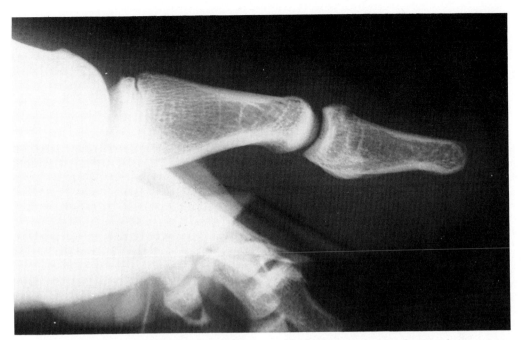

Figure 11.32.   A type III Salter-Harris fracture with displacement of the fracture fragment.

Impacted Fracture

In this type of fracture, one fragment is usually driven into the other fragment. It can be a very difficult type of fracture to see radiographically, because the fracture line is not readily apparent. The fracture appears as an increased bone density, possibly with deformity in the continuity of the bone (Figs. 11.17 and 11.18).

Potts Fracture

A Potts fracture is a fracture of the lower end of the tibia and fibula. This is otherwise known as a bi-malleolar fracture. A tri-malleolar or cot-ton fracture involves both the medial and lateral malleoli, as well as the posterior portion of the tibial plafont. This fracture generally implies that a complete dislocation of the ankle has occurred in addition to the fracture.

Jones Fracture

A Jones fracture is a fracture of the fifth metatarsal (Fig. 11.33).

Gosselin's Fracture

A Gosselin's fracture is a V-shaped fracture of the distal end of the tibia, which may extend into the ankle joint.

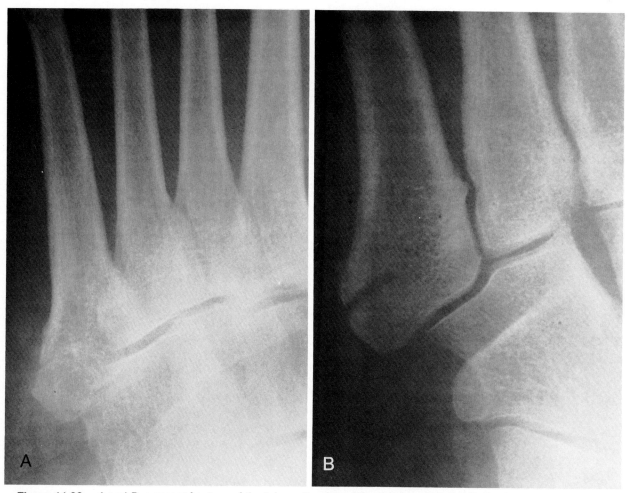

Figure 11.33. *A* and *B*, a recent fracture of the tuberosity of the fifth metatarsal. *C* and *D*, the fracture ends of the bone are resorbed before the new bone fills in the fracture site. *E* and *F*, the fracture site is now being filled in by new bone. Eventually, the defect will completely disappear if healing is complete.

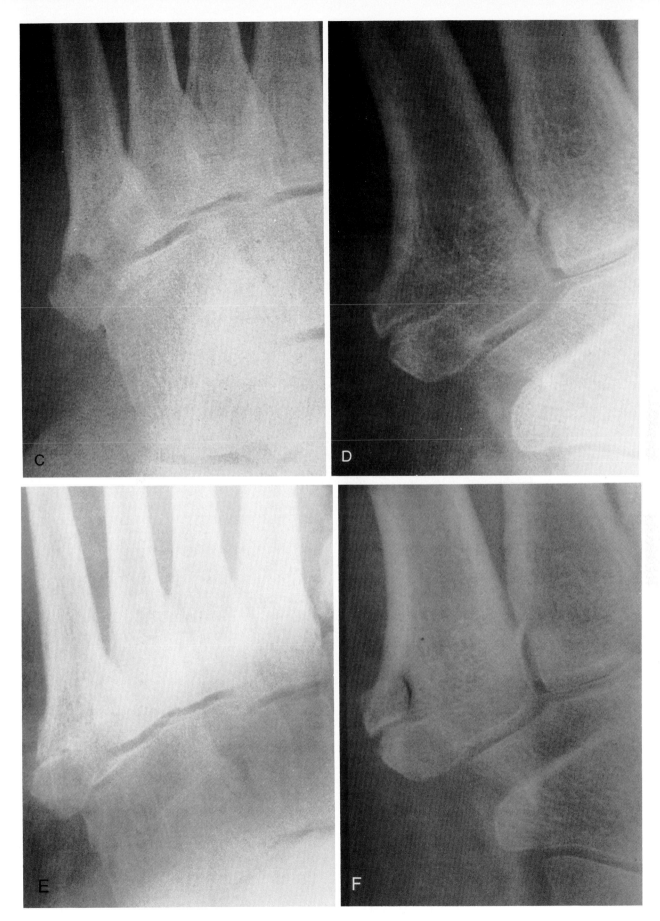

Figure 11.33. *(C–F)*

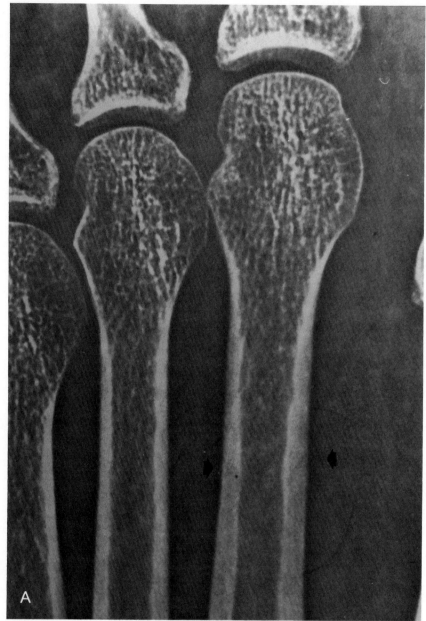

Figure 11.34.   Stress fracture of the second metatarsal. *A,* this xeroradiograph was taken one day after the fracture occurred. A very faint line can be seen *(arrows). B,* two weeks later, the fracture can now be clearly seen. *C,* one month following fracture. *D,* two months following fracture the healing is maturing.

Stress Fractures

Stress fractures can occur in normal or abnormal bone that is subjected to repeated minimal trauma. This trauma is usually less than that which would cause an acute fracture of the bone, but when this occurs repeatedly, microscopic fractures in the bone will eventually occur. There are two general types of stress fractures, including: a *fatigue fracture*, which results from the application

of abnormal stress to a normal bone,[3] and an *insufficiency fracture*, in which normal stress is placed on a bone with deficient elastic resistance.[3] Fatigue fractures usually occur when activity is being performed that is new to the patient. The activity usually will be strenuous and usually will have been repeated many times. This may involve a person who does not usually take long walks, who takes a long hike and then presents with a pain in a metatarsal bone. The causes of insuffi-

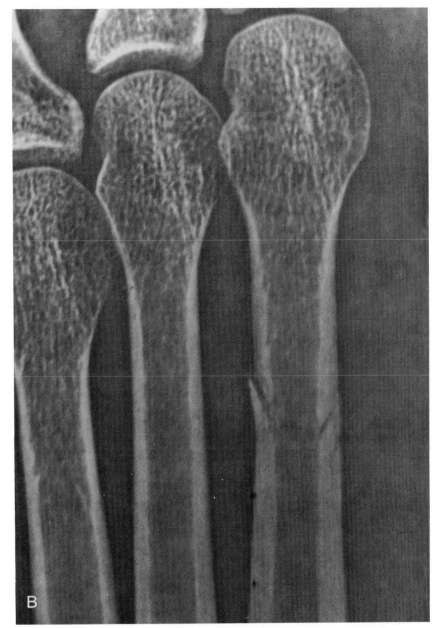

Figure 11.34. (*B*)

ciency fractures are diverse, and include many systemic diseases, including rheumatoid arthritis, osteoporosis, Paget's disease of bone, osteomalacia, renal osteodystrophy, osteogenesis imperfecta, etc.[3]

When a bone is stressed, under normal circumstances, osteonal remodeling takes place, in which resorption of the lamellar bone occurs and more dense osteonal bone is laid down. During this process, a certain period of vulnerability occurs in which the cortical bone has been weakened and not yet restrengthened (Figs. 11.34, 11.35, and 11.37).[3]

Further stress to this area will result in a microfracture. The stress fracture usually begins as a very small cortical crack, which then progresses as the stress continues, and eventually becomes a complete fracture. The clinical findings in the patient with the previously mentioned history will include the cardinal showings of inflammation and pain to palpation. The pain will usually be exacerbated by activity and relieved by rest.

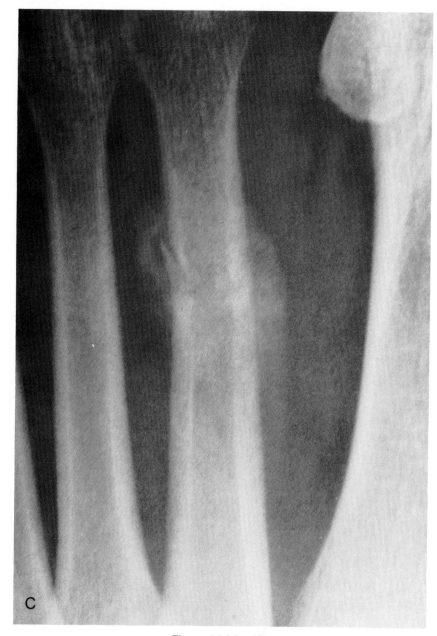

C

Figure 11.34. (C)

In the diaphyseal area, a stress fracture usually cannot be picked up on x-ray for 2–3 weeks. After this time, the initial stages of bone callus are observed and can confirm the diagnosis that has been suspected. At that time, the actual radiolucent line running through the shaft can be observed. Stress fractures can be diagnosed much more quickly, however, using a technetium bone scan (see Chapter 14). This scan will show a hot spot in a matter of hours following the fracture. In either an epiphyseal location or in a cancellous bone, a stress fracture will appear as an area of focal or linear sclerosis, representing a condensation of the trabeculae.

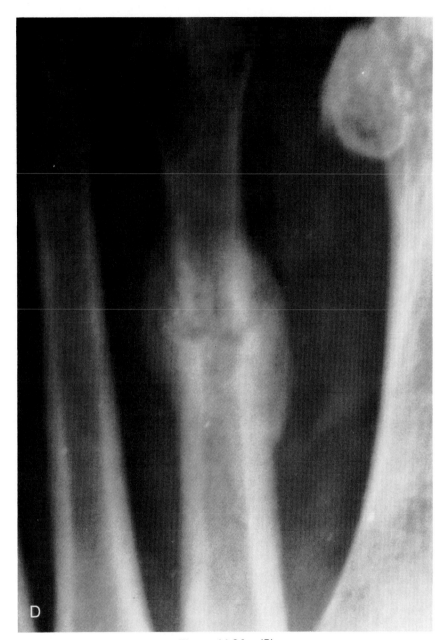

Figure 11.34. *(D)*

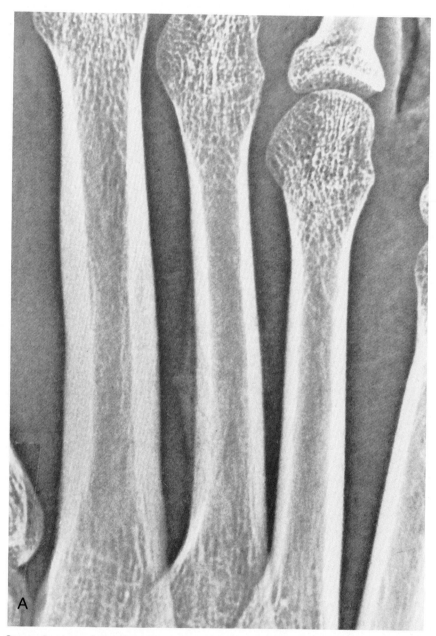

Figure 11.35. Stress fracture. *A,* twelve hours after the stress fracture occurred, this xeroradiograph showed a defect in the periosteum of the third metatarsal. A very tiny crack can be observed in the shaft of the bone. *B* and *C,* three weeks following the fracture healing is occurring. *D* and *E,* five weeks post-fracture the bone callus is maturing.

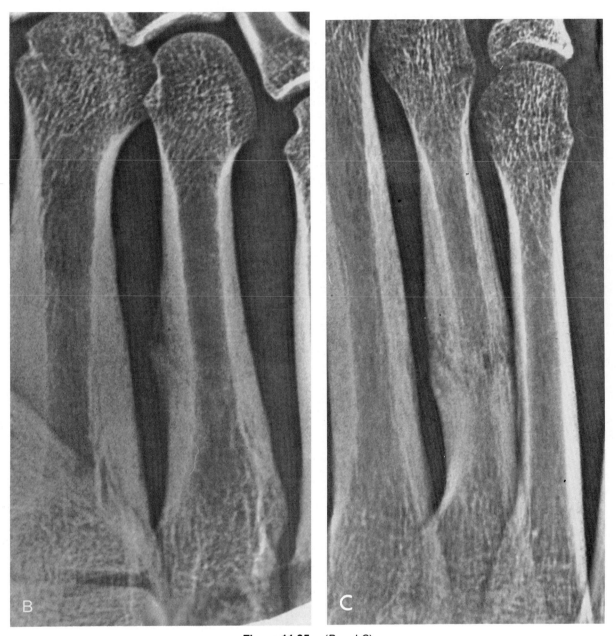

Figure 11.35. (*B* and *C*)

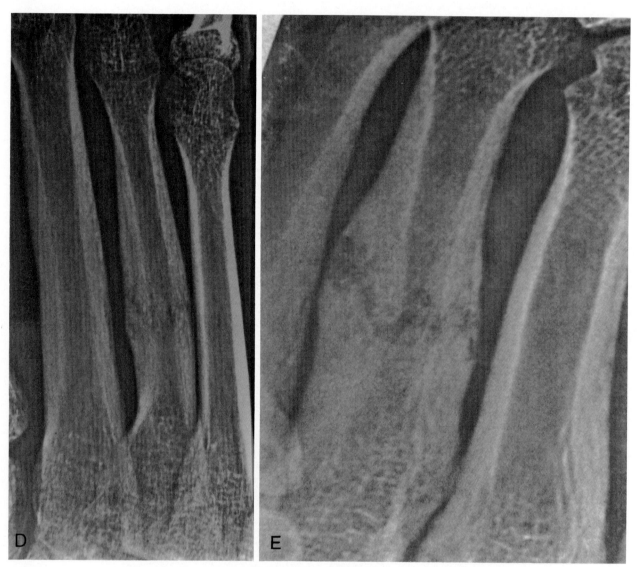

Figure 11.35.   (*D* and *E*)

Pathologic Fractures

A pathologic fracture is one in which the bone is disrupted at a site of preexisting abnormality,[3] such as a bone tumor. Frequently, the stress causing a pathologic fracture would not fracture a normal bone. Pathologic fracture is differentiated from an insufficiency fracture in that it usually occurs at the sight of tumorous lesion (Fig. 11.36).[3]

FRACTURE REPAIR

At the time of fracture, the stage is set for its repair. The very first step is the bleeding that occurs from the damaged ends of the bones, and from the damaged soft tissues in the area. A hematoma will be formed encompassing the medullary canal, the cortex, periosteum, and the fracture ends. During this time period, occasionally, a physiological anesthesia will occur, in which the patient will feel no pain from the trauma. This is a physiological response of the body to the severe trauma, and can be quite dangerous because the patient may hurt himself even further, not realizing that a fracture has occurred. During this inflammatory stage of healing, there will be a vasodilitation, exudation of plasma and leukocytes, and infiltration of the area, by the neutrophils, histocytes, and mast cells (Figs. 11.33 to 11.35).

During the next phase of fracture healing, the reparative phase organization of the hematoma will occur. Fibrovascular tissue will begin to replace the clot, and collagen fibers and bony matrix will be laid down connecting the two bone ends. Vascular budding will occur as the area is revascularized. There will be a differentiation and proliferation of osteogenic cells from the periosteum and endosteum. It might be said that a cellular bridge will have been built across the fracture gap. This is called a primary cellular callus. This callus

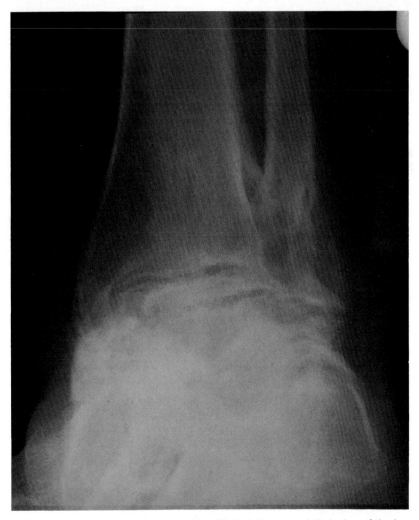

Figure 11.36. Pathologic fracture of the fibula following a lytic lesion of the bone.

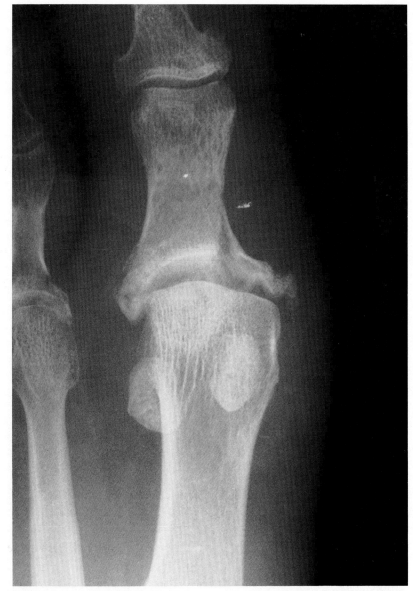

Figure 11.37. A spontaneous fracture of the proximal phalanx of the hallux.

will eventually envelop the bone ends and produce increased stability at the fracture site. During this process of repair, the dead bone at the fracture site will be resorbed and replaced. At least 2 weeks following the fracture, ossification of the primary cellular callus will occur. In this stage, the osteoid crystals are deposited in the preformed cellular elements.

The final stage in healing of a fracture is reorganization and remodeling of primary bone. By the process of remodeling, the internal and external callus is completely resorbed, trabeculae will have been proliferated along the lines of stress,

and the bone will take on a "normal" appearance.[4]

PRIMARY *VERSUS* SECONDARY FRACTURE HEALING

Fracture healing takes place in generally two different forms, depending on which bone and where in the bone the fracture has occurred.

Primary fracture healing generally involves the short bones, which are composed primarily of cancellous bone. Similar healing also occurs in the epiphyses of long bones, which are primarily cancellous. In this process, an internal callus is

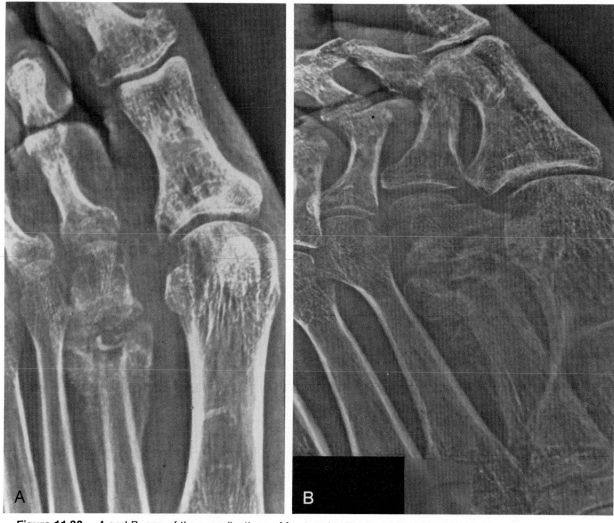

Figure 11.38. *A* and *B*, one of the complications of fracture healing is a non-union. There is exhuberant bone callus about the fracture of the second metatarsal, but healing has never occurred.

formed. There is very sparse, if any, exocallus formed in primary bone healing.

Secondary fracture healing occurs in long bones, and usually in the diaphyseal portion of the bone. This occurs primarily where the bone is cortical in nature. External or secondary bone callus forms, and this is the typical bone callus that is seen following most fractures. The long bones can be stimulated to heal by primary healing rather than secondary, by internal compression, and possibly by electrical stimulation.[4]

CONDITIONS EFFECTING BONE HEALING

Many factors, both local and systemic, can modify the healing process. Local factors that can change the process include the degree of trauma, the position of the fragments, the degree of torsion of the fragments, the degree of shortening of the

bone due to muscle contraction, the degree of bone loss, the type of bone involved, the extent of immobilization, the presence of infection, and the presence of underlying bone pathology (neoplastic, metabolic, etc). Systemic factors influencing bone healing include: old age, abnormal edema, poor circulation, faulty calcium supply and metabolism, extensive osteoporosis, and osteomalacia.[5]

COMPLICATIONS OF FRACTURE HEALINGS

Complications of fracture healing include: delayed union, non-union, mal-union, shortening, arrested epiphyseal growth, aseptic necrosis, and infection. Many of these factors, of course, depend upon which bone has been fractured and where in the bone the fracture occurs, e.g., in an open epiphyseal area. Delayed unions and non-unions

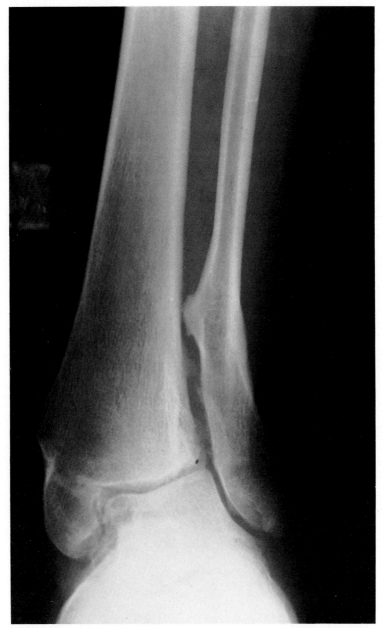

Figure 11.39.   This ankle fracture was improperly reduced and healed in a valgus position.

are thought to be caused by weakness and instability at the fracture site, improper immobilization, or possible overlying systemic disease. Symptoms would include an unnecessary prominance that should not be present, or other such deformity, and tenderness to palpation at the site of the fracture. Some bones are prone to non-unions, such as fractures in the neck of the femur, and the mid-shaft area of the tibia.

The x-ray features of a delayed union include the following. The ends of the bone will have a woolly, moth-eaten-type appearance. There will be no evidence of sclerosis at the fracture ends, and the medullary canal will seem to be open at both fracture ends. The fracture line will be wide and clearly visible, and bone callus will be either minimal, delayed, or completely absent, at a time when it should be present and the fracture should be showing signs of adequate healing (Figs. 11.38 to 11.41).

The x-ray features of a non-union must be documented with a serial set of x-rays. Usually, at least 6 months, and possibly 9 months are necessary before a fracture can be considered "non-union." A non-union will be characterized by pseudoarthrosis and sclerosis with rounding of the fracture ends. Little to no bone callus will be present.[5,6]

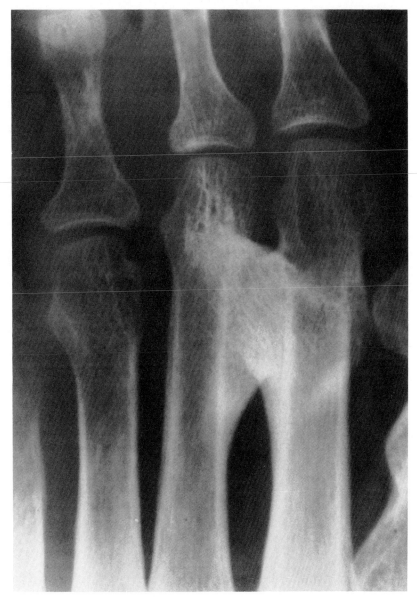

Figure 11.40. Bony bridging occurred between these two metatarsals following an osteotomy of the second metatarsal.

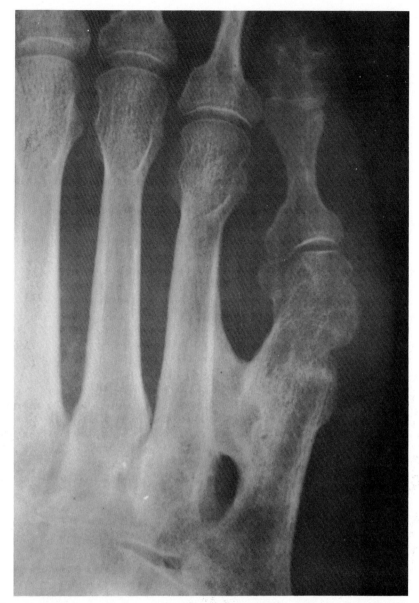

Figure 11.41. Bony bridging occurred following a fracture of the fifth metatarsal. Radiograph compliments of Dr. Ronald J. Strauss.

BOEHLER'S ANGLE

Boehler's angle is an important consideration in fractures of the calcaneus. In a fall from a height, the areas of the body that are most prone to fracture are the calcaneus and the lower spinal column. When x-raying the calcaneus, a lateral film should be taken and Boehler's angle should be considered. Boehler's angle which normally is between 25°–45° will be decreased in a calcaneal fracture, and may even become a negative angle. Bilateral films must be taken and must be compared to determine if Boehler's angle has been changed (Fig. 11.42).

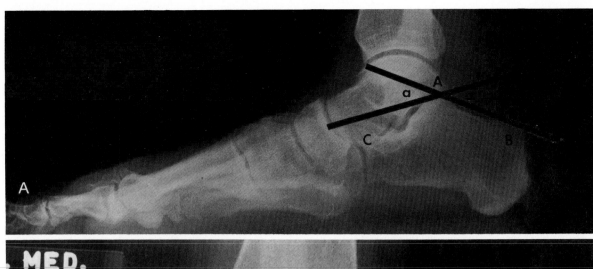

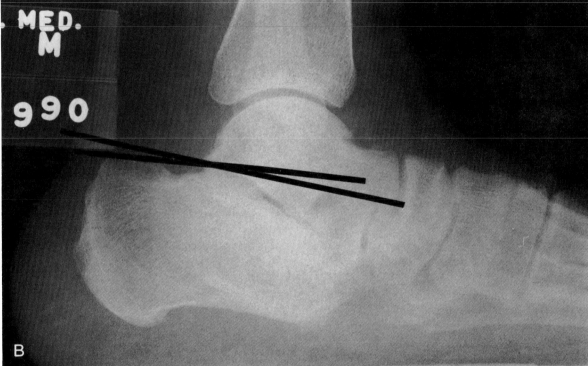

Figure 11.42. *A,* a normal calcaneus showing Boehler's angle. Boehler's angle is constructed by connecting *points A* and *B* and then connecting *points A* and *C*. The angle *a* is measured and should be between 25° and 45°. This angle becomes significant in a fracture of the calcaneus in which it decreases, as can be seen in *B.*

REFERENCES

1. VISSER, H. J., OLOFF, L. M., AND JACOBS, A. M.: Lateral ankle stabilization—Procedures: criteria and classification. J. Foot Surg., **10:** 74, 1980.
2. SALTER, R. B., AND HARRIS, W. R.: Injuries involving the epiphyseal plate. J. Bone Jt. Surg., **45A:** 587, 1963.
3. RESNICK, D., AND NIWAYAMA, G.: *Diagnosis of Bone and Joint Disorder,* W. B. Saunders, Philadelphia, 1981, vol. 3.
4. GREENFIELD, G. B.: *Radiology of Bone Disease,* 3rd Ed, J. B. Lippincott, Philadelphia, 1980.
5. DEPALMA, A. F.: *The Management of Fractures and Dislocations, An Atlas,* 3rd Ed, edited by J. C. Connelly, W. B. Saunders, Philadelphia, 1981.
6. CAMPBELL, W. C.: *Operative Orthopaedics,* 6th Ed, C. V. Mosby, St. Louis, 1980, vol. 3, p. 87.
7. LICHTENSTEIN, L.: *Diseases of Bone and Joints,* 2nd Ed, C. V. Mosby, St. Louis, 1975.
8. VAN MOPPES, F. I., AND VAN DER HOOGENBARD, C. R.: The significance of the peroneus tendon sheath in ankle arthrography. Fortschr. Rontgenstr. **132:** 572, 1980.
9. KAVANAUGH, J. H., ET AL.: The Jones fracture revisited. J. Bone Jt. Surg., **60-A:** 776, 1978.

CHAPTER 12

Tumors of the Foot*

LOUIS P. ZULLI, D.P.M.

The use of radiology in the diagnosis of bone neoplasms is unquestionably valuable. This text will outline some of the established principles of conventional radiographic diagnosis and some possible pitfalls, and will then briefly describe the value of newer techniques that have come to fall under the realm of diagnostic radiology.

In an attempt to improve the radiographic diagnosis of bone neoplasms, a set of criteria by many authors has been developed over the years, based partially on the accumulated experience of proven cases, and partially on the relatively predictable response of bone tissue to any type of injury. This radiographic approach emphasizes the combination of clinical data (age, sex, race, symptoms, family history, blood studies, etc.) and radiographic parameters, including anatomical location, character of lesion margins, nature of periosteal reaction, and the presence of a demonstrable neoplastic matrix, etc.

The value of this approach is unquestionable and has greatly contributed to increased diagnostic accuracy. At the same time, however, it has also resulted in some degree of oversimplification and an overemphasis on diagnosis, so that the formulation of a diagnosis or differential diagnosis frequently becomes an end in itself, and represents the end of radiology's role.

However, when bone tumors are diagnosed and treated with a team approach, the true value of radiology becomes most apparent. This involves the close cooperation of surgeons, oncologists, pathologists, radiation therapists, and radiologists. In such a group, the radiologist participates in the original diagnosis tentatively. The radiologist may also contribute to the decision of how to best

secure biopsy tissue by the surgeon, which in turn is handed over to pathologists and/or oncologists for definitive tissue diagnosis. Once diagnosis has been established, surgeon and/or radiation therapist or oncologist begins treatment.

When the podiatrist is confronted with a bone lesion, the possibility of a non-neoplastic process must be eliminated first. The clinical history and laboratory data are always important (e.g., history of trauma, presence of high serum calcium, blood dyscrasias, etc.). The presence of single and/or multiple lesions should be established initially, since this might determine the approach to diagnosis.

Once it has been established that the lesion is isolated and does not represent a secondary manifestation of an underlying disease, one then must address the question of the nature of the neoplasm.

The value of the patient's age has been amply stressed in the literature. It must be understood, however, that age alone must not be a deterrent to a particular diagnosis if all other features of a lesion are present at an uncommon age. Also, considerable overlapping of age occurs, since the majority of primary bone tumors (the osteosarcomas: osteoblastic, chondroblastic, osteolytic) develop between the 2nd and 4th decades of life; but many are also found much earlier in life.

The *exact anatomic location* is also important, and some parameters must be specifically analyzed. First, it should be determined whether the lesion is *epiphyseal* (e.g., in giant cell tumor, chondroblastoma), *metaphyseal* (e.g., in central osteosarcoma, aneurysmal bone cyst), or *diaphyseal* (e.g., in Ewing's sarcoma). It should also be determined if the lesion is central or eccentric. Finally, an attempt should be made to determine whether the lesion originates from the medullary cavity or

* Figures in this chapter appear on pages 286–319.

from the cortex of the bone, and whether the bone lesion is secondary to a soft tissue process. These parameters are important since each type of tumor tends to have some relatively constant location. Chondroblastoma is classically located within the unfused epiphysis of bone; the giant cell tumor extends almost invariably to the articular surface, and the adamantinoma is nearly always confined to the tibia or the lower jaw bone.

All tumors are composed of characteristic tissue components and, therefore, have, by definition, a *tumor matrix*: osteoid and cartilaginous. The cartilaginous tissue must become calcified to be radiographically demonstrable. Therefore, only two types of tumor matrix, osteoid and cartilaginous, are to be separated radiologically.

Cartilage is classically formed by individual lobules of tissue; and calcifications, therefore, take the form of isolated dots, ringlets, and C-shaped structures radiographically. Their size varies, but the pattern is usually constant. Cartilaginous (calcified) matrix can be recognized within the bone marrow (as in Ollier's disease, which is characterized by the presence of multiple enchondromas and diaphyseal enchondromas, both of which may significantly resemble chondrosarcomas radiographically), or outside the medullary cavity (as in a periosteal chondroma). Cartilage matrix seen over an osseous pedicle projecting away from a joint is characteristic of an osteochondroma. A very large cartilage component, or a change in size of a previously stable one, favors the diagnosis of a chondrosarcoma. Location in other than small bones is unusual for enchondroma, and a diameter over a few centimeters is very uncommon. Large, proximal femoral lesions with central cartilage matrix and buttressing of the bony cortex should be considered chondrosarcomatous until proven otherwise.

Osseous tissue calcifies in a confluent, cloudy form, varying from faintly to heavily dense. Interpretation of an osteoid matrix is more difficult than that of the cartilage type. Osteoid formation is a more universal response of bone to damage than is cartilage formation. The presence of a fluffy, cotton type of osteoid matrix within the medullary canal of bone should not be interpreted as diagnostic of tumor osteoid, since reactive and neoplastic osteoid have almost identical radiographic features. Only when osteoid matrix calcification projects outside the bone into the soft tissues is a tentative diagnosis of osteosarcoma justified.

The absence of a recognizable radiographic matrix limits the capacity of radiological diagnosis.

Therefore, *indirect data* now play an important role. The nature of the margins of the lesion are of special diagnostic importance. Since radiographic evidence of bone destruction is only a reflection of the balance between tumor destruction and bone regeneration, the margins of the tumor are a direct reflection of the relative aggressiveness of the process. A thick, well-defined sclerotic rim represents a slowly progressive lesion and, therefore, usually indicates a benign process. At the other extreme, an ill-defined, indistinguishable margin usually indicates an extremely progressive lesion which can be malignant. There is a spectrum between these two extremes of margins and radiographic judgment should prevail.

Permeated patterns in bone and "*moth-eaten*" *patterns* of bone should also be considered in diagnosing bone tumors. The difference between the two is one of gradation, with the moth-eaten pattern having larger and better defined lytic components, varying from a few millimeters to slightly below a centimeter. These patterns are characteristic of small round-cell tumors of bone. Of these, the paramount example is Ewing's tumor. It must be remembered always that an extremely aggressive benign process may strongly resemble permeated and moth-eaten patterns. The most common example of this is osteomyelitis and occasionally rapidly occuring osteoporosis. Extraosseous soft tissue masses with underlying permeated patterns in bone is almost an assurance of the presence of a malignancy.

Periosteal reactions are another important feature in diagnosing bone tumors. Periosteal reactions are divided into two categories: uninterrupted and interrupted. *Classic uninterrupted periosteal reaction* is a well-defined line of periosteal density representing calcification of the tissue formed by the cambium layer of the periosteum in response to an injury. Homogenous, usually thickened (not always), occasionally granular and variable in length, it is seen classically in infectious processes and with such benign tumors as osteoid osteoma, osteoblastoma, eosinophilic granuloma and many others. Occasionally, benign-looking periosteum is seen in malignant tumors, e.g., fracture of a malignant tumor may produce areas of benign periosteal reaction.

Interrupted periosteal reactions are more complex, consisting of many varieties and can be placed into three main classes: lamellated, broken, and spiculated. For the most part, an interrupted periosteum is an indication of an aggressive (and frequently malignant) lesion.

A *lamellated* or "onion skin" reaction of periosteum results from a phasic (on and off) progression of a benign and/or malignant aggressive process. It may be seen in Ewing's sarcoma, eosinophilic granuloma, infection, and osteoid osteoma.

A *broken* periosteal reaction, usually known as "Codman's triangle," merely indicates an aggressive process causing bone destruction faster than the capacity of the periosteum to regenerate. If the extent of periosteal calcification is sufficient, a triangle is formed by the cortex of the bone.

A *spiculated* periosteal reaction represents the most aggressive of the periosteal reactions. It is composed of calcified linear structures progressing perpendicularly from the bony cortex. It is most likely related to the deposition of osteoid tissue, primarily malignant or reactive to a malignant process along periosteal vessels, when the periosteum is elevated. The vessels extend from the cortex to the elevated periosteum, and when bone is deposited around them they produce the classic individual spicules ("starburst" pattern). Spiculated periosteal reactions are not necessarily specific to primary bone tumors; it is also observed in metastatic disease but with less frequency.

Cortical Expansion

Under certain circumstances, the balance between bone destruction and bone production is such that any expanding neoplastic mass may be successfully encapsulated by periosteal calcification. The result is an increased diameter of the involved bone. This can occur in any part of a long or flat bone such as giant cell tumor, aneurysmal bone cyst, and metastatic lesions (especially of renal and thyroid primaries).

So far we have demonstrated that on the basis of x-ray findings from conventional roentgenograms we can determine some definite characteristics of bone neoplasms, e.g., malignant or benign changes, possible nature of the lesion, provided we have a demonstrable matrix.

A REVIEW OF BONE TUMORS AND TUMOR-RELATED LESIONS

General Considerations

VALUE OF X-RAY EXAMINATION AND INFORMATION OBTAINED

In the diagnosis of bone tumors, the x-ray examination is of great importance and may reveal or indicate:

1) whether or not a tumor arising from or connected with bone is present;
2) whether the tumor is benign or malignant.
3) the extent of the involvement;
4) in most cases, the actual type of tumor present, according to its histologic character.

The diagnosis should be made upon all of the findings, i.e., age, sex, history, physical findings, etc., in addition to the x-ray findings. The latter should be classified and analyzed and the diagnosis arrived at by elimination. *Except for the biopsy,* the radiograph is, no doubt, the most important single means of diagnosis.

TEN POINTS OF VALUE IN VIEWING A FILM OF A BONE TUMOR AND FOR CLASSIFICATION

Radiograph may reveal:
1) the origin of growth: medullary, cortical, or periosteal. This can frequently be determined in the early stages and depends upon the location of the lesion or upon the part of the bone most affected;
2) whether or not there is production of new bone and, if present, its character;
3) whether or not there is destruction of bone;
4) whether the tumor invades the soft tissues and neighboring parts;
5) whether it extends up and down the shaft or is expansile;
6) whether there is a sharp line of demarcation between the normal bone and the area of the tumor;
7) whether it ruptures the cortex;
8) the location, i.e., which bone and what part of the bone;
9) whether the lesion is single or multiple, both as to the number of bones involved and the number of lesions in one bone;
10) rapidity of growth, determined either by repeated examinations or by estimation of the character of the growth.

In describing bone tumors, those of the above characteristics which are of importance in each case will be tabulated by the corresponding number.

Benign Tumors

EXOSTOSES

Small projections from the cortex of the long bone, which may be pencil-shaped, flat-topped, or rounded:
1) Cortex;
2) Production;
3) Not applicable;

4) Not invasive;
5) Not applicable;
6) Sharply circumscribed;
7) No rupture;
8) Long bones near their ends;
9) Usually multiple bones and lesions, but may be single;
10) Slow growing.

MULTIPLE CARTILAGINOUS EXOSTOSES (FAMILIAL TYPE)

Similar to above except that they are always multiple and are near joints. The shadows are not seen in early life until they ossify. Marked deformity of the bones may occur due to disturbance in growth.

OSTEOMATA

Very similar to exostoses except that they are larger, tend to be predunculated, and may appear cystic due to areas of cartilage within the tumor mass. They are usually single. Their structure is similar to that of normal bone.

OSTEOCHONDROMATA

These are a combination form of osteoma and chondroma which give a picture similar to osteoma except that they tend to be larger and to show more of the large areas of rarefaction within the dense mass of bone. These areas of lessened density are due to islands of cartilage (Figs. 12.10, 12.11, 12.28, and 12.37).

OSTEOCHONDROMATOSES

These are cartilaginous tumors lying within the joints, free from the bone, which resemble osteomata very closely after they become calcified.

ENCHONDROMATA OR CHONDROMATA

Cartilaginous deposits within the shafts of bones, usually multiple and most frequent in the phalanges, give the appearance of cystic areas because the cartilage is of such low density that it produces a defect in the bone. Pathologic fractures are common and frequently the tumors are first discovered as a result of the fracture.

In many cases, such chondromata are a part of the picture of the familial type described above (Fig. 12.14).

Bone Cysts

These have somewhat the appearance of enchondromata except that they are larger, are usually medullary in origin and location, appear in the long bones, extend up and down the shaft, and may be single. Pathologic fractures are common and often lead to their discovery. They may be single or multiple, but the latter may be related to parathyroid tumors. The single lesions are often indistinguishable from localized osteitis fibrosa (Figs. 12.15, 12.16, 12.31, and 12.32).

Benign Giant Cell Tumors (Giant Cell Sarcoma) (Figs. 12.6, 12.21, and 12.33)

1) always medullary;
2) no production but show trabeculation within; the rarefied area;
3) bone destruction;
4) not infrequently invade soft tissues;
5) extend up and down;
6) sharply demarcated;
7) rarely ruptures cortex, but expands it markedly;
8) long bones, almost always in the epiphysis or end of bone;
9) single;
10) slow growing.

Careful observation will reveal a dense area of bone extending around and delineating the soft tissue mass which is very striking. Pathologic fractures are common. It is probable that these tumors are of the same nature as localized osteitis fibrosa, but, in occasional instances, malignant changes occur which are indicated by rupture of the cortex and invasion of soft tissue.

Benign Angiomata

Similar in appearance to benign bone cysts except that they often show trabeculae of bone within the area of decreased density and are more expansile.

Ossifying Hematomata

While not properly tumors, these must be differentiated from benign neoplasms.

1) periosteal;
2) production;
3) no destruction;
4) no invasion;
5) extension is lateral, not in the long axis of the shaft;
6) sharply circumscribed;
7) no rupture;
8) any bone;
9) single;
10) slow growing.

FIBROUS DYSPLASIA OF BONE (JAFFE-LICHTENSTEIN AND ALBRIGHT'S SYNDROME)

Fibrous dysplasia of bone is a disturbance in the intramedullary bone replacement process so that normal bone undergoing lysis is replaced by an abnormal proliferation of fibrous tissue. This disease may be monostotic or polyostotic.

Histologically, the main feature is a fibro-osseous metaplasia. It is possible that occasional cases of fibrous dysplasia may undergo change to fibrosarcoma.

Radiographically, all types of bones may be affected, although there is a large predilection for the large bones of the extremities. The osseous lesions may be radiolucent or radiopaque, but they are always covered by a thin shell of bone (ossified periosteum). The cortex is always eroded from within, while the periosteum attempts to compensate by laying down a thin shell of normal bone. These lesions are always expansile in nature. Associated deformities are common. The areas of bone involved do not tend to reossify and there is a tendency for slow distal progression. These lesions may not be recognized until a pathologic fracture occurs either in childhood or early adult life.

OSTEOID OSTEOMA (BENIGN NEOPLASM)†

1) Osteoblastic, connective tissue origin (usually cortical);
2) new bone production (residual central nidus surrounded by compact bone);
3) some destruction and resorption of bone;
4) non-invasive;
5) expansile;
6) a sharp sclerotic margin of demarcation;
7) does not rupture cortex;
8) tibia, fibula, vertebrae, humerus, and phalanges (any part of these bones, along the diaphyses);
9) usually singular;
10) slow growing.

Malignant Tumors: Primary

OSTEOGENIC SARCOMA (FIVE TYPES)
(Fig. 12.2 to 12.5)

a) Medullary, round cell, or telangiectatic type
   1) Medullary;

2) no bone production;
3) much bone destruction;
4) invades soft tissue;
5) expansile;
6) not sharply circumscribed;
7) ruptures and destroys cortex;
8) usually long bones nearer ends, but may be any bone;
9) single, both bone and lesion;
10) very rapid growth.

The complete destruction of all bone in its path, the rapid development of the soft-tissue tumor, and the complete lack of bone regeneration even though the cortex is attacked; all are characteristics of this tumor. Pathologic fractures are very common.

b) Periosteal type (Fig. 12.27)
   1) Periosteal and cortical;
   2) bone production laid down perpendicularly to the shaft;
   3) moderate bone destruction;
   4) invades soft tissue;
   5) expands cortex early;
   6) not sharply circumscribed;
   7) destroys cortex;
   8) long bones, usually near ends;
   9) single;
   10) rapid growth.

The excessive, irregular, and unlimited production of bone with fine, needle-like projections extending out perpendicularly to the shaft of the bone is the characteristic of this tumor. Lifting up of the periosteum at either end of the tumor is a common manifestation. Pathologic fractures occur.

c) Mixed type
   Combines many of the features of the above two.

d) Sclerosing type
   Similar to the periosteal except that there is little destruction and the newly found bone tends to be dense and to originate in the cortex. The bone is marble-like in density.

e) Chondrosarcoma type
   Located usually near the joints, chiefly destructive, but may show productive areas and are similar to the mixed type in their x-ray appearance.

EWING'S SARCOMA, ENDOTHELIAL MYELOMA, RETICULOSARCOMA GROUP
(Figs. 12.8, 12.19, 12.23, and 12.24)

May be single, involving one bone, or multiple, involving more than one bone. The tumor resembles a periosteal type of sarcoma and also osteo-

---

† Osteoid osteoma is not be be confused with the "giant osteoid osteoma" which is a synonym for the benign osteoblastoma (Figs. 12.25, 12.26, and 12.36).

myelitis, from both of which it must be distinguished.

1) medullary and peripheral;
2) bone production both parallel to shaft (like osteomyelitis) and transverse to shaft with fine needles of bone (like sarcoma);
3) some bone destruction;
4) invades soft tissue;
5) extends up and down;
6) not sharply demarcated;
7) destroys the cortex;
8) most common in long bones and in the middle of the shaft;
9) single or multiple (different from osteogenic sarcoma);
10) fairly rapid growth.

This tumor tends to lay down numerous layers of bone like an "onion skin" in appearance. It responds to irradiation more rapidly than osteogenic sarcoma.

HEMANGIOENDOTHELIOMA

Usually multiple but may be single.
1) Medullary;
2) little bone production;
3) bone destruction which may have a sclerotic border;
4) invades the soft tissue;
5) expands the cortex;
6) not sharply demarcated;
7) destroys the cortex;
8) may occur in any bone;
9) usually multiple;
10) rapid growth.

This tumor resembles hypernephroma metastases when multiple. May show bone production in fine needles transverse to the shaft which tends to distinguish it from metastases. It appears to be common in the spine and pelvis.

MYELOMA

1) Medullary;
2) no bone production;
3) bone destruction in small rounded, punched-out areas;
4) invades soft tissue late;
5) expands cortex early;
6) sharply demarcated early;
7) ruptures cortex late;
8) most common in sternum, ribs, skull, and lumbar spine, but may be in any bone;
9) always exceedingly multiple as to lesion and usually as to bone;
10) slow growing.

The most characteristic lesions are often found in the skull. Occasionally, extreme cases of multiple myeloma may produce a diffuse osteoporosis of all the bones, resembling osteomalacia and difficult to distinguish from it. Rarely, single lesions are found, particularly in the spine. Such cases commonly eventuate into the multiple form.

Malignant Tumors: Metastatic (Secondary)

CARCINOMA

Osteoclastic

Secondary to carcinoma of any organ, but rarely the prostate. Most common from the breast, pelvic organs, and thyroid. Pathologic fractures are frequent (Fig. 12.22).

1) Medullary;
2) no production;
3) marked bone destruction either in small irregular areas or large ragged-edge areas;
4) invades soft tissues, but does not produce much soft tissue tumor;
5) does not expand;
6) not sharply demarcated;
7) ruptures and destroys cortex;
8) any bone, most common in pelvis and lumbar spine;
9) always multiple lesions, usually multiple bones;
10) rapidly growing.

Osteoblastic

Produces bone by irritation of tumor mass. May or may not be accompanied by osteoclastic type. Most common from carcinoma of the prostate (Fig. 12.17), but may be secondary to carcinoma of the breast and, rarely, of thyroid and other organs (Figs. 12.29 and 12.30).

1) Medullary;
2) Bone production within the confines of the bone, i.e., there is increased density but usually no bone produced along the periosteum or beyond the margins of the bone;
3) May have some destruction;
4) No invasion;
5) No expansion;
6) Not sharply demarcated;
7) No rupture;
8) Usually lower lumbar spine and pelvis but may involve other bones later;
9) Always multiple, bones and lesions;
10) Slow growing.

The radiological findings are very characteristic. Frequently, the diagnosis of metastasis from a carcinoma of the prostate, to the pelvis, is possible before there are any prostatic symptoms or signs. The presence of a rather homogeneous area of increased density in which the normal trabeculae of a flat bone are not visible and which is not sharply demarcated from its surrounding normal bone is characteristic.

Hypernephroma (Kidney-Adrenal Tissue)

Has much the same characteristics as osteoclastic carcinoma except that it is slower growing and may be more sharply demarcated. Tends to occur above the elbows and knees but not necessarily so. Frequently single lesions occur and, occasionally, they may seem to originate in the cortex alone.

Neuroblastoma in Children (Neurocytoma, Hutchinson's Tumor, Immature Embryonic Neuroma)

A characteristic type of metastasis is produced which shows numerous tiny areas of rarefaction in the metaphysis of the long bones, frequently periosteal proliferation from subperiosteal infiltration, and characteristic ray-like bone spicules projecting, either from the long bones or, more commonly, from the skull. Occasionally, large destructive areas can be found.

HODGKIN'S DISEASE (Lymphatic Tissue, Liver, Spleen, and sometimes Kidneys)

This may invade the bones either by direct extension or by distant metastasis. The appearance suggests most strongly carcinomatous metastases, usually osteoclastic, but not rarely osteoblastic. Occasionally the earliest findings are a diffuse rarefaction of the involved bones.

LEUKEMIA (Lymphatics, Spleen, Bone Marrow)

Rarely invades bones, but may produce a diffuse, widespread rarefaction with many minute areas of destruction and, particularly in children, periosteal proliferation.

PAGET'S DISEASE OR OSTEITIS DEFORMANS

This may be inflammatory, but it is classified with tumors. It is characterized by a special kind of bone production, increased trabeculation of bones, great thickening of their shafts, some destruction, bowing of the pelvis and femora, increased size of the involved bones, and flattening of the skull—a general distrubtion. It resembles somewhat osteoblastic carcinoma, but shows, in addition, small cysts. The most characteristic feature is the coarse, thick, irregular trabeculae of the flat bones.

OSTEITIS FIBROSA CYSTICA AND PARATHYROIDISM

Multiple bone cysts and, in addition, increased trabeculation with bone sclerosis and generalized distribution occur. Pathologic fractures are common. It is probably due to hyperparathyroidism or parathyroid tumors. With abnormalities of the parathyroid secretion, diffuse decalcification of bones may also occur without any typical cysts. Characteristic of this condition is the subperiosteal absorption of cortical bone shown particularly well in the skull and the phalanges. The bones take on a granular appearance and the cortex becomes very thin.

FIBROSARCOMA OF BONE AND SECONDARY INVOLVEMENT FROM TUMORS OF SOFT PARTS

Destruction of bone may occur from extension into it of tumors arising in soft parts contiguous to it. This is frequent, for example, in the mandible where carcinoma of the floor of the mouth may erode the mandible. A similar process occurs in the other facial bones (Figs. 12.9, 12.12, and 12.35).

Fibrosarcoma arising in the soft tissues may invade the bone in such a way as to appear to be primary in the bone itself. These types of tumors are characterized by:
1. destruction of bone;
2. irregularity of surface of the invaded area;
3. local character of the growth corresponding to the position of the soft tissue lesion (Figs. 12.7, 12.13, and 12.18).

SUMMARY OF BONE TUMOR FINDINGS

1. Origin
   a) Medullary
      Enchondroma, bone cyst, giant cell tumor, round cell osteogenic sarcoma, myeloma, carcinoma, hypernephroma, osteitis fibrosa cystica, and angioendothelioma.
   b) Cortical and periosteal
      Osteoma, enchondroma, ossifying hematoma, periosteal and sclerosing osteogenic sarcoma, osteitis fibrosa cys-

tica, osteitis deformans, and Ewing's sarcoma of diffuse type (Fig. 12.38).

2. Bone production
Osteoma, ossifying hematoma, periosteal and sclerosing types of osteogenic sarcoma. Ewing's sarcoma of diffuse type, osteoblastic carcinoma. Giant cell tumor and bone cysts may show bone production after fracture or treatment.

3. Bone destruction
All malignant tumors and all benign tumors *except* osteoma, osteochondroma, and exostosis.

4. Invasions of the soft tissue
All malignant tumors tend to invade the soft tissues, particularly those primary in bone. Benign tumors of the productive type, such as osteoma, extend out into the soft tissues but are sharply demarcated from them and do not invade them. Giant cell tumors invade the soft tissues but are sharply encapsulated by a shell of bone.

5. Cortex expanded with invasion up and down the shaft
Enchondroma, bone cysts, and giant cell tumor.

6. Not sharply demarcated
All malignant tumors and rarely benign giant cell tumors.

7. Rupture cortex
All malignant tumors and occasionally giant cell tumors.

8. Location
Metastatic lesions to middle of bones, sarcoma nearer ends. Giant cell tumor at very end of bones. Hypernephroma above knees and elbows. Osteoblastic carcinoma to pelvis and spine. Ewing's sarcoma, diffuse type, in middle of shaft of long bones.

9. Multiplicity
a) Usually single
Giant cell tumor, osteogenic sarcoma
b) Usually multiple
Myeloma, osteitis fibrosa cystica, osteoblastic carcinoma, exostoses or familial type.

10. Special findings
a) Giant cell tumor
Trabeculations within cystic area of destruction, location in epiphysis, layer of bone over soft tissue tumor.
b) Periosteal type of osteogenic sarcoma
Ray-like bone production, fine spicules transverse to shaft.
c) Myeloma

Round, sharply defined, very multiple areas of destruction; best seen in skull.
d) Ewing's sarcoma
Multiplicity of malignant primary tumors in bone. Resemblence of the diffuse type to osteomyelitis.
e) Osteoblastic carcinomatous metastases
Irregular areas of increased density, particularly in the pelvis, often with a markedly increased density of many bones.

Finally, let us take a look at some additional modalities at our disposal today: tomography, xeroradiography, computed tomography, and arteriography.

Tomography is used in bone tumor diagnosis to eliminate spurious shadows of overlying structures. Normal or standard x-ray studies may make it difficult to determine the true nature of some lesional margins (especially with benign, cystic-type lesions, where a progressive thinning wall may resemble an ill-defined margin). Tomography clearly determines (in cartilaginous tumors) that the calcifications are of the individual ringlet type and located through the entire lesion predominantly centrally, whereas in the case of bone infarction they are situated peripherally. Tomography is important in demonstrating the difference (radiographic) between a fibrous dysplasia of bone, and/or a lytic osseous lesion, and/or whether there is a nidus present in an osteoid osteoma, which may not be clearly evident in a normal x-ray study.

Xeroradiography has no significant advantage over plain x-ray film in the evaluation of bony tumors and their detail; however, because of its edge enhancement characteristics, xeroradiography is capable of defining soft tissue planes and soft tissue to better advantage, thereby improving accuracy in detecting soft tissue mass components.

Arteriography's main contribution is in assessing the extent of vacularity of a tumor. It does not contribute in tissue diagnosis, especially since malignant and benign lesions may have identical vascularity. Arteriography, however, is important when undertaking limb-salvaging surgical procedures.

Computed tomography (CT) has been an invaluable aid since its introduction in clinical diagnosis and in the radiographic evaluation of bone tumors. It contributes in five basic categories.

1. In determining the extent of the disease or lesion (because of its capacity for separating soft tissue planes that are even minimally of different densities);

2. in evaluating the result of treatment;

3. in determining the nature of the disease or lesion conventional radiographs are sometimes non-specific. The presence of a well-defined lytic lesion in bone may represent a simple bone cyst, fibrous dysplasia, enchondroma, or ocassionally a malignant lesion with benign characteristics. CT in this case may determine the true nature of the disease by demonstrating the "absorption coefficient" value of the lesion;

4. to detect presence of pathology. Sometimes a lesion is too small for x-ray to demonstrate;

5. to plan radiation therapy.

BIBLIOGRAPHY

BEGG, A. C.: The vascular pattern as an aid to the diagnosis of bone tumors. J. Bone Jt. Surg., **37**: 371, 1955.

DAHLIN, D. C.: *Chondrosarcoma in Bone Tumors*, 3rd Ed, Charles C. Thomas, Springfield, 1978.

DE SANTOS, L. A.: *The Radiology of Bone Tumors: Old and New Modalities*, American Cancer Society, 1980.

DE SANTOS, L. A., BENARDINO, M. E., AND MURRAY, J. A.: Computed tomography in the evaluation of osteosarcoma. Am. J. Radiol., **132**: 535, 1979.

EDEIHEN, J., AND HODES, P. J.: *Roentgen Diagnosis of Diseases of Bone*, 2nd Ed, Williams & Wilkins, Baltimore, 1975.

GAMBLE, F. O., AND YALE, I.: *Clinical Foot Roentgenology*, Williams & Wilkins, Baltimore, 1966.

GREENFIELD, G. B.: *Radiology of Bone Disease*, 2nd Ed, J. B. Lippincott, Philadelphia, 1975.

JAFFE, H. L.: *Tumors and Tumorous Conditions of the Bones and Joints*, Lea & Febiger, Philadelphia, 1958.

KAHN, L. B.: Chondrosarcoma. Cancer, **37**: 1365, 1976.

LEWIN, P.: *The Foot and Ankle*, Lea & Febiger, Philadelphia, 1949.

LEWIS, M. R.: *Roentgen Foot Diagnosis*, Von Schill Memorial Press, Chicago, 1952.

LEWIS, M. R.: *Atlas of Foot Roentgenology*, Edwards Brothers, Ann Arbor, 1964.

LICHTENSTEIN, L.: *Diseases of Bone and Joints*, C. V. Mosby, St. Louis, 1970.

LICHTENSTEIN L: *Bone Tumors*, 5th Ed, C. V. Mosby, St. Louis, 1977.

LODWICK, G. S.: *The Bones and Joints: Atlas of Tumor Radiology*, Yearbook Medical Publishers, Chicago, 1971.

MESCHAN, I.: *Roentgen Signs in Clinical Practice*, W. B. Saunders, Philadelphia, 1968, vol. 1.

SAVERKIN, N. G.: Fibrosarcomata. J. Bone Jt. Surg., **61B**: 366, 1979.

SPJUT, H. J., DORFMAN, H. D., FECHNER, R. E., ET AL.: Tumors of bone and cartilage. *Atlas of Tumor Pathology*, Armed Forces Institute of Pathology, Washington, D. C., 1971.

WEINSTEIN, F.: *Roentgenology of the Foot*, Warren H. Green, St. Louis, 1974.

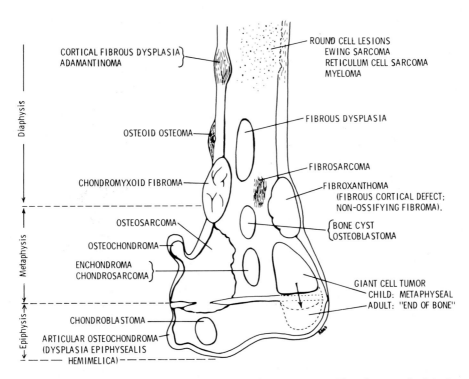

Figure 12.1. Composite diagram illustrating frequent sites of bone tumors. The diagram depicts the end of a long bone which has been divided into the epiphysis, metaphysis, and diaphysis. The typical sites of common primary bone tumors are labeled. Bone tumors tend to predominate in those ends of long bones which undergo the greatest growth and remodeling, and hence, have the greatest number of cells and amount of cell activity (shoulder and knee regions). When small tumors, presumably detected early, are analyzed, preferential sites of tumor origin become apparent within each bone, as shown in this illustration. This suggests a relationship between the type of tumor and

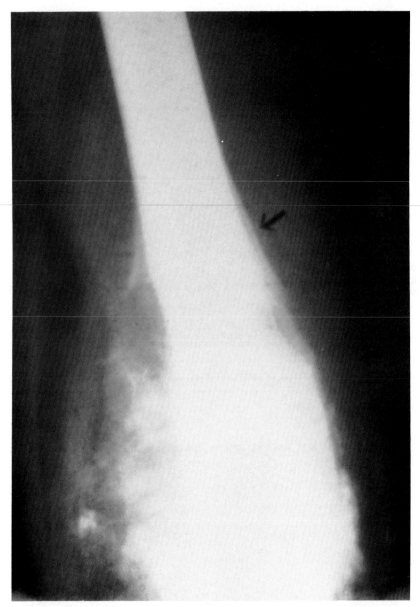

Figure 12.2.   Osteosarcoma involving the distal end of the femur in an 11-year-old female; a common site. Extensive radiating destruction beyond normal confines of the femur with associated periosteal and subperiosteal reaction and extensive destruction are present. Numerous layers of calcified periosteum are visible, giving us the "onion skin" appearance. Medullary and cortical destruction and proliferation are also present. An amputation was performed. Patient expired with pulmonary metastases.

the anatomic site affected. In general, a tumor of a given cell type arises in the field where the homologous normal cells are most active. These regional variations suggest that the composition of the tumor is affected or may be determined by the metabolic field in which it arises. (From THEROS, E. G.: Radiologic and pathologic analysis of solitary bone lesions, part I. Radiol. Clin. North Am., **19:** 716, 1981, with permission.)

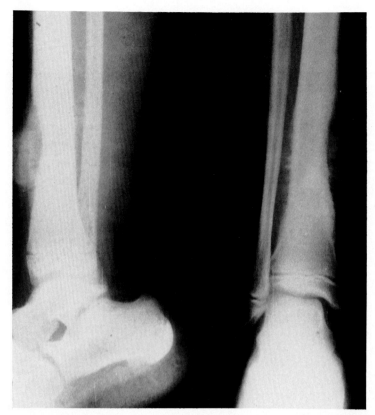

Figure 12.3. Osteosarcoma in a 10-year-old female. Note the concave defect on the medial aspect of the tibia (an operative biopsy defect). Numerous ray-like spicules of bone may be seen extending out from the anterior and medial margins of the distal end of the tibia. A soft tissue mass and subperiosteal reaction are evident. The biopsy reported an osteogenic sarcoma.

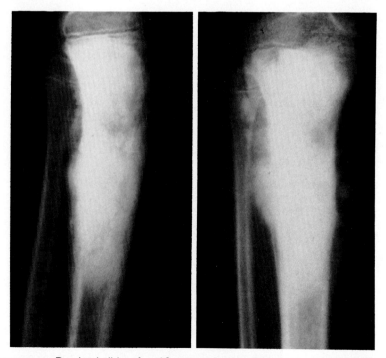

Figure 12.4. Osteosarcoma. Proximal tibia of a 10-year-old male. The area appears dense and sclerotic with associated areas of bone destruction invading into the cortex and medullary canal. Elevated proliferative calcified periosteal reactions throughout the lesion are present. Ossifications also radiate into the soft tissues.

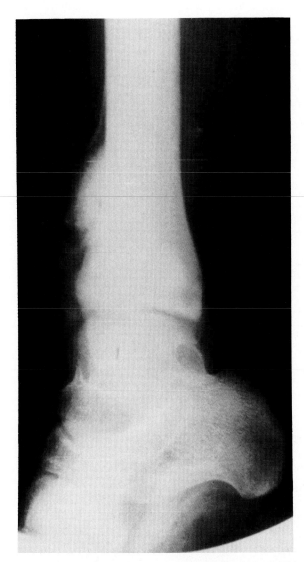

Figure 12.5.   Osteosarcoma a 14-year-old female x-rayed for a painful swollen ankle of 2 months duration. A firm mass, tender, not hot; no fever and no leukocytosis were present. X-rays reveal proliferative lesions involving the anterior and lateral aspects of right ankle (distal tibia). Extensive ossification is noted extending beyond the normal confines of the bone and into the soft tissues. Extensive calcified periosteum extends up the tibial shaft. Sclerotic changes rather than destructive changes are predominant. A Codman's triangle is present. A biopsy confirmed osteosarcoma and an amputation was performed. Five months later, there was metastasis into the lungs, abdomen, and scapula.

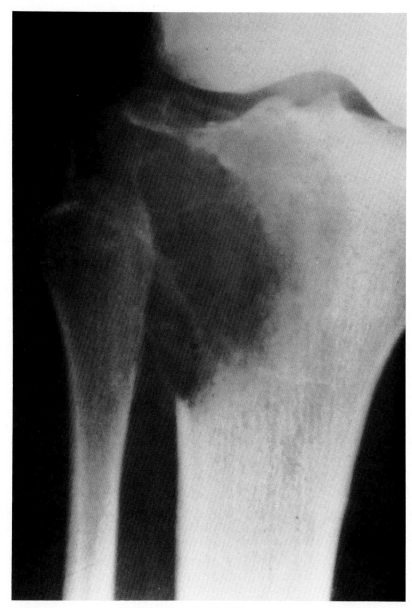

Figure 12.6.   Giant cell tumor in a 38-year-old female. The lesion is on the proximal tibia, a common site. There is expansion and ballooning of the cortex with a thin, interrupted shell of bone remaining. The lesion appears trabeculated with an ill-defined margin and little to no bony reaction. The histological diagnosis was a benign giant cell tumor. Currettage and packing with bone chips were performed.

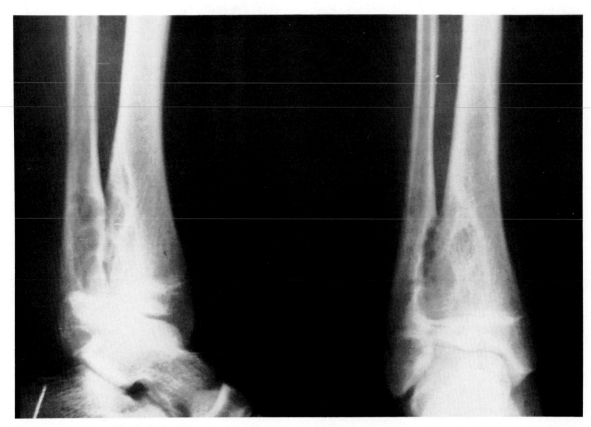

Figure 12.7.   Fibrosarcoma in a 15-year-old male. The destructive process is at the distal end of the tibia and adjacent fibula. Histologically, the diagnosis was a fibrosarcoma with invasion by direct extension. The cortices are destroyed over the posterior and lateral aspects of the tibia and medial aspect of adjacent fibula. The treatment was block resection of the involved areas of bones.

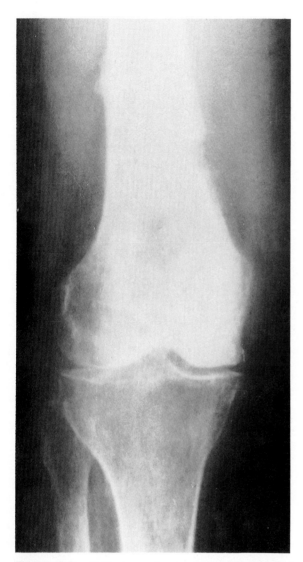

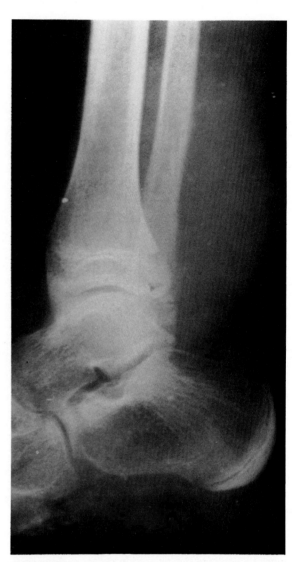

Figure 12.8.   Reticulum cell sarcoma in a 70-year-old female. Pain was present in the knee for several years prior to this study. Irregular, mottled areas of destruction and sclerosis are present involving the distal femur, especially at the region of lateral condyle. Some periosteal new bone formation is evident. A cortical defect in the supracondylar region is biopsy-produced.

Figure 12.9.   Malignant synovioma. An irregular area of destruction of the cortex of the distal fibula and a large associated soft tissue mass posteriorly are present. Patient is a 10-year-old female. This is the second most common site for a malignant synovioma, the knee being the first.

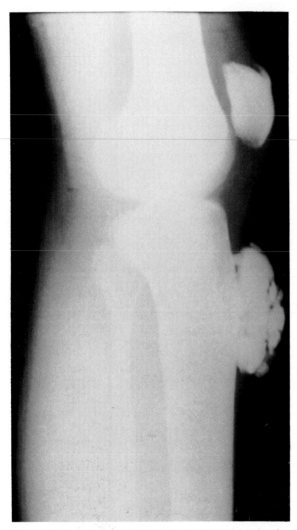

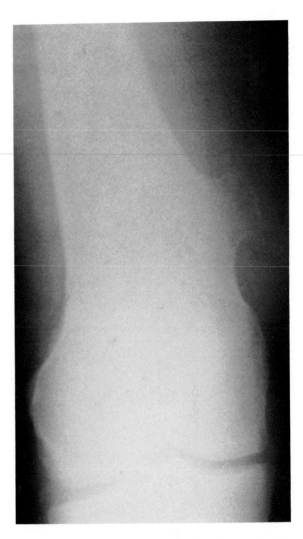

Figure 12.10. Osteochondroma (benign) eminating from tibial tubercle.

Figure 12.11. Osteochondroma (benign) eminating from the medial side of the distal one-third of the femur.

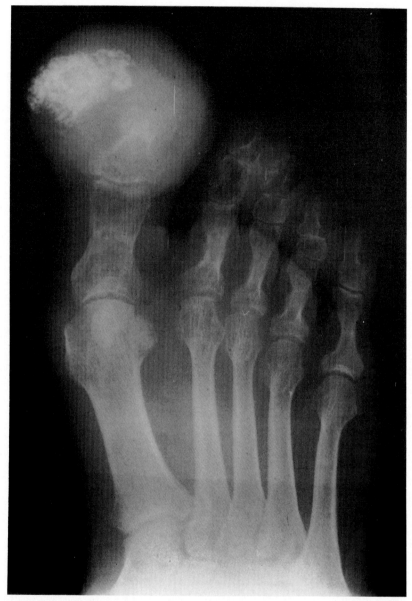

Figure 12.12.   Malignant synovioma. A bulky, irregular (patchy) soft tissue mass is evident distally, right hallux. This mass is frequently evident with malignant synoviomas. These tumors tend to spread through the lymphatics and this patient also had two large 4–5 cm nodes in the inguinal region, which were biopsied and proven to be synovioma metastasis. The hallux was amputated at the MP joint level and 4000 roentgens in air were delivered to the inguinal nodes. The patient has been free of cancer for the past 10 years. However, these tumors have been known to metastasize even after this long a period.

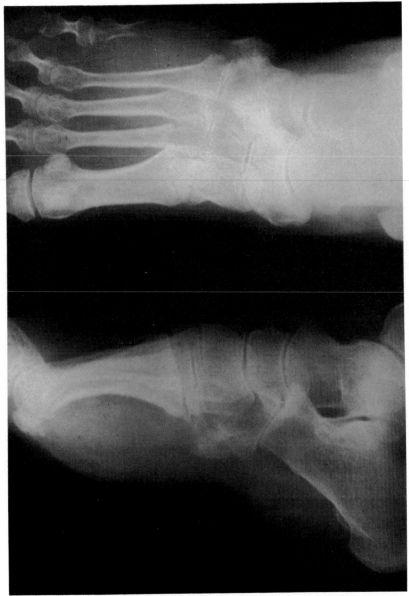

Figure 12.13.   Fibrosarcoma in a 29-year-old female. This study was obtained 2 years after the original diagnosis, indicating the rather indolent nature of this tumor. There is extensive destruction of the fifth metatarsal with only a thin shell of cortical bone persisting. There is a prominent soft tissue mass plantarly in this region. There is usually no proliferative bone reaction with fibrosarcoma. Confirmed by biopsy.

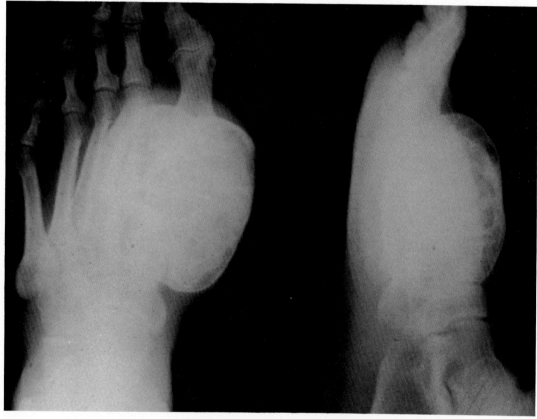

Figure 12.14.   Enchondromata. A large, partially calcified mass overlying the entire left first metatarsal bone is seen. There is a sharp, smoothly contoured shell of sclerotic bone well demarcating the lesion. Biopsy confirmed a benign enchondroma.

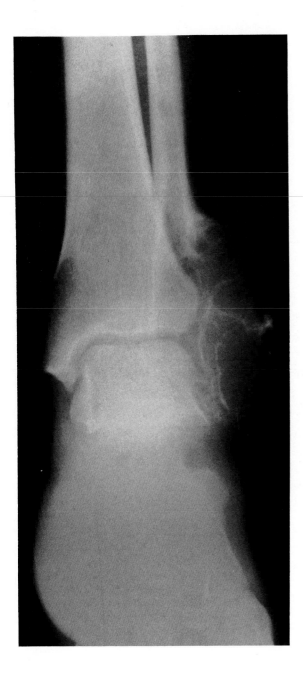

Figure 12.15. Aneurysmal bone cyst. An expansile lesion of the distal fibula which balloons out to a considerable extent beyond the normal fibular contours is present. The lesion is covered over by a thin cortical shell with numerous fine osseous trabecular septae in evidence. There is no associated destruction of the adjacent tibia and talus bones. Surgery of this area revealed a shell-like protrusion of cortical bone from the fibula surrounding a soft tissue mass of convoluted vascular channels. The blood vessels were in direct communication with normal circulation. Biopsy confirmed a benign cyst.

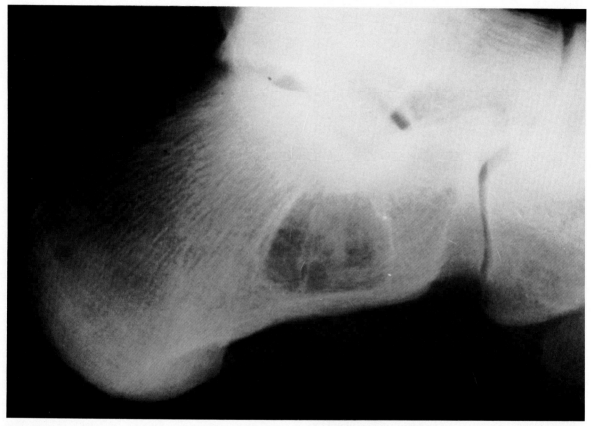

Figure 12.16.   Unicameral bone cyst, differentiated from neutral triangle of the calcaneus. Note the sclerotic borders and distended internal trabecular pattern.

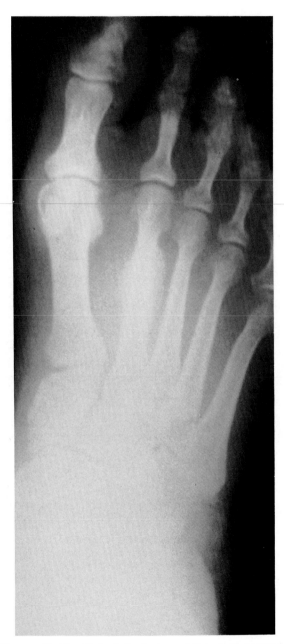

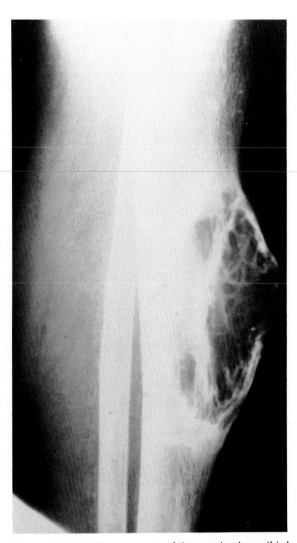

Figure 12.18. Fibrosarcoma of the proximal one-third of tibia in a 65-year-old male. These lesions can begin centrally or in the periosteum. This probably represents a central lesion that has destroyed, ballooned, and eroded through the cortex. Very little reactive proliferative bone reaction is seen. Biopsy confirmed malignant.

Figure 12.17. Metastatic lesion of the right second metatarsal shaft. This patient's primary lesion was in his prostate (prostatic carcinoma), to be differentiated from a typical bone callus formation.

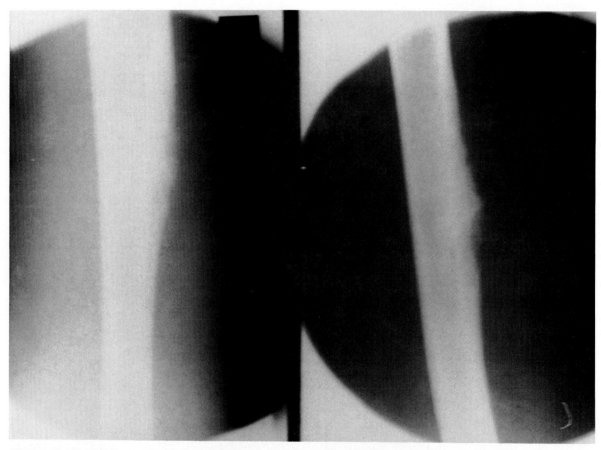

Figure 12.19.   Ewing's tumor (endothelial myeloma), to be differentiated from osteomyelitis and periosteal sarcoma. This case involves the distal third of the femur. Note the periosteal new bone formation, and cortical thickening, involving the posterior and lateral aspect of the femur with subsequent destruction of newly laid down periosteal bone, giving a laminated or "onion skin" appearance, frequently associated with Ewing's. In this case an amputation was done, but the patient developed widespread osseous metastasis, which also affected the lungs, and death ensued.

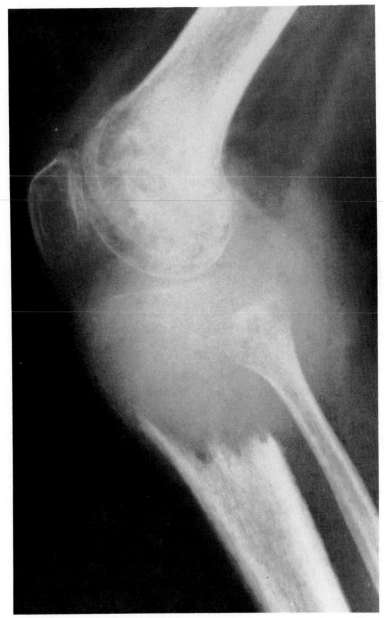

Figure 12.20.   Giant cell tumor (malignant). Proximal tibia of a 43-year-old male. These tumors are unusually seen before age 20, and rarely in childhood and adolescence. Extensive destruction of proximal tibia, and irregular invasive margins with no intact cortical shell are seen. Note the considerable demineralization of the adjacent femur. A large soft tissue mass is also evident. Biopsy confirmed malignancy.

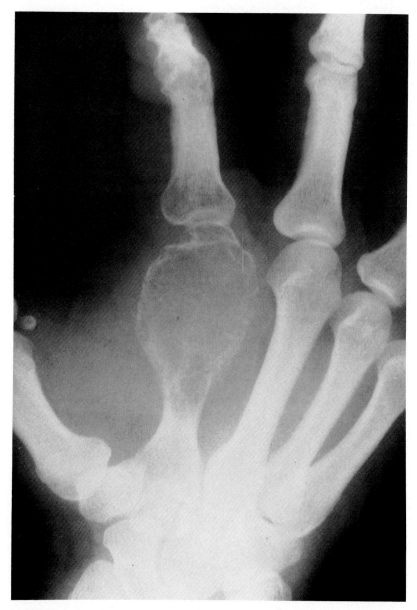

Figure 12.21. Giant cell tumor (malignant), 31-year-old male. A large destructive expansile lesion in the distal two-thirds of the second metacarpal is present. Intact shell of a bone and numerous small trabeculae are evident. This is not a common site. The entire second ray was amputated; no recurrence in 9 years.

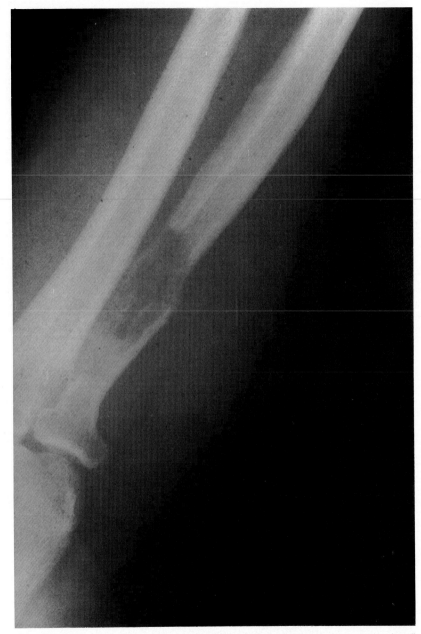

Figure 12.22.   Metastatic bone tumor. A poorly marginated destructive lesion in the proximal radius within no bony proliferation is present. Original CA in this case was the kidney. Metastatic bone tumors are by far the most common bone tumors with about one-fourth of CA patients eventually showing skeletal metastasis.

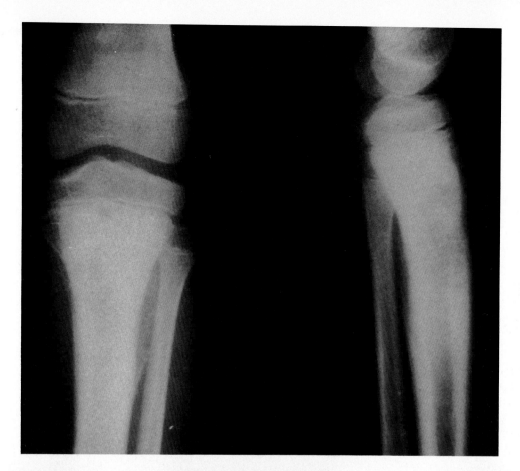

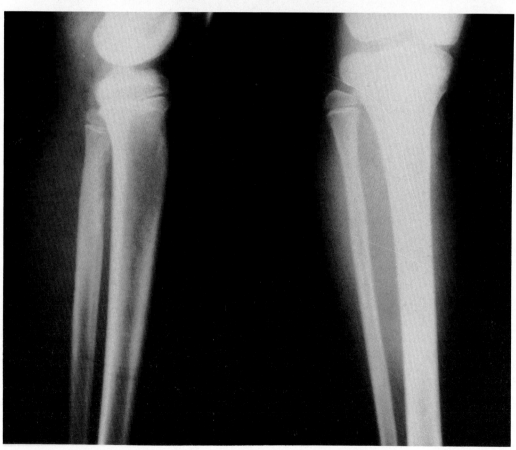

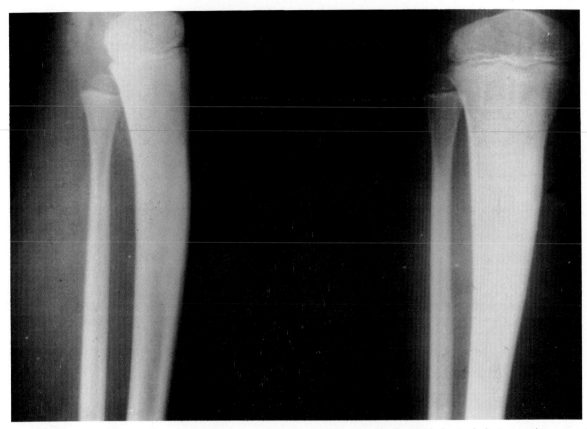

Figure 12.25. Osteoid osteoma. This patient is a 6-year-old male. Usually diagnosis is made between the ages of 10 and 30, but no age group is immune. Males are affected twice as often as females. Fifty per cent occur in the lower extremity; the tibia following the femur as a most common site. The small radiolucent nidus of osteoid tissue within the sclerotic bone about the lesion is evident. At times a calcified nidus is present within the lucency, but not in this case.

Figure 12.23 (*upper left*). Ewing's tumor. Endothelial myeloma in a 10-year-old male, x-rayed because of pain and swelling immediately below the knee for a few months and getting worse. X-rays show an irregular bone proliferation producing a dense sclerotic metaphyseal region. Periosteal new bone formation about the proximal tibia with a characteristic laminated appearance is present. Clinically, a soft tissue mass was also evident as is usually the case with Ewing's tumor.

Figure 12.24 (*lower left*). Ewing's tumor. A 9-year-old female with clinical picture of osteomyelitis: fever, leukocytosis, and a painful swollen and hot left lower leg. There is a destructive lesion involving primarily the anterior aspect of the proximal fibula and periosteal reaction extending down to almost the entire length of the fibula, especially anteriorly. There are four linear streaks of periosteal new bone separated by lucent lines producing the "onion skin" effect. Biopsy confirmation is mandatory to differentiate from osteomyelitis.

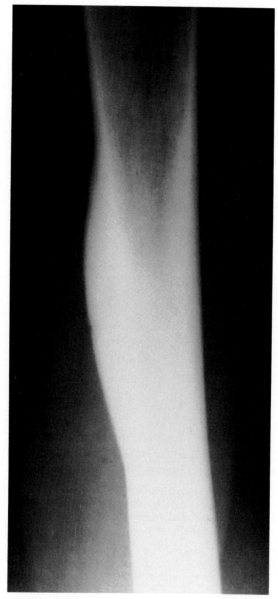

Figure 12.26. Osteoid osteoma. This patient is a 26-year-old female. A small radiolucent defect is evident with a dense area of new bone formation producing a mound of bone along the medial aspect of the femur. These lesions occur in any part of bone and are not limited to the metaphyses; they have been reported in the epiphyses.

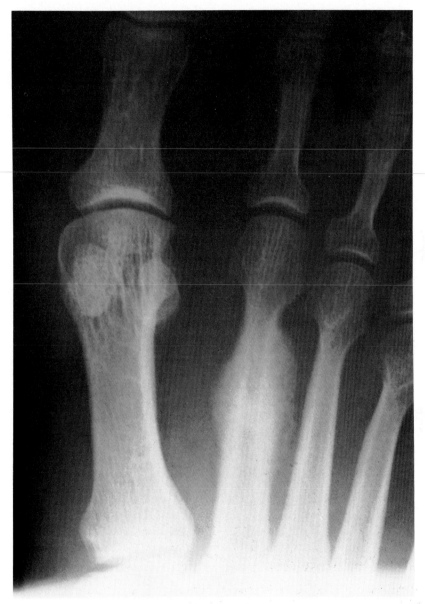

Figure 12.27.   Osteogenicsarcoma (periosteal type) of the second metatarsal shaft. Note the periosteal-cortical origin with cortical destruction, rupture, and expansion.

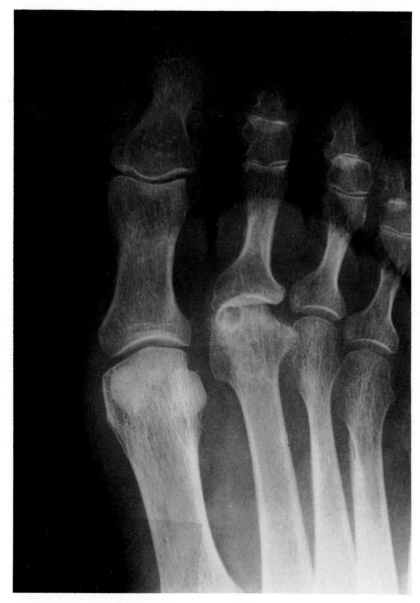

Figure 12.28.   Osteochondroma effecting the left second metatarsal head principally. A well-demarkated sclerosed central lesion is noted at the distal medial portion of the head; note expansion of the entire head, as well as the expansile reaction of the proximal portion of the proximal phalanx of this joint.

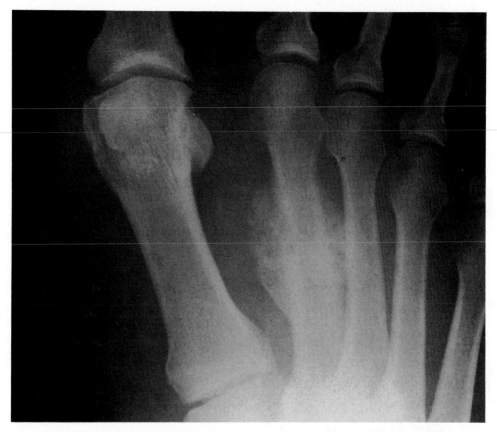

Figure 12.29.   Carcinoma (secondary) osteoblastic type of the second metatarsal shaft, secondary to a prostatic carcinoma. Note its medullary origin in the midshaft with irregular bony proliferation and uncommon involvement of the periosteum with cortical rupture.

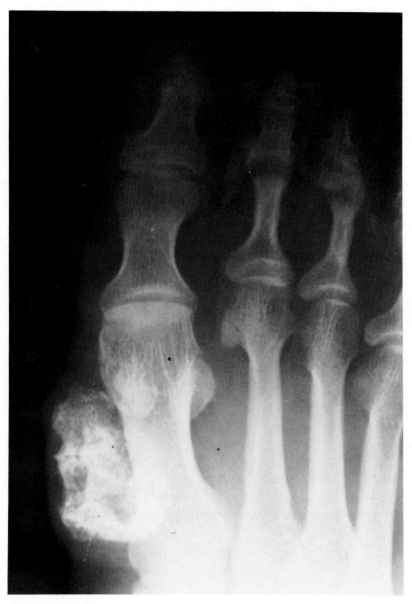

Figure 12.30.   Calcified (unclassified) mass. A partially calcified osseous mass medial to the first metatarsal head partially overlying, but not attached, to the proximal one-third of the first metatarsal shaft is present. Pathology report: benign bony and cartilagneous nodule of unknown etiology.

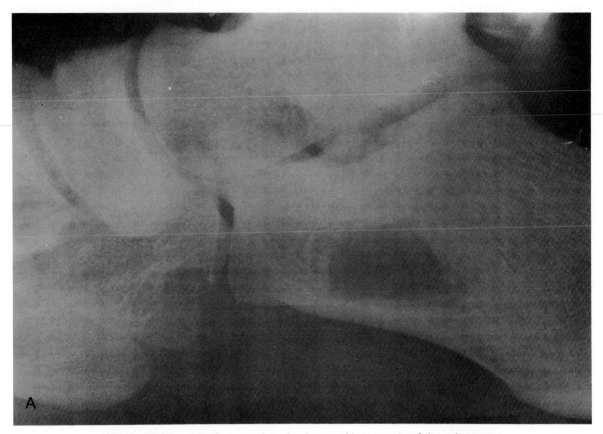

Figure 12.31. *A* to *C*, examples of unicameral bone cysts of the calcaneus.

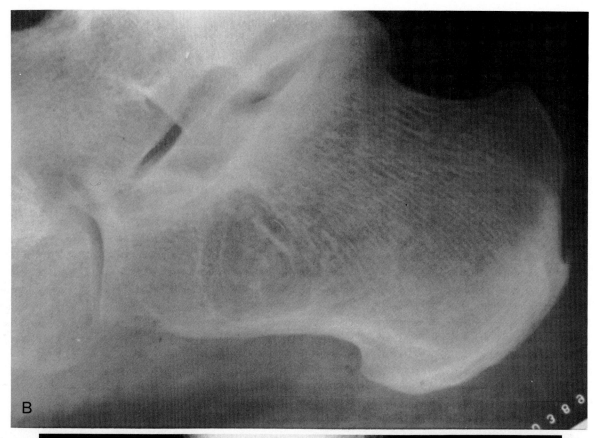

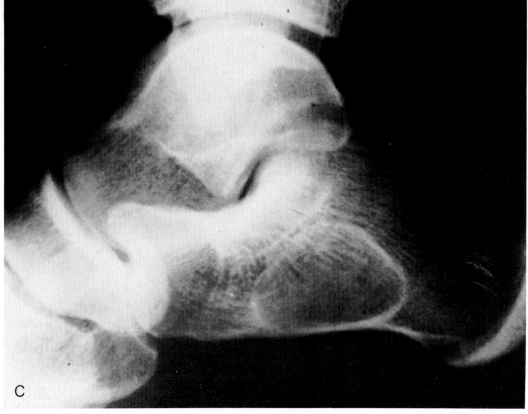

Figure 12.31.   (*B* and *C*)

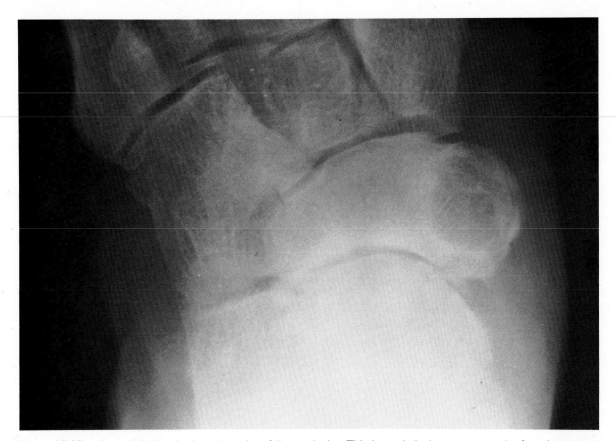

Figure 12.32.   A cystic lesion in the tuberosity of the navicular. This is a relatively uncommon site for a bone cyst.

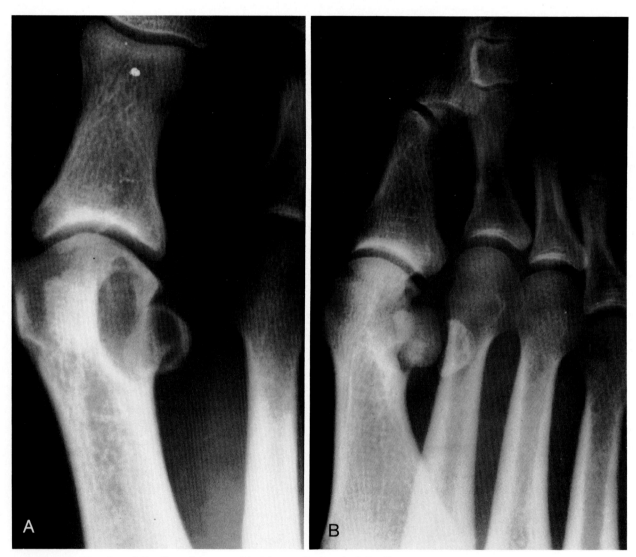

Figure 12.33. *A* and *B*, villonodula synovitis (giant cell tumor) of the first metatarsal. Note the erosion of the first metatarsal and involvement of the fibular sesamoid.

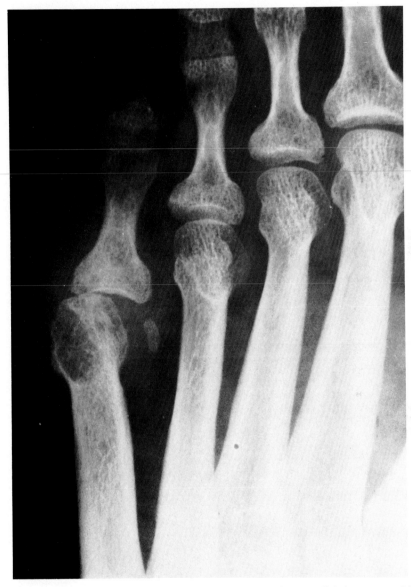

Figure 12.34.   Giant cell tumor of the fifth metatarsal head. There is a large radiolucent area within the head of the fifth metatarsal. A soft tissue mass is present in the tissues around the fifth metatarsophalangeal joint and causing a subluxation of the joint.

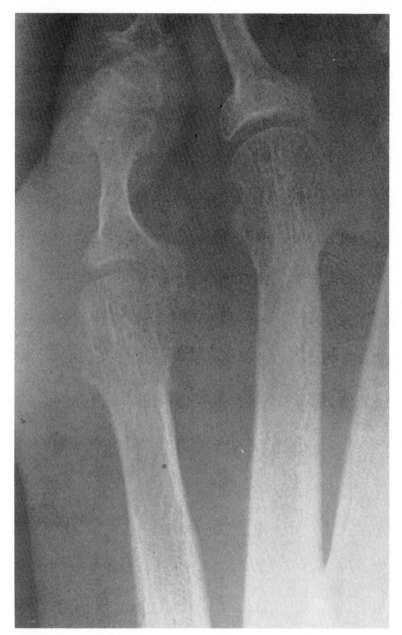

Figure 12.35.   A large soft tissue mass lateral to the fifth metatarsal head causing erosion of the lateral aspect of the head.

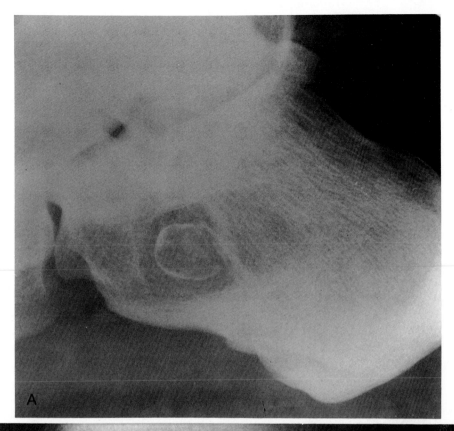

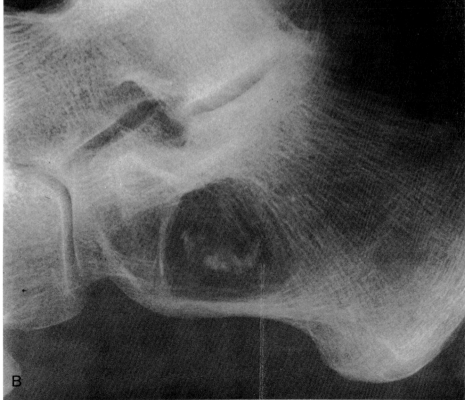

Figure 12.36.   *A* and *B*, osteoid osteomas of the calcaneus. This is a fairly common site for an osteoid osteoma.

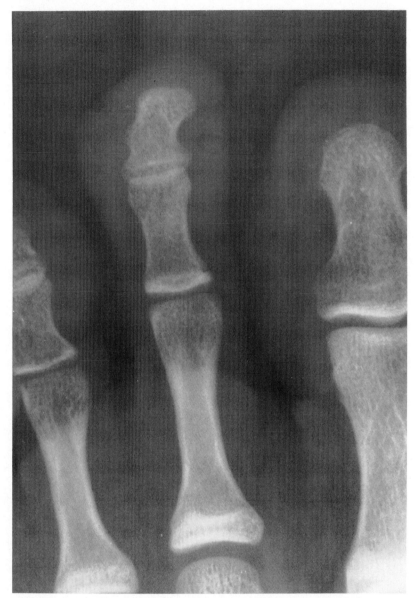

Figure 12.37. Osteochondroma of the distal phalanx of the second toe. This lesion caused a deformity of the nail and considerable pain.

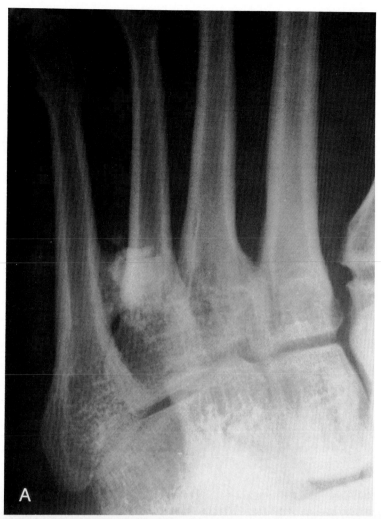

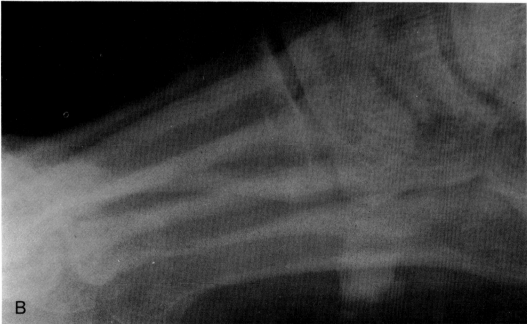

Figure 12.38.   *A* and *B*, a periosteal myositis ossificans extending into the soft tissues beneath the fifth metatarsal.

CHAPTER 13

Systemically Induced Changes in Skeletal Structure

ROBERT VAN DERSLICE, M.D.

The number of systemic diseases leading to radiographically detectable bone and joint changes is legion, and obviously a detailed description and discussion of all such possible conditions are beyond the scope of this text. Some disorders (notably the arthritides), while qualifying as diseases with protean systemic manifestations, will be discussed elsewhere in this text and will not be repeated here. Other disorders (e.g., achondroplasia), while not representing diseases per se, are included for the sake of completeness, and due to their relative frequency and their interesting radiographic characteristics. Included in this chapter are a number of selected conditions, some commonly seen and some relatively infrequently encountered, which can be classified for convenience into the following categories:

1. Endocrinologic
2. Metabolic
3. Hematologic and reticuloendothelial
4. Dysplastic
5. Neoplastic and paraneoplastic
6. Miscellaneous

I. ENDOCRINOLOGIC
(Figures appear on pages 325–341.)
Acromegaly and Gigantism

Acromegaly and gigantism result from the excessive secretion of growth hormone (somatotropin) from eosinophilic or chromophobe adenomas of the pituitary gland. When the condition occurs before closure of the epiphyseal growth centers of the skeleton, gigantism results; after epiphyseal closure, the resulting clinical syndrome is known as acromegaly. The physiologic effects of growth hormone are multiple and varied, with hypersecretion resulting in an increased size and mass of bone, cartilage, muscle, connective tissue, and soft tissue viscera. Clinically, the patient with acromegaly may show enlargement of the hands and feet, jaw, forehead, and tongue. The chest becomes enlarged, also due to elongation of the ribs, with evidence of a dorsal kyphosis. The presence of the pituitary tumor may lead to headaches, visual disturbances, amenorrhea in women, and decreased libido in men. A variety of rheumatologic complaints also occur in acromegalics, including backache, arthropathy of the knees, shoulders, and hips, the carpal tunnel syndrome, and a proximal muscle myopathy. Concommitant dysfunctioning of other endocrine glands may accompany the primary disorder with evidence of coexistant diabetes mellitus or hyperthyroidism.

RADIOLOGY

The radiographic findings in acromegaly reflect the anabolic effect of growth hormone on bone, cartilage, and soft tissue. In the skull (Fig. 13.1), enlargement of the frontal and maxillary sinuses is characteristic, as is enlargement, elongation, and thickening of the mandible leading to clinically evident prognathism and dental malocclusion. The cranial vault may also appear thickened, particularly in the area of the occipital protuberance. Enlargement of the sella turcica may also be noted due to the presence of the intrasellar tumor.

In the spine, the vertebral bodies may appear enlarged (due to apposition of bone on the anterior and lateral aspects of the vertebral body) with evidence of superimposed degenerative change (osteophytosis and bony sclerosis) which may be prominent (Fig. 13.4). The height of the intervertebral disc spaces may be increased due to hypertrophy of the discal soft tissues. An interesting finding in the spine, particularly in the lumbar area, is scalloping of the posterior aspects of the vertebral bodies as noted on lateral spinal radiographs, a finding of unclear pathogenesis, but which may reflect the effect of increased bone resorption which seems to occur concommitantly with bone deposition in acromegalics (Fig. 13.7). A kyphosis of the thoracic spine is also characteristic.

Multiple abnormalities of the hands and feet are noted in this disorder. These bony parts, due to the large number of articulations found here, will show the greatest amount of enlargement due to cartilaginous proliferation at these articulations. The tufts of the terminal phalanges enlarge, assuming the characteristic "spade-like" configuration (Fig. 13.2). Small bony excrescences may be seen at the sites of tendinous attachment to bone with typically small, beak-like projections arising from the heads of the metatarsals and metacarpals which may be enlarged and squared. Small, degenerative bony ossicles may also be noted around the articulations of the hands and feet. Widening of these articulations, particularly the metatarsophalangeal and metacarpophalangeal joints, may also be seen owing to cartilage proliferation. In the foot, thickening of the metatarsal shafts with narrowing of the shafts of the proximal phalanges is characteristic (Fig. 13.6). The calcaneus may also demonstrate multiple bony excrescences at the various sites of tendinous attachment. Lateral radiographs of the foot also demonstrate thickening of the soft tissues inferior to the calcaneus due to connective tissue hyperplasia and collagen deposition (Fig. 13.3). This thickening of the foot's "heel pad," while not being totally diagnostic of acromegaly, can be used to suggest the diagnosis. A value of greater than 23 mm in males and 21.5 mm in females should arouse suspicion of this entity, but obviously these absolute values do not take into account such factors as overall body habitus, race of the patient, and localized skin conditions responsible for heel thickening such as infection and edema, all factors which could affect this measurement. The soft tissues of the fingers and toes also thicken.

Chondrocalcinosis (due to deposition of calcium pyrophosphate dihydrate crystals) may also be observed in some patients with acromegaly,

Table 13.1.
Conditions Associated with Chondrocalcinosis

1. Hyperparathyroidism
2. Pseudogout and calcium pyrophosphate arthropathy
3. Acromegaly
4. Wilson's disease
5. Ochronosis
6. Hemochromatosis
7. Degenerative joint disease
8. Diabetes

particularly at the knee (Fig. 13.5). This radiographic feature occurs in a wide variety of other conditions as well, which are ennumerated in Table 13.1.

Cushing's Disease

Cushing's disease represents a clinical syndrome created by an excess production of glucocorticoids that may be the result of hyperplasia of the adrenal glands, adrenal adenomas, or adrenal carcinomas. Non-endocrine tumors occasionally are responsible, including such neoplasms as bronchogenic carcinomas, thymomas, and bronchial adenomas (which may secrete polypeptides having biochemical activity similar to ACTH). Long-term exogenous steroid administration can also lead to the Cushing syndrome (Fig. 13.8).

Clinically, patients with this disorder may exhibit the typical Cushing's body habitus with truncal obesity, a "moon" facies, and a "buffalo hump" in the interscapular region, findings which reflect the deposition of adipose tissue at various sites in the body. Adipose tissue may also be deposited within the mediastinum (leading to mediastinal widening on chest x-ray) and abdomen. Patients are most commonly hypertensive as well and may exhibit weakness and personality change (including depression, irritability, confusion, etc.). Other features of the syndrome include hirsutism, cutaneous striae, acne, amenorrhea, ecchymoses, polyuria and polydypsia, and edema. Osteoporosis of the skeletal structures, representing an important complication that can result in pathologic fractures, reflects the metabolic effects of increased bony resorption and decreased bone deposition attendant to this disorder.

RADIOLOGY

Generalized osteoporosis and demineralization of the skeleton is one of the radiologic manifestations of this disorder. This is frequently most pronounced in the spine where pathologic compression fractures are a common sequelae of the weakened osteoporotic bone (Fig. 13.9). The collapsed, biconcave vertebral bodies may show a narrow rim of increased radiodensity along their superior and inferior borders, these areas of marginal condensation representing hypercallosis along the fractured vertebral end-plated. The propensity to develop extensive and exuberant callus formation at sites of fracture is one of the interesting features of Cushing's disease and may not only be seen in this manner in the spine, but can also be noted surrounding healing pathologic fractures of the extremities. Fractures through the pubic rami and ischiae may also be seen in association with thick callus formation. Rib fractures are also common.

Another characteristic of Cushing's disease is the complication of osteonecrosis, a complication which may also follow long-term exogenous corticosteroid therapy (for collagen vascular disease, asthma, etc.) (Figs. 13.10 and 13.11). This osteonecrosis of hypercortisolism most frequently affects the femoral heads, although involvement may also involve the humeral heads and other sites, including the talus and metatarsal heads (Table 13.2). The radiographic features of aseptic necrosis of bone include subchondral collapse and fragmentation of bone, cystic formation, bone sclerosis, and a relatively normal and intact articular space.

Hyperthyroidism

Due to an excess of the thyroid hormones thyroxine and triiodothyronine, hyperthyroidism is most commonly the result of toxic diffuse goiter (Grave's disease) or toxic nodular goiter (Plummer's disease). Occasionally, patients with these disorders will show generalized osteoporosis reflecting the presence of excessive bone metabolism and turnover and a negative calcium balance. The resulting hyperthyroid osteopathy is most common in a chronic state of hyperthyroidism, usually in patients having the disease for more than 5 years (Fig. 13.13).

RADIOLOGY

The important x-ray feature of hyperthyroid bone disease is that of diffuse skeletal demineralization affecting the spine, skull, pelvis, hands, and feet. In the spine, compression fractures can occur which may result in a kyphotic spinal curvature. Pathologic fractures may also occur in the long bones and in the shorter tubular bones of the hands and feet, which demonstrate an increased

Table 13.2.
Conditions Causing Aseptic Necrosis of the Femoral Heads

1. Steroid therapy and Cushing's disease
2. Collagen vascular disease
3. Sickle cell anemia
4. Gaucher's disease
5. Pancreatitis
6. Alcoholism
7. Caisson disease
8. Diabetes mellitus
9. Post-fracture of femoral neck

Table 13.3.
Conditions Associated with Generalized Periostitis of Bone

1. Hypertropic (pulmonary) osteoarthropathy
2. Thyroid acropachy
3. Hypervitaminosis A
4. Chronic venous stasis
5. Fluorosis
6. Scurvy
7. Trauma ("battered child")
8. Pachydermoperiostitis
9. Rickets, healing
10. Leukemia
11. Polyarteritis nodosa
12. Disseminated osteomyelitis
13. Infantile cortical hyperostosis (Caffey's disease)
14. Widespread bone infarction (e.g., hand-foot syndrome of sickle cell anemia)

radiolucency of bone with medullary trabecular lysis and fine intracortical radiolucent striations.

Thyroid Acropachy

This unusual condition represents a rare complication of treated hyperthyroidism, seen in patients having had thyroid ablation with radioactive iodine or surgery anywhere from several weeks to several years before the onset of the disorder. Patients are usually euthyroid or hypothyroid when they present clinically, but the condition has rarely been recognized as a direct complication of hyperthyroidism occurring while the patient is in the hyperthyroid state. The clinical findings of thyroid acropachy are exopthalmos, soft tissue swelling, pretibial myxedema, and digital clubbing.

RADIOLOGY

The important radiograph abnormality seen in this condition is disseminated periostitis (Table 13.3) which most commonly affects the metatarsals, metacarpals, and phalanges, with the diaphyses of long bones being involved less frequently. In the foot, the first metatarsal and the proximal phalanges of the toes are more commonly affected. The periostitis is often asymmetric in distribution and may be dense and thick, or occasionally spiculated (Fig. 13.12). Surrounding soft tissue swelling is usual. Soft tissue masses of the lower extremities may, on occasion, be noted as well.

Hypothyroidism and Cretinism

Congenital hypothyroidism is known as cretinism and is important in producing retardation of skeletal maturity.

RADIOLOGY

A delayed appearance and fusion of all growth centers is characteristic, with the developing epiphyseal ossification centers showing irregular deformity and an occasional fragmented or stippled appearance (Fig. 13.15), particularly of the capital femoral epiphysis (Fig. 13.14). This leads to a flattened femoral head with a broad femoral neck and a resultant coxa vara deformity. Slipping of the capital femoral epiphysis may also occur.

Other findings include a thick calvarium with a brachycephalic skull, open fontanelles with wormian bone (sutural bone) formation, delayed dental development, vertebral body flattening, thoracolumbar gibbus deformity, and a diffuse increase in bony density.

Primary Hyperparathyroidism

Primary hyperparathyroidism may result from a parathyroid adenoma, hyperplasia of the parathyroid glands, or, rarely, from primary parathyroid carcinoma. Ectopic secretion from certain bronchogenic carcinomas represents an unusual etiology. Increased levels of parathormone directly affect osseous tissue throughout the body with an increased osteoclastic and osteocytic osteolytic activity that promotes calcium liberation from bone into blood. The other end-organ of significance for parathormone is the kidney where the hormone inhibits tubular resorption of phosphate, thus increasing urinary phosphorous excretion. Biochemically, patients with primary hyperparathyroidism (and no significant renal disease) will characteristically have an elevated serum calcium level and a decreased serum phosphorous level.

The signs and symptoms of hyperparathyroidism are varied. They may be related to the genitourinary system (renal colic secondary to calculi, (Fig. 13.16), hematuria, polyuria), the skeletal system (vague skeletal pains, pathologic fractures), the gastrointestinal system (anorexia, constipation, vomiting, ulcer symptoms), or central nervous system (headaches, somnolence, hallucinations). It should be noted that the extensive and severe skeletal changes of hyperparathyroidism once seen are usually not encountered presently due to earlier detection and treatment of this condition.

RADIOLOGY

The skeletal abnormalities of hyperparathyroidism are directly related to the effects of parathormone on bone, specifically the ability of the hormone to incite bone resorption (Fig. 13.18). The classic and pathognomonic x-ray finding is subperiosteal resorption of bone, a finding best identified in the small bones of the hand, particularly the middle phalanges of the second and third digits (Fig. 13.17). The smooth outer cortical margin of the bone is lost, replaced by a finely irregular and spiculated border that is the result of osteoclastic activity here activated by the parathormone stimulus. This same subperiosteal resorptive change is encountered at other sites, including the phalanges of the feet, the inner borders of the proximal femora and tibiae, the ribs, and distal radius. Resorption of the tufts of terminal phalanges (acroosteolysis; see Table 13.4) is also occasionally seen. Elevated parathormone levels will also cause bone resorption at sites other than subperiosteal locations. Subchondral bone resorption is also identified, an example being the erosive changes at the sacroiliac joints which can lead to radiographic findings simulating the sacroiliitis of such inflammatory conditions as ankylosing spondylitis, Reiter's disease, and psoriatic arthritis (with widening, irregularity, and erosions of these articulations). Similar changes occur at the acromioclavicular and sternoclavicular joints, as well as at the symphysis pubis and discovertebral junctions of the spine. Subligamentous resorption of bone represents another form of bone lysis, detectable on the inferior surface of the calcaneus, at the femoral trochanters, at the humeral tuberosities and ischial tuberosities, and at the inferior aspect of the distal clavicle (Fig. 13.22). The loss of the lamina dura surrounding tooth sockets is classically described in hyperparathyroidism but is not specific for this disorder, being also identified in osteomalacia, Cushing's disease, Paget's disease, scleroderma, and dental infections.

Table 13.4.
Conditions Causing Acroosteolysis

1. Hyperparathyroidism
2. Psoriatic arthritis
3. Raynaud's disease
4. Scleroderma
5. Frostbite
6. Thermal and electrical injury
7. Gout
8. Leprosy
9. Neurotrophic disease
10. Drug therapy (dilantin, phenobarb, ergot)
11. Sarcoid
12. Diabetic gangrene
13. Chemical osteolysis (vinyl chloride)
14. HPO

A peculiar and interesting feature of hyperparathyroidism are brown tumors (or osteoclastomas), focal lytic bone lesions resulting from intraosseous hemorrhage and eventual replacement with fibrous tissue and giant cells (Figs. 13.19 to 13.21). The lesions may be single or multiple, occurring in both the appendicular and axial skeleton and have been discovered in the small bones of the hands and feet. While characteristically lytic, non-calcified, and non-expansile, they may on occasion be dramatic radiographically, being grossly expansile and multi-locular in appearance. When multiple, they must be differentiated from metastatic disease. These lesions are also noted in secondary hyperparathyroidism but are more common in the primary form.

As the disease progresses, the skeleton will become demonstrably demineralized due to the resorption of cortical and medullary bone. This resultant osteoporosis can lead to skeletal deformities with vertebral compression fractures and thoracic kyphosis, basilar invagination of the skull (a "settling" of the softened skull into the upper cervical spine), and pathologic fractures of the extremities.

Another characteristic of primary hyperparathyroidism is soft tissue calcification secondary to metastatic calcium deposits within blood vessel walls, hyaline and fibrocartilage of joints, joint capsules and other periarticular soft tissues, and soft tissue viscera such as the kidneys (nephrocalcinosis). Chondrocalcinosis (typified by involvement at the knee), represents the deposition of calcium pyrophosphate dihydrate crystals within both hyaline (e.g., articulating) cartilage and fibrocartilage (e.g., menisci). Soft tissue calcifications are more common in the secondary form of hyperparathyroidism than in the primary variety.

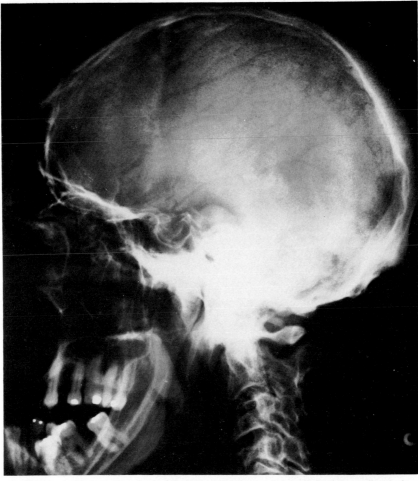

Figure 13.1. Acromegaly: lateral skull radiograph demonstrating enlargement of the sella turcica due to a pituitary tumor, enlargement of the frontal sinuses, mandibular enlargement and elongation, and thickening of the cranial vault, particularly in the occipital area.

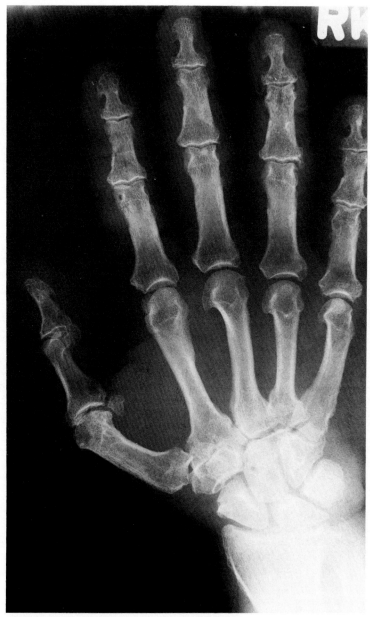

Figure 13.2. Acromegaly: PA hand examination. Radiographic features include prominence of the metacarpal heads (which also demonstrate small osteophytic excrescences), a small degenerative ossicle in the third metacarpophalangeal joint, thickening of the cortices of the metacarpals, and slight widening of the metacarpophalangeal joints. Degenerative appearing change is seen at the wrist and interphalangeal joints. The tufts of the terminal phalanges are enlarged and spade-like (a tuft-breadth value greater than 12 mm in men and 10 mm in women is characteristically seen in acromegalics).

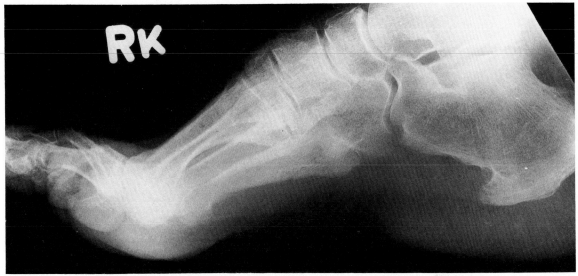

Figure 13.3.   Acromegaly: lateral foot examination. Observe the thickened soft tissues inferior to the calcaneus which on the original radiograph measured 27 mm (positive heel-pad sign, see text). A large, bulky inferior calcaneal hyperostotic "spur" is also evident.

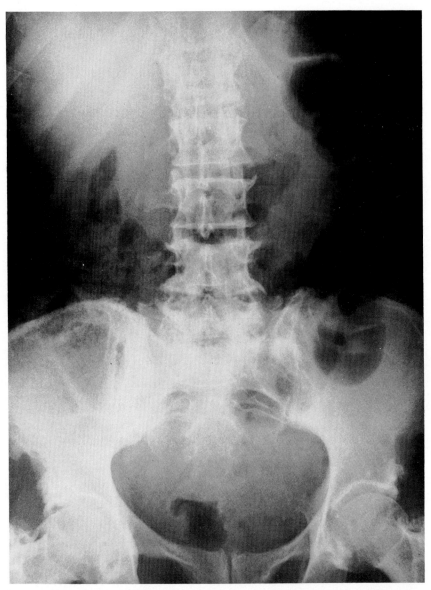

Figure 13.4. Acromegaly: abdominal radiograph demonstrating degenerative osteoarthritic changes in the lumbar spine with osteophytic and paraspinal bone production. Observe the multiple bony excrescences around the pelvis, representing hyperostotic bone proliferation at sites of ligamentous and tendinous attachment.

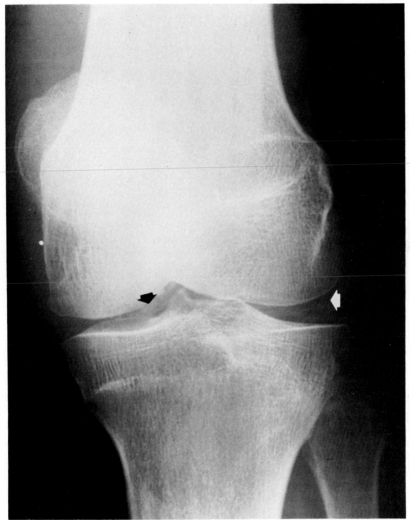

Figure 13.5.   Acromegaly: AP knee radiograph demonstrating curvilinear calcific deposits (arrows) within the medial and lateral joint spaces of the knee. This chondrocalcinosis is due to the deposition of calcium pyrophosphate dihydrate (CPPD crystal deposition) within the hyaline-articulating cartilage and fibrocartilaginous menisci of the knee. This finding is not specific for acromegaly, also seen in many other conditions (Table 13.1).

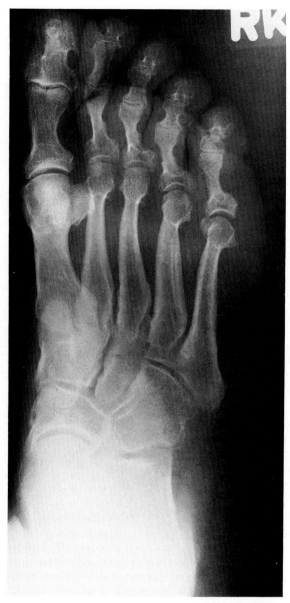

Figure 13.6.   Acromegaly: abnormalities of the foot. Observe bony excrescences arising from the metatarsal heads and terminal phalanges, thickening of metatarsal cortices, tuftal prominence, and irregularities of the articulations of the mid-foot.

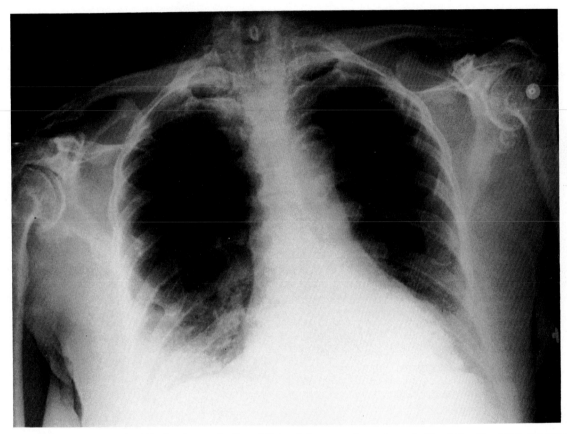

Figure 13.7.   Acromegaly: PA chest examination. Bilateral degenerative osteoarthritis of the shoulders is noted in this acromegalic.

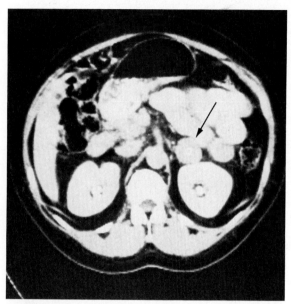

Figure 13.8. Cushing's disease: abdominal CAT scan. Computerized axial tomographic section through the level of the left adrenal gland demonstrating a 2.6-cm round adrenal mass above the left kidney (*arrow*) in a 35-year-old female patient with Cushing's disease. Surgical resection yielded an encapsulated adrenal adenoma.

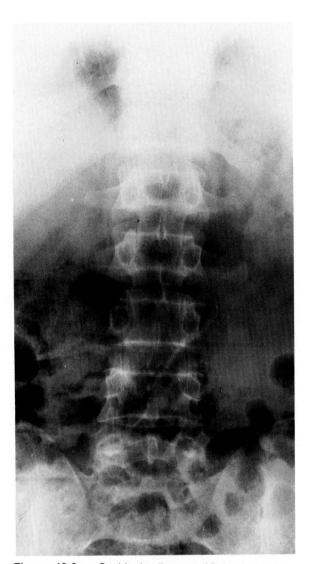

Figure 13.9. Cushing's disease: AP lumbar spine. 35-year-old female with osteoporosis of the lumbar spine. The vertebral end-plates may demonstrate some early sclerotic change which is occasionally prominent in patients with Cushing's disease, reflecting hypercallosis of the fractured end-plates (see text).

Figure 13.11. Cushing's disease. Advanced aseptic necrosis of the left hip in a patient on long-term steroid therapy.

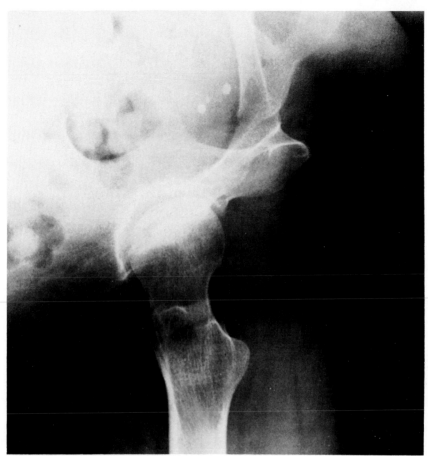

Figure 13.10. Complication of exogenous steroid therapy. Forty-eight-year-old male patient on long-term steroid therapy for asthma demonstrating changes of aseptic necrosis of the right hip with sclerosis, subchondral fracture, and flattening of the femoral head. Such change may be noted at other sites, such as humeral heads, condyles of the femora, talus, and metacarpal and metatarsal heads.

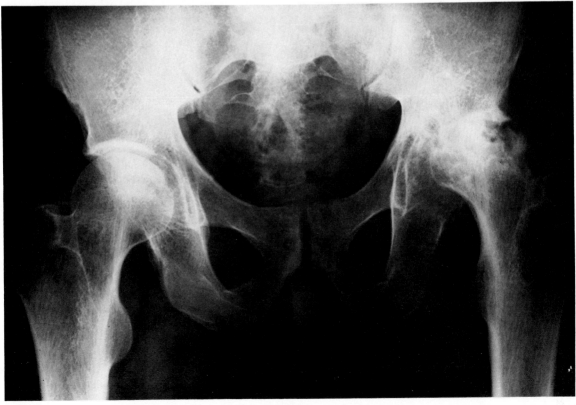

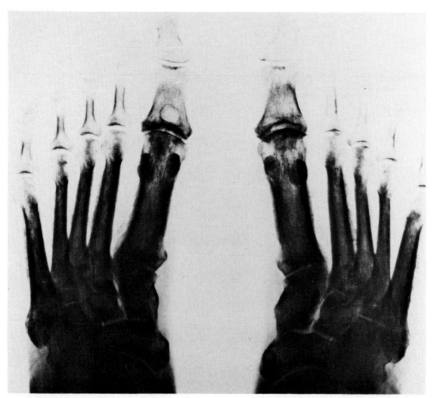

Figure 13.12.   Thyroid acropachy. Foot examination demonstrating thickened, irregular, somewhat lobulated periosteal proliferation in the metatarsals bilaterally.

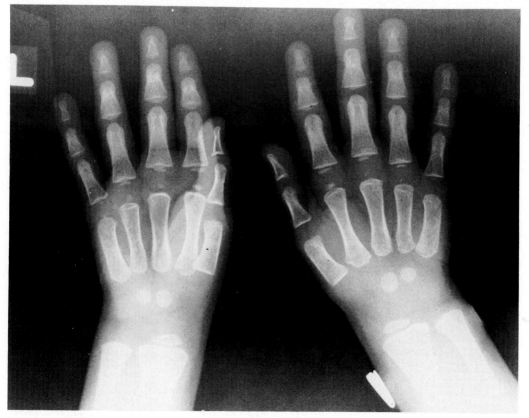

Figure 13.13.   Hypothyroidism. Bilateral hand examination of a 7-year-old female with growth retardation and a bone age of approximately 18 months.

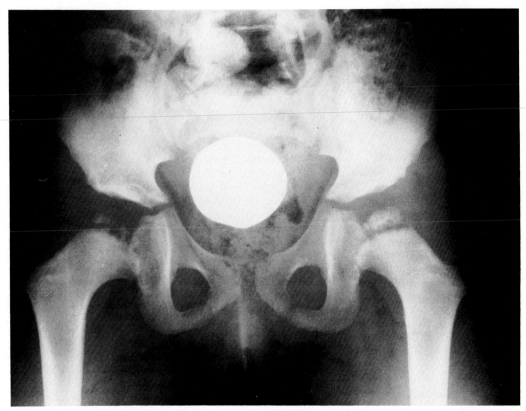

Figure 13.14.   Hypothyroidism. AP pelvis examination showing stippled appearance of the femoral capital epiphyses.

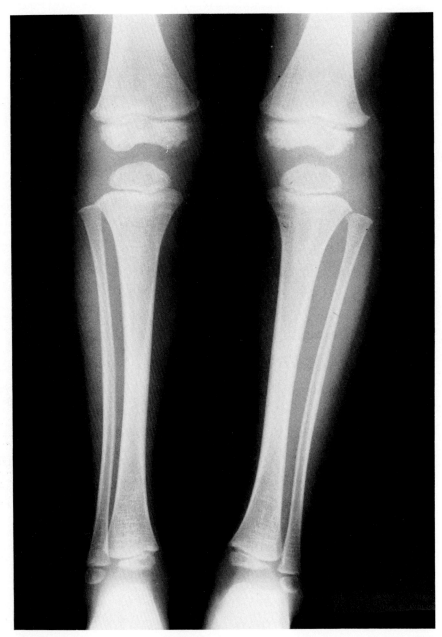

Figure 13.15. Hypothyroidism. AP leg examination demonstrating irregular appearance of the distal femoral epiphyses which have formed from multiple sites of ossification.

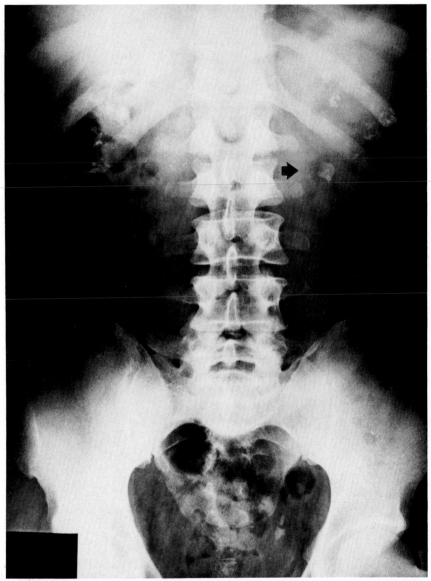

Figure 13.16. Hyperparathyroidism: nephrocalcinosis. Abdominal radiograph demonstrating bilateral upper abdominal calcifications due to deposits of calcium in the renal parenchyma (nephrocalcinosis) in a 43-year-old patient with primary hyperparathyroidism. The larger calcification on the left (*arrow*) probably represents a renal calculus (nephrolithiasis) in the collecting system of the left kidney. The bones appear normal.

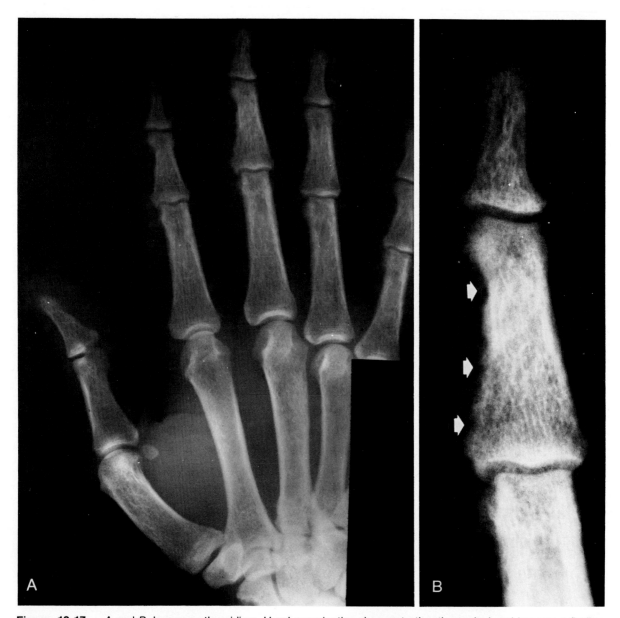

Figure 13.17. *A* and *B*, hyperparathyroidism. Hand examination demonstrating the typical and important finding of subperiosteal bone resorption. Observe the irregularity and loss of normal smooth cortical outline, especially along the radial sides of the middle phalanges (*arrows*). Intracortical tunneling and medullary trabecular prominence are also seen.

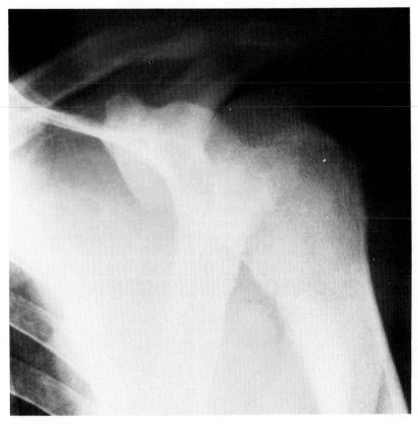

Figure 13.18.   Hyperparathyroidism: AP shoulder. Lack of definition and irregularity along the proximal inner aspect of the humerus representing change due to subperiosteal bone resorption. The acromioclavicular joint is widened, due to resorption of bone, particularly of the distal clavicle.

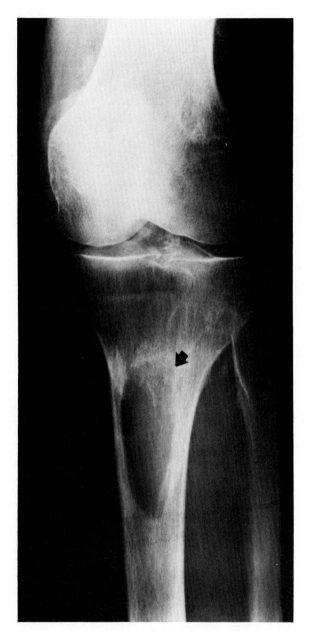 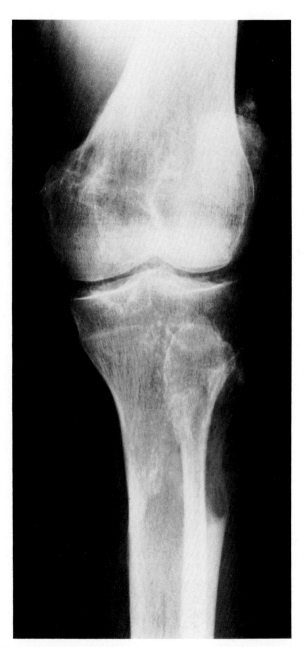

Figures 13.19 (*left*) and 13.20 (*right*).   Hyperparathyroidism. A large, lytic lesion (*arrow*) oriented along the long axis of the tibial shaft representing a brown tumor with a characteristic lack of bone sclerosis and internal calcification. These lesions can be found anywhere in the bony skeleton. Also observe chondrocalcinosis in the knee joint and amorphous soft tissue calcification above the knee, probably representing calcium deposited in the synovial lining of the knee joint. The fibula demonstrates bone resorption with prominent lucent striations and lack of corticomedullary definition.

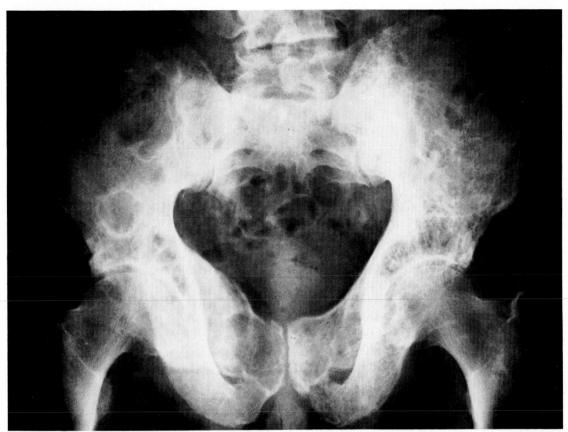

Figure 13.21. Hyperparathyroidism: AP pelvis. Multiple radiolucent lytic defects in the pelvic bones (especially in the pubic rami which are expanded) represent multiple brown tumors. Marked trabecular prominence around the left acetabulum and in the left ilium represent bone resorption due to abnormal elevated parathormone levels.

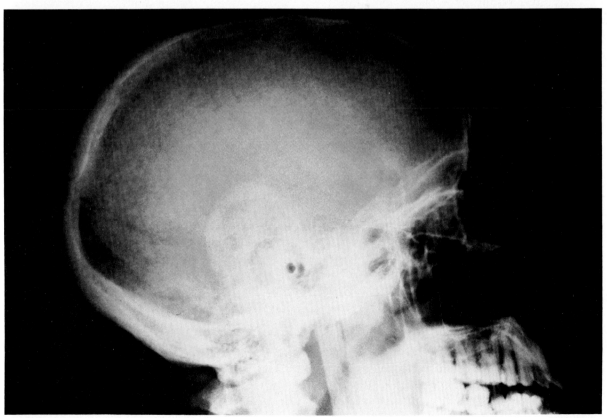

Figure 13.22. Hyperparathyroidism: lateral skull exam. Observe the granular, mottled texture of the cranial vault reflecting bone resorption due to hyperparathyroidism ("salt and pepper" skull).

II. METABOLIC
(Figures appear on pages 346–358.)

Osteomalacia and Rickets

Osteomalacia refers to a qualitative abnormality of bone, a condition where an overabundance of osteoid is associated with a deficient amount of mineralization; the condition is known as rickets when it involves the growing skeleton. A variety of disorders can lead to osteomalacia, with renal tubular disorders representing important etiologies. These conditions include vitamin D-resistant rickets or osteomalacia, renal tubular acidosis, and Fanconi's syndrome. Dietary deficiency of vitamin D represents the classic etiology of rickets which, due to vitamin D fortification in foods, is less common a cause in the United States. Other conditions such as malabsorption states (pancreatic disease, inflammatory bowel disease, biliary tract obstruction), enzyme deficiencies (hypophosphatasia), and long-term use of anti-convulsant medications (vitamin D antagonists) can all lead to osteomalacia. Patients with osteomalacia may demonstrate muscular weakness, non-specific skeletal pains, and skeletal deformity.

RADIOLOGY

There are basically three radiographic abnormalities encountered in osteomalacia: pseudofractures, decreased bony density, and bone deformity. Pseudofractures (also known as looser's zones) represent incomplete horizontal fractures thought to occur through areas of stress. On x-ray they appear as short radiolucent bands, sometimes with sclerotic margins, that are characteristically bilateral and symmetrical in distribution with the common sites of involvement being the inner proximal margins of the femora, scapular margins, pubic rami, ribs, clavicles, and radii and ulnae. Pseudofractures may also occur in the metatarsals of the feet.

Due to the softness of the undermineralized bone, bony deformity may result. Bowing of the long bones of the lower extremity and pelvis, protrusio actabuli deformity of the hips, kyphoscoliosis of the spine, and basilar invagination of the skull may all result (Fig. 13.25).

The skeleton appears undermineralized radiographically due to the presence of non-calacified osteoid. Cortical margins may become thinned and indistinct and the medullary portions of bone may acquire a somewhat coarsened texture due to prominence of secondary trabeculae and a smudged appearance reflecting the large proportion of non-mineralized osteoid.

The radiographic manifestations of rickets are characteristic and are most marked at the major sites of growth in the growing skeleton, these areas being the knees, wrists, shoulders, ankles and costochondral junctions of the ribs (Fig. 13.26). Impairment of mineralization at the zone of provisional calcification of the epiphyseal growth plate results in disappearance of this zone and the characteristic finding of widening of the radiolucent epiphyseal plate, the extent of this widening reflecting the severity and chronicity of the rachitic process (Figs. 13.23 and 13.24). The metaphyses assume a frayed, indistinct and irregular appearance with an eventual and characteristic cupping deformity with metaphyseal widening. The osseous structures are generally undermineralized with thinning of the cortices. Bowing deformities of the weight-bearing bones of the lower extremities are common, while pseudofractures, a finding of osteomalacia, are unusual in rickets. Greenstick fractures, however, may be occasional complications.

Secondary Hyperparathyroidism and Renal Osteodystrophy (Uremic Osteopathy)

The pathophysiology of secondary hyperparathyroidism and renal osteodystrophy is complex and incompletely understood. A full discussion of the physiological and biochemical intricacies of these conditions is beyond the scope of this text. Suffice it to say, secondary hyperparathyroidism represents a response of the parathyroid glands to a chronic state of hypocalcemia resulting from renal glomerular disease (which results in a reduced renal clearance of phosphate and a secondary drop in serum calcium concentration). As a consequence of serum hypocalcemia, a feedback mechanism of homeostasis is triggered with stimulation of the glands and release of parathormone resulting in the various skeletal changes discussed in the section on primary hyperparathyroidism. Other pathophysiologic processes also come into play with chronic glomerular renal disease. With decreased functioning renal mass, a resistance to vitamin D results; this resistance increases as the severity of the renal disease progresses with the kidney becoming less and less capable of producing the active metabolite of vitamin D (1,25-dihydroxycholecalciferol). Vitamin D resistance results in signs of osteomalacia (rickets in children) due to decreased calcium absorption from the gut and from the lack of vitamin D's direct effect on osteoid mineralization. Thus, the major radiographic features of renal osteodystrophy are a combination of signs due to hyperparathyroidism and osteomalacia. A third important feature of renal osteodystrophy, osteosclerosis, further complicates the x-ray picture. The pathogenesis of this abnormality remains in question; while once being thought to represent change due to the anatagonistic activity of calcitonin, this is probably not the case, and this sclerosis may actually represent a direct effect of parathormone itself on bone.

Soft tissue calcification represents an important radiographic feature of secondary hyperparathyroidism and renal osteodystrophy, such calcifications occurring more frequently than in the primary form.

RADIOLOGY

As noted above, the radiographic findings in renal osteodystrophy consist of a combination of signs of hyperparathyroidism and osteomalacia (or rickets), with signs of the former characteristically dominating. The specific x-ray features of hyperparathyroidism are discussed in the section on primary hyperparathyroidism and the radiography of osteomalacia is discussed in that section.

The propensity toward osteosclerosis helps distinguish the primary form of hyperparathyroidism from the secondary form where it is more common. This osteosclerosis most commonly affects the base of the skull, pelvis, ribs, and vertebral column, where selective areas of radiodensity are characteristically located along the superior and inferior aspects of the vertebral body, producing the classic "rugger-jersey spine" (Figs. 13.30 and 13.31). Occasionally, the sclerosis is diffuse, involving all bones, the condition then having to be differentiated from the other causes of diffuse bony sclerosis (Table 13.5).

Periosteal reactive change is sometimes noted, with the metatarsals and pelvis being most commonly involved. The long bones are less frequently affected with this change.

Soft-tissue calcification is characteristically widespread and prominent with calcifications occurring in blood vessel walls, within cutaneous and subcutaneous tissues, and within soft tissue viscera. (This calcification, while pathologically present as metastatic deposits, may not always be radiographically detectable, however.) Occasionally, large calcific masses are identified surrounding joints. These "tumoral" calcific masses, appearing as cloud-like, lobulated deposits, are due to deposits of calcium hydroxyapatite and resemble in all respects the masses of idiopathic tumoral

Table 13.5.
Conditions Associated with Generalized Osteosclerosis

1. Renal osteodystrophy
2. Paget's disease
3. Osteoblastic metastases
4. Osteopetrosis
5. Myelosclerosis
6. Sickle cell anemia
7. Fluorosis
8. Lymphoma
9. Multiple myeloma (very rare)
10. Sarcoidosis (very rare)

calcinosis. Chondrocalcinosis is characteristically more commonly seen in the primary form than the secondary form of hyperparathyroidism. Likewise, brown tumors seem to be more common in the primary variety but are noted occasionally in secondary hyperparathyroidism and uremic osteopathy (Figs. 13.27 to 13.29).

Osteoporosis

While osteomalacia refers to a qualitative abnormality of bone, osteoporosis refers to a quantitative abnormality, reflecting an overall decrease in bone mass. Osteoporosis is obviously a complication of innumerable disease processes, including congenital conditions such as osteogenesis imperfecta (Fig. 13.32), conditions associated with bone marrow hyperplasia with resultant bone resorption such as chronic anemias and leukemia, endocrine disorders like Cushing's disease, rheumatologic conditions such as rheumatoid arthritis, and neurologic abnormalities such as muscular dystrophy. Of concern here is the primary form of osteoporosis known as senile (or involutional) osteoporosis, representing the most common metabolic disease of bone. Occurring in women following menopause and in elderly men, it undoubtedly reflects an abnormality due to the changing hormonal status associated with aging, as well as being associated with dietary factors, decreased physical activity, and decreased intestinal absorption of calcium. Other factors, many unknown, also undoubtedly contribute to a state of negative calcium balance and the development of senile osteoporosis.

Clinically, senile osteoporosis can lead to nonspecific bone pain, particularly back pain. Osteoporotic bone is particularly susceptible to fracture, often with minimal insulting trauma. Serum calcium and phosphorus levels are usually normal unless there is immobilization (which elevates serum calcium).

A specific form of osteoporosis, termed disuse osteoporosis (Figs. 13.34 and 13.35), follows prolonged immobilization that may follow fracture with casting or which may be seen with paralysis secondary to neuromuscular abnormality. This represents a localized form of osteoporosis which demonstrates the importance of mechanical stresses in maintaining normal bone integrity.

Sudeck's atrophy (Fig. 13.36), also known as the reflex sympathetic dystrophy syndrome, represents a special form of localized osteoporosis which is encountered following trauma ranging from minor to severe injury. The osseous structures distal to the site of injury participate in a severe, often spotty osteoporosis which is associated with surrounding soft tissue swelling and edema. The process is characteristically painful. Although the exact etiology of this condition is unknown, it is most likely due to a neurocirculatory disturbance.

RADIOLOGY

Radiographically, a generalized loss of bone density is seen in senile osteoporosis with thinning of cortices and a "washed-out" appearance of the medullary spaces due to thinning and loss of bony trabeculae. (It should be mentioned that it is believed that 30–40% of bone must be lost before being recognized by conventional radiography.) The osteoporosis is characteristically most marked in the axial skeleton, including the vertebral column, ribs, pelvis, and proximal humeri and femora. In the spine, wedging of vertebral bodies (particularly in the thoracic spine), biconcave vertebral bodies, and pathologic fractures are common (Fig. 13.33). Pathologic fractures at other sites, especially the hips, proximal humeri, wrists, metatarsals, and ribs, represent common complications (Fig. 13.37).

Hypervitaminosis A

Both acute and chronic forms of vitamin A intoxication are recognized clinically. The acute variety is important in its capability of producing increased intracranial pressure, while the chronic form, usually a condition recognized in the pediatric age group, results in pruritis, hair loss, hepatosplenomegaly and jaundice, and tender swelling of the extremities.

RADIOLOGY

The important radiologic findings are encountered in the chronic variety of hypervitaminosis A with the production of a generalized periostitis of bone. It is seen initially as a thin, often wavy radiodense line paralleling the underlying bony cortex of involved bones; with time, this periosteal reactive change can merge with the underlying cortex to produce an appearance of cortical thickening. These changes are usually noted in the diaphyseal areas of the bone with sparing of the metaphyses and epiphyses. The most commonly involved bones are the ulna and the metatarsals, with involvement seen less frequently in the clavicles, tibiae, fibulae, metacarpals, and other tubular bones.

Hypervitaminosis D

An unusual disorder resulting from the excessive intake of vitamin D, the condition is important in its ability to produce hypercalcemia and the various clinical and radiologic features attendant to this biochemical aberration. With chronic vitamin D poisoning, symptoms of anorexia, polyuria, polydypsia, abdominal pain, and vomiting may be experienced by the patient. Renal failure may eventually result due to the deposition of metastatic calcification in renal parenchyma.

RADIOLOGY

The important radiographic features are due to metastatic calcification, with calcific deposits identifiable within blood vessel walls, periarticular soft tissue structures, muscles, and other soft tissues. It should be mentioned that such metastatic calcification can also be encountered in a variety of other disorders, including hyperparathyroidism, sarcoidosis, milk-alkali syndrome, multiple myeloma, and other entities characterized by prolonged states of hypercalcemia. Occasionally, large bulky cloud-like masses of calcification are seen surrounding joints. In children, the condition may lead to metaphyseal bands of increased radiodensity due to dense calcification of proliferating cartilage here, and in the adult, the condition may produce a generalized osteoporosis of bone.

Scurvy

Scurvy is due to a chronic deficiency of vitamin C (absorbic acid) which leads to a form of osteoporosis that is most marked and clinically most apparent in infancy (infantile scurvy). Vitamin C is necessary for normal collagen synthesis, as well as for normal osteoblastic activity and bone mineralization, and the deficiency of the vitamin results in abnormal bone development in the growing skeleton. There is also a tendency to hemorrhage, probably relating to a lack of intercellular cement within capillaries. The condition is usually manifest between the ages of 6 months and 2 years, with infants demonstrating pale skin and petechial hemorrhages, swollen inflamed gums, hematuria and melena, and a failure to thrive.

RADIOLOGY

Generalized demineralization of the osseous structures is observed with cortical thinning and a washed-out appearance of medullary bone. Due to a failure of normal proliferation of cartilage cells at the zone of provisional calcification of the growth plate, this portion of the bone becomes more heavily calcified than normal, leading to the so-called "white line" of scurvy at the metaphysis; a similar white line forms around developing epiphyses (as well as at the tarsus and carpus), producing what are known as "ring epiphyses" (Wimberger's sign of scurvy) (Figs. 13.38 and 13.39). The zone of provisional calcification may not only appear denser than normal, but also wider, form-

ing small, laterally directed, spur-like excrescences. On the metaphyseal side of bone beneath the dense zone of provisional calcification, there may be a narrow band of decreased radiodensity representing the area of bone where active bone formation is not normally progressing. It is through this weakened portion of bone, known as the scurvy zone, that pathologic fractures may occur with resultant displacement of the adjacent epiphysis. Subperiosteal hemorrhage is encountered in long tubular bones, notably the femur, tibia, and humerus, and can lead to diffuse periosteal proliferative change surrounding the diaphysis.

With healing, the bones will regain normal mineralization and radiodensity, the scurvy zone will become calcified, the thickened zone of provisional calcification will migrate into the shaft of the bone, and the subperiosteal new bone will merge with the underlying bony cortex (Fig. 13.40).

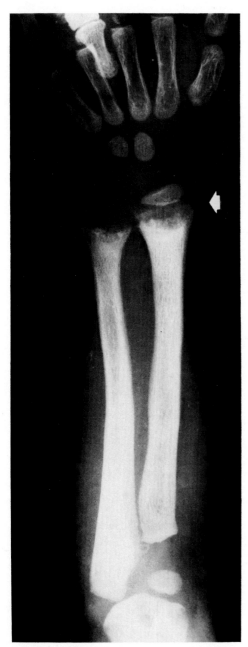

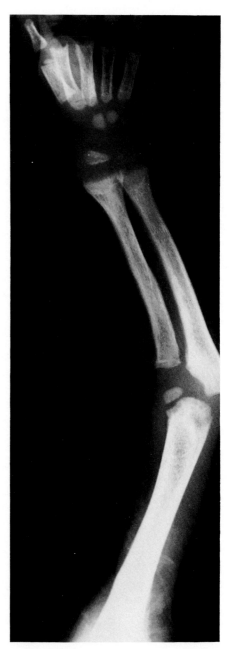

Figure 13.23. Rickets: AP forearm examination. Observe the widened distal radial epiphyseal growth plate with fraying (''paintbrush'' appearance) of the metaphysis (*arrow*). The distal ulnar metaphysis is also frayed and splayed in appearance. The bones of the forearm are demineralized with trabecular prominence.

Figure 13.24. Rickets. AP forearm examination in another patient with nutritional rickets demonstrating findings similar to those in Figure 13.23.

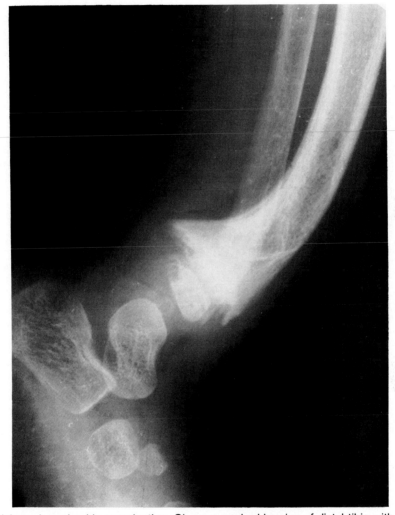

Figure 13.25.   Rickets: lateral ankle examination. Observe marked bowing of distal tibia with flaring of the distal tibial metaphysis. Bony texture is coarsened.

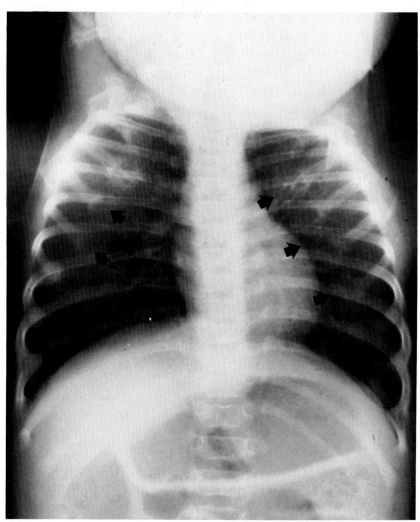

Figure 13.26. Rickets. AP chest examination demonstrating flaring and widening of the anterior growing ribs (*arrows*).

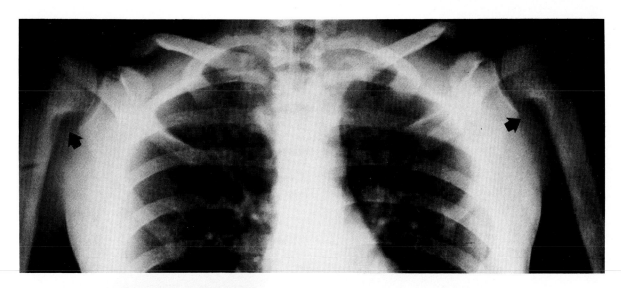

Figure 13.27 (top). Renal osteodystrophy: 22-year-old male patient with chronic glomerular renal disease and secondary hyperparathyroidism. Observe areas of bony lysis along proximal inner aspects of humeri (*arrows*) representing subperiosteal bone resorptive change.

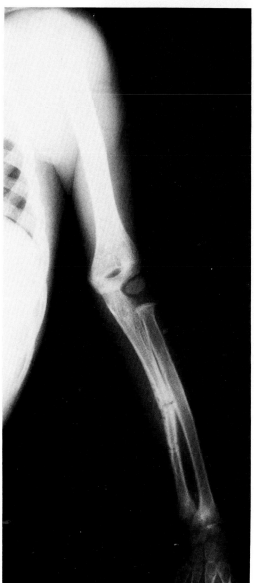

Figure 13.28. Renal osteodystrophy. Arm examination of a child with chronic renal disease demonstrating pseudofractures of the mid-ulnar shaft, rachitic metaphyseal changes at the wrist, and osteoporosis.

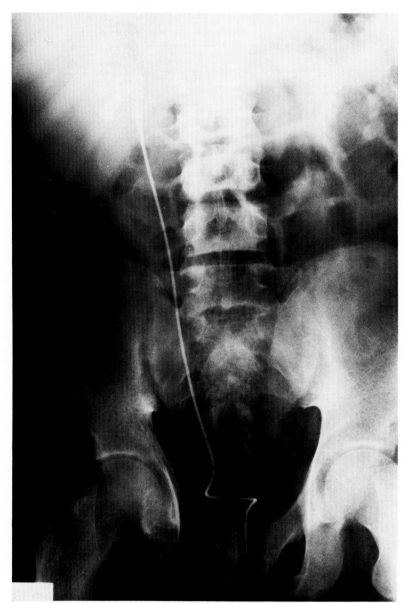

Figure 13.29.   Renal osteodystrophy. Supine abdominal radiograph demonstrating a catheter in the right ureter with radio-opaque contrast filling of a small chronically diseased right kidney (the left kidney demonstrated similar findings on retrograde pyelography). The sacroiliac joints are widened and indistinct due to the subarticular bony resorptive effects of hyperparathyroidism in this patient with chronic renal disease.

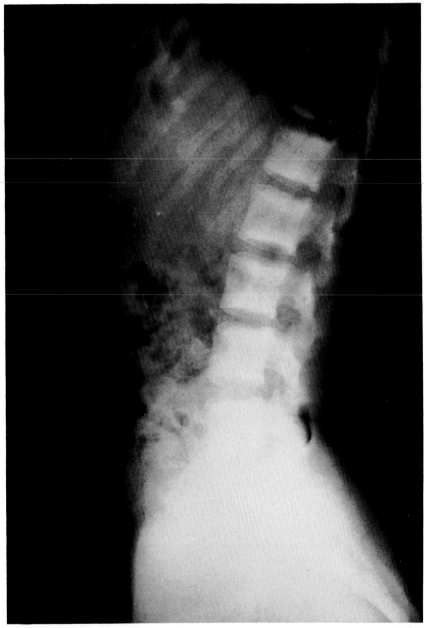

Figure 13.30.   Renal osteodystrophy: lateral lumbar spine examination. Osteosclerotic change along the inferior and superior vertebral body margins (''rugger-jersey'' spine) in a patient with chronic glomerular disease.

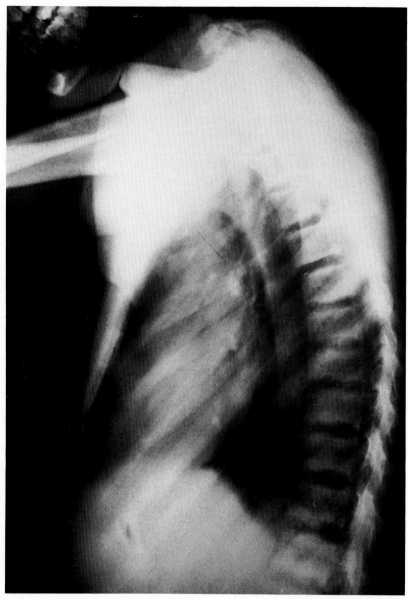

Figure 13.31. Renal osteodystrophy. Lateral thoracic spine with similar "rugger-jersey" appearance.

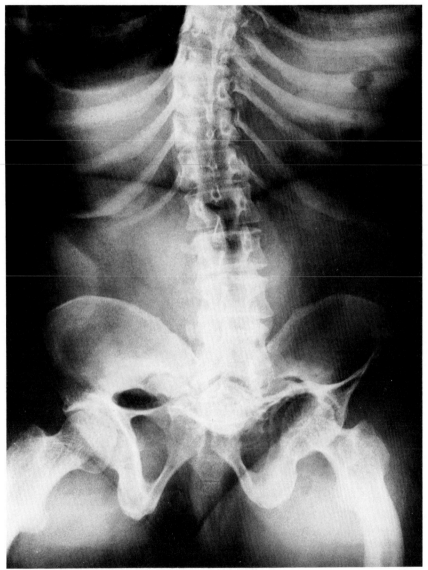

Figure 13.32. Osteogenesis imperfecta. Abdominal and pelvic radiograph demonstrating osteoporosis and marked bony deformity of the pelvis, proximal femora, and ribs in this patient with osteogenesis imperfecta congenita.

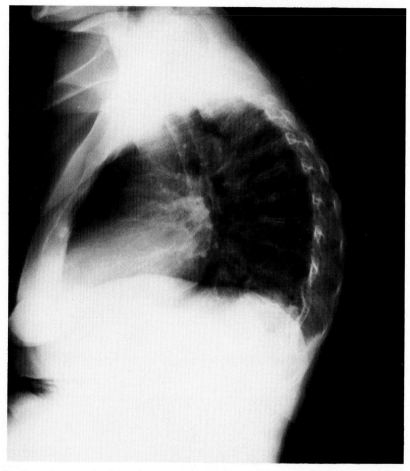

Figure 13.33. Senile osteoporosis: lateral chest examination. Marked decreased bony density of the thoracic vertebral bodies. The mid-thoracic vertebrae demonstrate anterior wedging and compression which has resulted in a kyphotic spinal deformity.

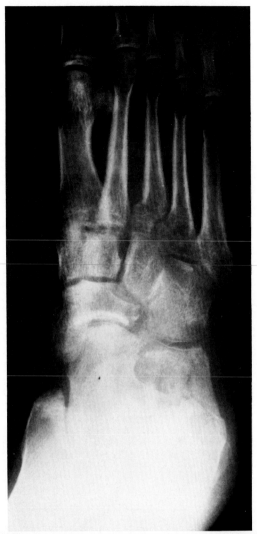

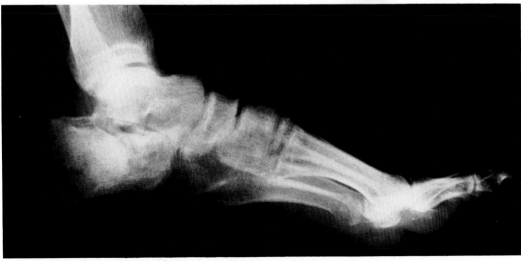

Figures 13.34 (*top*) and 13.35 (*bottom*).   Disuse osteoporosis: immobilization of the foot following calcaneal fracture resulting in osteoporosis of disuse. The osteoporosis is most marked around joint articulations, notably in the mid-foot. Note calcaneal fracture on lateral view.

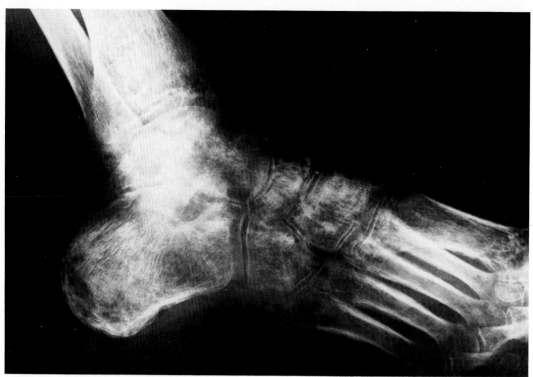

Figure 13.36. Sudeck's atrophy (reflex sympathetic dystrophy syndrome): spotty osteoporosis of an advanced degree in a patient having sustained lower extremity trauma several weeks before the current foot exam. The osteoporosis is most marked in subarticular, subchondral bone. X-ray examination must be correlated with clinical findings for definite diagnosis (soft tissue swelling, vasomotor disturbances, hyperesthesia, and skin changes).

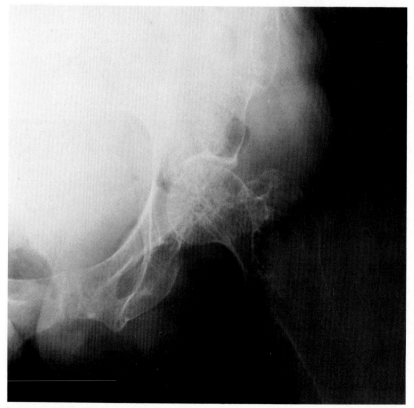

Figure 13.37. Osteoporosis: left hip examination. Marked osteoporosis of the hip in a patient with a neuromuscular disorder. Observe prominence of the residual primary trabecular structures following resorption of secondary trabeculae.

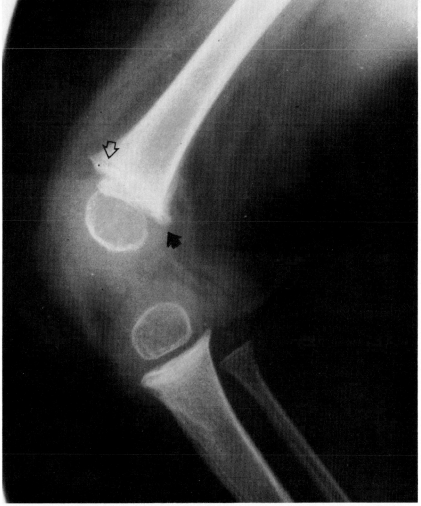

Figures 13.38 (*top*) and 13.39 (*bottom*). Scurvy: lateral knee examination. Observe the classic ring epiphyses (Wimberger's sign of scurvy), the zone of decreased radiodensity beneath the dense zone of provisional calcification (scurvy zone, *open arrow*) and the beak-like excrescences (Pelken's sign) representing lateral marginal extensions of the zone of provisional calcification (*solid arrow*).

357

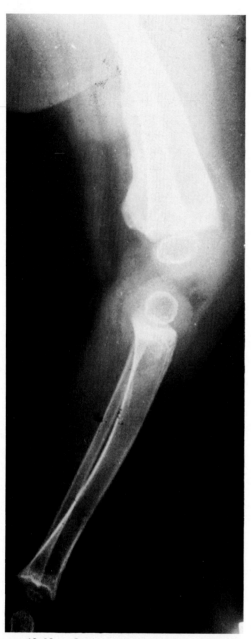

Figure 13.40. Scurvy: lower extremity. Observe exuberant cloaking periosteal new bone formation surrounding the femur in this child with healing scurvy. This reactive new bone formation has followed extensive subperiosteal hemorrhage.

III. HEMATOLOGIC AND RETICULOENDOTHELIAL

(Figures appear on pages 361–378.)

Sickle Cell Anemia

Sickle cell anemia represents an hereditary hemoglobinopathy in which the amino acid valine is substituted for glutamic acid at the sixth position of the beta chain of the hemoglobin molecule. This abnormality can lead to sickling of the red blood cell with a resultant decreased life span of the abnormal cell. The condition may be manifest as homzygosity (Hb S-S, sickle cell disease), heterozygosity (Hb A-S, sickle cell trait), or in combination with another abnormal hemoglobin (e.g., Hb S-C). Patients with sickle cell disease demonstrate the most severe clinical findings and have the greatest degree of bone abnormality on x-ray. They may experience episodes of extremity pain frequently beginning during the second and third years of life, as fetal hemoglobin (Hb F) is replaced by the abnormal hemoglobin (Hb S). These "crises" are secondary to ischemia produced by the sickled cells which clog small vessels leading to stasis, thrombosis, and eventual infarction and osteonecrosis. The crises may be accompanied by fever, soft tissue swelling, and an increased white cell count. Ischemia of abdominal viscera and the central nervous system will also result in painful abdominal crises, headaches, convulsions, hemiplegia, and other clinical abnormalities.

RADIOLOGY

The radiologic findings of sickle cell disease are basically due to two pathologic processes, marrow hyperplasia and vascular occlusion. These pathologic processes are translated to the radiographic as observable and recognizable abnormalities. Hyperplasia and expansion of the bone marrow results in widening of the medullary spaces and cortical narrowing, loss of internal trabeculation with prominence and thickening of residual, nondestroyed trabeculae, and a resultant increased radiolucency of the skeleton. These changes are most notable in the axial skeleton, the skull often showing characteristic changes with diploic space widening and thickened perpendicularly oriented internal trabeculation producing the so-called "hair-on-end" or "crew-cut" pattern (this finding is more commonly seen in thalassemia, however) (Fig. 13.41). Spinal osteoporosis results from marrow hyperplasmia which may produce an appearance of trabecular prominence, the thickened residual trabeculae aligning themselves in a vertical orientation (Figs. 13.46 and 13.47). The vertebral bodies also commonly demonstrate a characteristically abnormal contour on their superior and inferior surfaces as seen on lateral radiographs. Smooth concave depressions result in the so-called "fish," "fish-mouthed," or "H" vertebrae, which are probably the result of compression of the adjacent intervertebral discs into weakened, osteoporotic vertebral bodies, as well as being secondary to ischemic changes in the vertebral end-plates, which causes an abnormality in osteogenesis here (Fig. 13.42).

The feature of sickle cell disease that allows radiologic differentiation of this anemia from other severe anemias is the presence of bone infarction and osteonecrosis. The earliest manifestation of this phenomenon often occurs as sickle cell dactylitis (Fig. 13.43), a disorder seen between the ages of 6 months and 2 years. The condition is also known as the "hand-foot" syndrome and is the result of bone infarction involving the small bones of the hands and feet. Early in the condition, soft tissue swelling of the digits is commonly observed. Bone changes can be seen within 1–2 weeks following onset of symptomatology with evidence of areas of medullary lucency involving the metacarpals, metatarsals, and phalanges, which may be surrounded by periosteal reactive change. Small ill-defined areas of sclerosis may be seen within the involved bones as well. It should be noted that the clinical and radiologic features of this syndrome mimic the findings of osteomyelitic dactylitis, another complication of sickle cell disease.

Bone infarction can be encountered at all ages in both diaphyseal and epiphyseal locations. Involvement of the capital femoral epiphyses, which is commonly bilateral, leads to aseptic necrosis with the radiographic findings of bone fragmentation and subchondral collapse of bone, flattening of the femoral head, bone sclerosis, and secondary degenerative change. Osteonecrosis of the capital femoral epiphysis of a growing child will mimic the changes of Perthes' disease. Changes of osteonecrosis may also occur at the proximal humeral epiphysis, as well as at other sites such as the talus, knee, and elbow. Diaphyseal infarctions are most commonly encountered in the femur, tibia, and humerus. The radiographic appearance of these infarcts is characteristic with patchy ill-defined areas of medullary radiolucency containing varying amounts of serpiginous calcification (Figs. 13.44 and 13.45). Periostitis may surround the area of bone infarction. Occasionally, bone sclerosis secondary to bone infarction with healing will be widespread in distribution throughout the skeleton, leading to diffuse blastic bone disease that must be distinguished radiographically from other conditions characterized by diffuse, dense bones (Table 13.5).

As a sequela of bone infarction, residual bone abnormality can result reflecting growth disturbances of bone. Shortening of bones may occur as a result of injury incurred by the epiphysis with early epiphyseal fusion. Tibiotalar slant at the ankle has been infrequently observed in sickle cell disease (as well as in hemophilia and juvenile rheumatoid arthritis), probably resulting from damage to the distal tibial growth plate with premature fusion of its lateral portion. Growth disturbance of the vertebral end-plates most likely contributes to the "H" deformity of the individual vertebral bodies.

Patients with sickle cell disease are also at risk of developing osteomyelitis, often due to Salmonella organisms. This complication must always be kept in mind in these patients as the radiologic findings of infection (bone destruction, periostitis, and soft tissue swelling) and infarction may be similar.

Thalassemia

Actually a group of disorders due to impaired hemoglobin synthesis, thalassemia is responsible for producing a severe hemolytic anemia which can produce striking skeletal change on radiographs. The abnormality in thalassemia results from a decreased production of either the α or β chain of the hemoglobin molecule. Homozygous and heterozygous states exist with the homozygous form of β thalassemia (known as Cooley's anemia or thalassemia major), producing the most severe anemia and the most marked bone changes.

The symptoms of thalassemia major are most commonly first encountered during the first year of life with findings of severe anemia and pallor, malaise, hepatosplenomegaly, facial deformity, and growth retardation. Patients require repeated blood transfusions for survival, but rarely do they survive beyond adolescence, succumbing from the severe anemia, infection, or complications of the recurrent transfusions.

RADIOLOGY

The radiographically detectable abnormalities seen in patients with thalassemia are primarily due to one pathologic process—marrow hyperplasia and expansion. As opposed to sickle cell disease, bone infarction plays virtually no role in the production of skeletal abnormality seen radiographically. Erythroid hyperplasia in thalassemia major is marked, leading to cortical thinning and expansion of the medullary cavities, osteoporosis due to resorption of secondary trabeculae (Figs. 13.51 and 13.53), and accentuation of residual trabeculae giving the texture of bone a characteristic "lace-like" appearance. Long and short tubular bones lose their normal biconcave contour, appearing rectangular and squared-off (Figs. 13.48 to 13.50). The distal metaphyseal ends of long bones may flare out, giving the bone the so-called "Erlenmeyer flask" deformity. In the skull, the hair-on-end pattern is commonly seen (Fig. 13.52), with the most marked change identified in the frontal area, while the inferior occipital area is characteristically spared. The paranasal sinuses (and mastoids) do not develop normally in these patients as the facial bones become sites of marrow hyperplasia. Maxillary involvement can lead to maxillary overgrowth, with malocclusion of the teeth, hypertelorism, and facial "swelling," features giving the patient a rodent-type facies. This propensity to facial bone involvement is almost unique to thalassemia, rarely being seen in other anemias.

Disturbances of growth may also be noted in thalassemia. In 10–15% of patients, premature fusion of the epiphyses in tubular bones of the extremities occurs most commonly at the distal femur and proximal humerus. Such epiphyseal involvement may lead to shortening and deformity of the affected limb.

Hemophilia

The radiographic bone and joint abnormalities identified in the hemophilias reflect changes due to hemorrhagic events characterizing these hereditary bleeding diatheses. Hemophilia A (classic hemophilia), due to a deficiency of clotting factor VIII, and hemophilia B (Christmas disease), due to a factor IX deficiency, represent sex-linked recessive disorders seen almost exclusively in males. In those patients with severe hemophilia, abnormal and relatively unprovoked bleeding episodes may occur subcutaneously, into deeper soft tissue structures, and notably into joints. This intraarticular bleeding leads to a severe inflammatory arthropathy, constituting one of the important clinical manifestations of this disease. Hemarthroses usually begin in early life, commonly beginning between the ages of 2 and 3 years, with the knee, ankle, and elbow being the most commonly affected joints, probably because these

joints are more susceptible to minor traumatic episodes. As the attacks of joint bleeding are repeated, a state of chronic hemarthrosis and inflammation results with bone and cartilage destruction, periarticular fibrotic change, joint contractures, and eventual muscle wasting. With increasing age, attacks of hemarthrosis tend to decrease in frequency and severity.

RADIOLOGY

The radiologic manifestations of joint disease in hemophilia depend on the number of bleeding episodes into a specific articulation and the chronicity of the process. Early, the only radiographic abnormality will be joint effusion due to the hemarthrosis. With repeated attacks, hemosiderin becomes deposited within the synovial lining of the joint, setting up an inflammatory reaction with increased vascularity of the synovium. This thickened, inflamed synovium may be radiographically detectable, sometimes appearing particularly dense due to the hemosiderin deposits within it. With further bleeding episodes, the inflammatory reaction worsens, the overgrown synovium, or pannus, now capable of producing cartilaginous and osseous erosions and destruction as it migrates across the joint in a manner similar to the pannus of rheumatoid arthritis. Radiographically, joint space narrowing, erosions and irregularity of subchrondral bone, and osteoporosis are seen (Fig. 13.57). The "end-stage" joint will demonstrate severe superimposed degenerative change with subchondral cysts, osteophyte formation, osteoporosis, and joint destruction.

The radiographic picture may be complicated by growth disturbances at the joint which are produced by the chronic state of hyperemia induced by hemarthrosis. Overgrowth of epiphyses and premature epiphyseal fusion in the growing skeleton may result in epiphyseal enlargement and such abnormalities as leg length discrepancy (Fig. 13.59). Uncommonly, epiphysiolysis is noted.

The most common site of involvement is the knee (Figs. 13.54 to 13.56). Radiographs may disclose enlargement of the distal femoral and proximal tibial epiphyses, reflecting accelerated maturation and growth of these centers. Depending on the stage of the disease, varying degrees of degenerative change will be demonstrated with joint effusion, irregularity of the joint, subchondral erosions, and osteophytosis. Specific radiographic features to the knee include widening of the intercondylar notch of the distal femur (which may be due to bleeding into the cruciate ligaments), squaring of the inferior aspect of the patella (a feature also seen in juvenile rheumatoid arthritis), and fixed flexion deformity of the knee.

At the ankle, tibiotalar slanting may be observed (Fig. 13.58), most likely reflecting a growth disturbance with premature fusion of the lateral aspect of the distal tibial epiphyseal plate with consequent overgrowth of the medial aspect of the distal tibia. Bony ankylosis of subtalar joints has also been recognized.

Periosteal reactive change secondary to subperiosteal hemorrhage is rarely seen in children. This finding has infrequently been noted in the phalanges of the hands and feet and in the long bones.

Occasionally, large lytic lesions of bone are seen in hemophiliacs representing the so-called hemophiliac pseudotumors. These represent lesions created by intraosseous or subperiosteal bleeding, resulting in medullary bone destruction, cortical expansion, and a resultant "blow-out" lesion of bone (radiographically resembling aneurysmal bone cysts). These "tumors" may be found in the long bones, jaw, and pelvis, and are occasionally found in the small bones of the hands and feet.

Gaucher's Disease

Gaucher's disease represents a relatively rare condition which is characterized by the accumulation of large, glucocerebroside-laden reticuloendothelial cells (Gaucher cells) in various parts of the body, including the liver, spleen, lymph nodes, and bone marrow. (The disorder is due to a defi-ciency of the enzyme glucocerebrosidase.) The condition varies in its severity. In an acute infantile form, CNS involvement often predominates, with death resulting in the first year of life. A chronic form of lesser severity may lead to patient presentation during the first decade of life or at anytime in later life, with symptoms of fatigue due to anemia or symptoms relating to the splenomegaly which may be marked.

RADIOLOGY

The bone changes in Gaucher's disease reflect the replacement of bone marrow with the abnormal histiocytes. There may be patchy, ill-defined areas of bone destruction or merely generalized bone demineralization. Cortical bone may be thinned with evidence of endosteal scalloping secondary to marrow expansion. Occasionally, bone is abnormally widened, resulting in contour defects of the affected bone (e.g., "Erlenmeyer flask" deformity of the distal femur) (Fig. 13.60). Periosteal reaction is also sometimes noted (Fig. 13.61).

Another x-ray feature seen in this disorder is bone infarction which may reflect marrow-packing with Gaucher cells which results in vascular compromise. Gaucher's disease represents one of the disorders responsible for ischemic necrosis of the femoral heads (Fig. 13.62) (Table 13.2). Aseptic necrosis also may affect the humeral heads.

With long-standing disease, the medullary areas of bone may become sclerotic, representing osseous metaplasia. Occasionally, this bony sclerosis is diffuse.

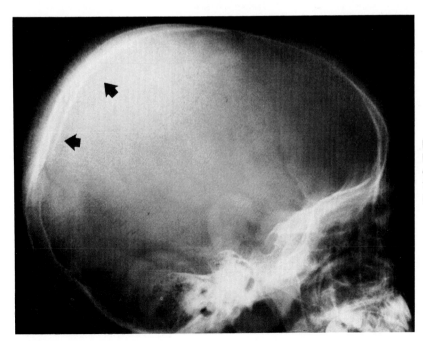

Figure 13.41. Sickle cell anemia: lateral skull examination. Thickening of the skull diploë with perpendicular trabecular striations in the parietal area ("hair-on-end" appearance).

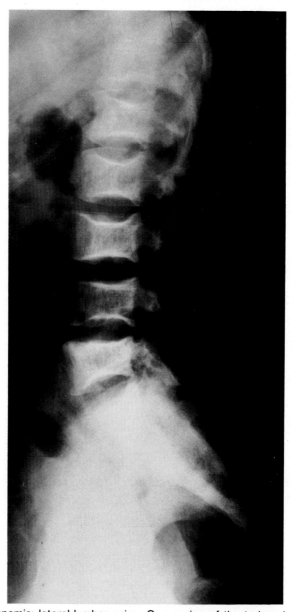

Figure 13.42.   Sickle cell anemia: lateral lumbar spine. Coarsening of the trabecular pattern representing spinal osteoporosis and biconcave deformities of the individual vertebral bodies are observed in this patient with sickle cell anemia.

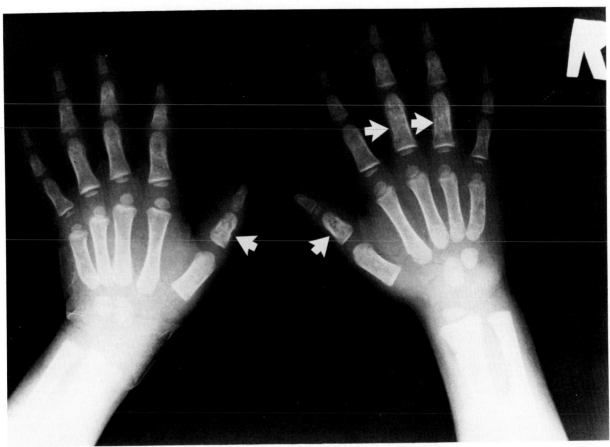

Figure 13.43.   Sickle cell anemia: "hand-foot" syndrome. Observe the dense, inhomogeneous appearance of the phalanges (*arrows*) in this infant with sickle cell anemia. Fine periosteal proliferation is also present in these infarcted bones.

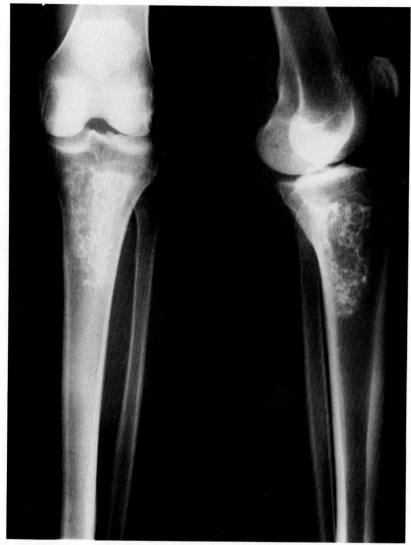

Figure 13.44. Sickle cell anemia: lower extremity examination. Serpiginous medullary calcification in proximal tibia (medullary cavity) representing healed bone infarct.

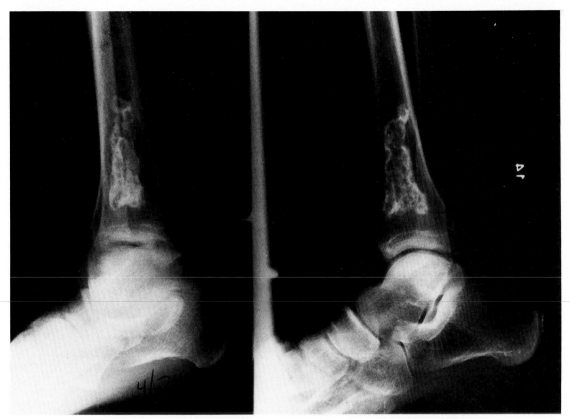

Figure 13.45. Sickle cell anemia. Healed medullary bone infarction in distal tibia.

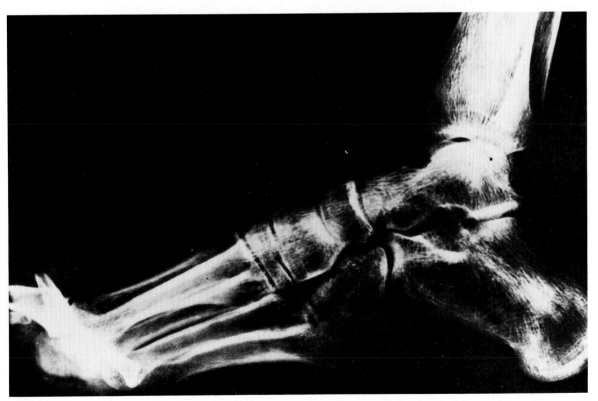

Figure 13.46. Sickle cell anemia. Marked osteoporosis of the osseous structures of the foot in a 30-year-old patient with sickle cell disease.

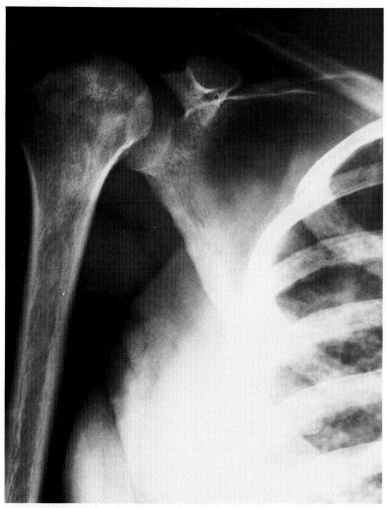

Figure 13.47. Sickle cell anemia: right shoulder examination. Radiographic findings including demineralization and trabecular prominence reflecting marrow hyperplasia and ill-defined sclerosis in the humeral head reflecting relatively early osteonecrotic change.

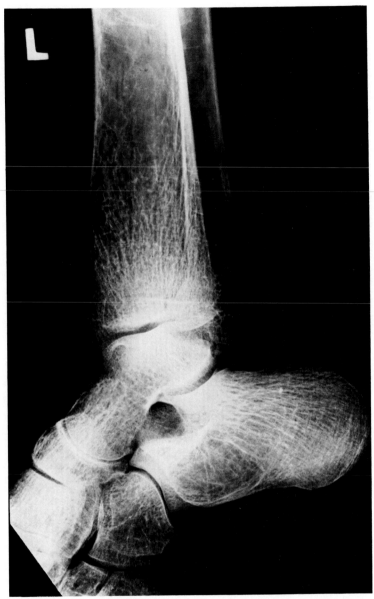

Figure 13.48. Thalassemia. Observe the marked trabecular prominence in the osseous structures comprising the foot and ankle in this patient with Cooley's anemia. The distal tibia is widened and rectangular in appearance (lack of tubulation). Both findings reflect the pathologic process of marrow hyperplasia.

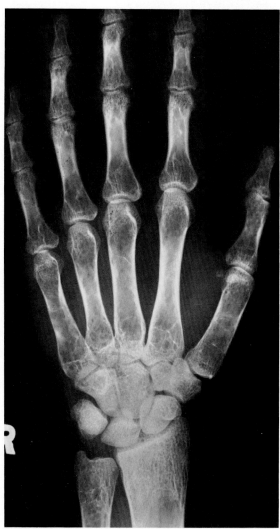

Figure 13.49. Thalassemia. Trabecular prominence of the small bones of the hand reflecting erythroid hyperplasia occurring here. Thalassemia represents one of the most severe of the hemolytic anemias.

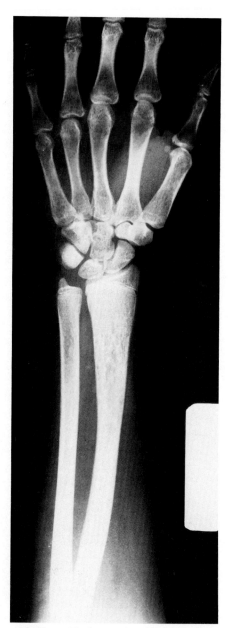

Figure 13.50.   Thalassemia: forearm examination. Observe trabecular prominence and lack of tubulation of the distal radius.

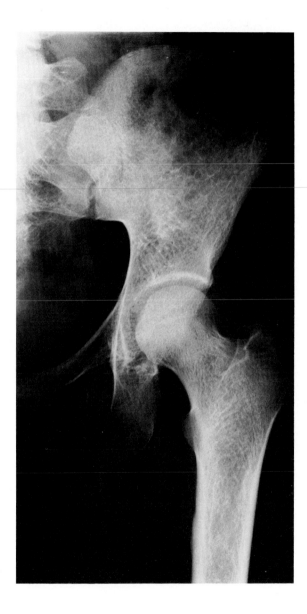

Figure 13.51. Thalassemia: AP examination of the left hip. The osseous structures comprising the hip are osteoporotic with pronounced trabecular prominence.

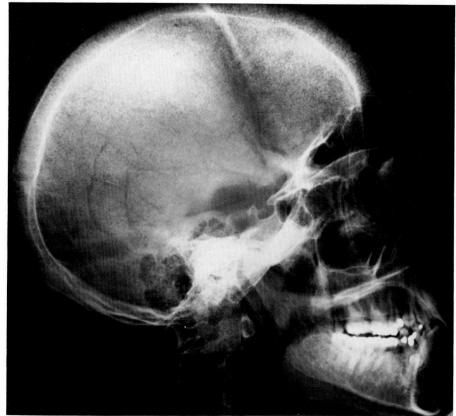

Figure 13.52. Thalassemia: lateral skull examination. Thickening of the diploic tables with a pattern of trabecular prominence (early "hair-on-end" appearance) reflects erythroid hyperplasia occurring in the calvarium. The sinsuses of this patient with thalassemia appear normally aerated.

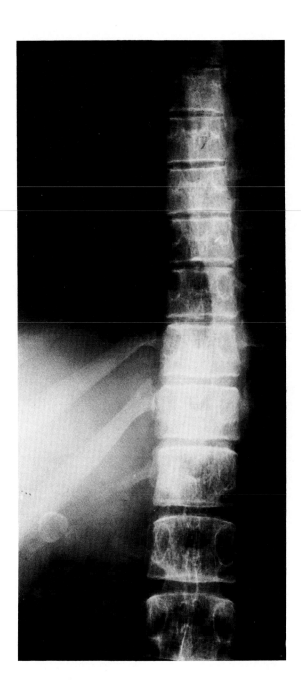

Figure 13.53. Thalassemia: AP spine examination. The spine is osteoporotic with accentuation of the trabecular structures. Observe the abdominal calcification representing a gallstone, a complication of the chronic hemolytic anemias.

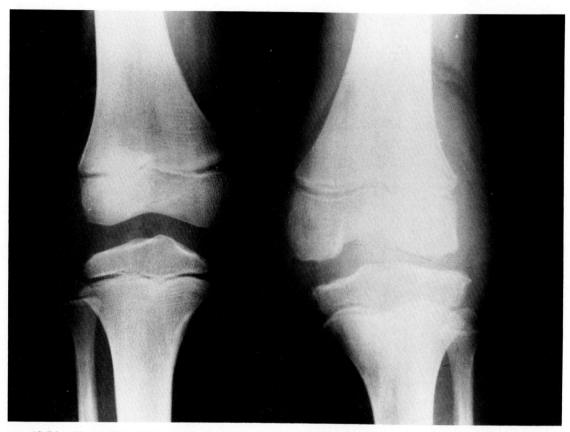

Figure 13.54.   Hemophilia: bilateral AP knee examination. The left knee is surrounded by marked soft tissue swelling representing hemarthrosis. The distal femoral epiphysis is somewhat larger and more irregular than the corresponding right epiphysis (see text).

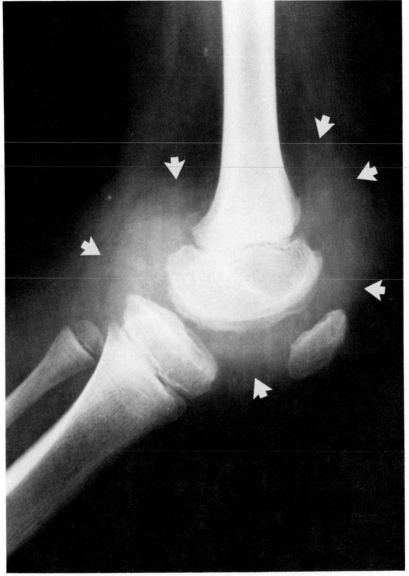

Figure 13.55. Hemophilia: lateral knee examination. An extensive bloody joint effusion in a hemophiliac child occurring after relatively minor trauma to the leg. The effusion is outlined in *arrows*. Observe also the irregular contour of the developing epiphyses.

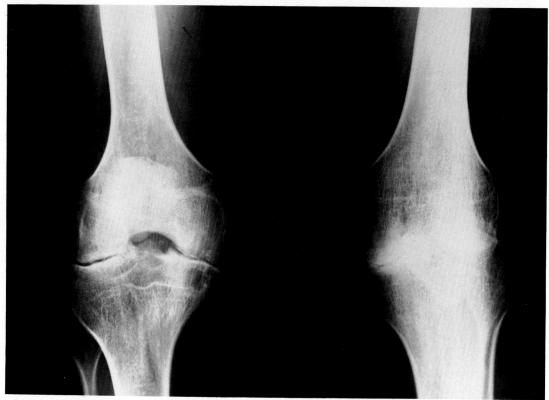

Figure 13.56. Hemophilia: bilateral AP knee examination. Postadolescent patient with hemophilia demonstrating advanced degenerative disease at the knees. The joint spaces of the knee are almost obliterated (particularly on the left). The bones are osteoporotic secondary to disuse. Observe the widened intercondylar notch of the distal right femur.

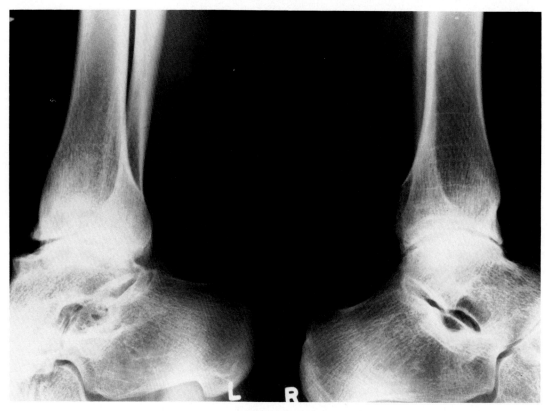

Figure 13.57. Hemophilia: bilateral ankles. Degenerative narrowing and joint space irregularity bilaterally is noted.

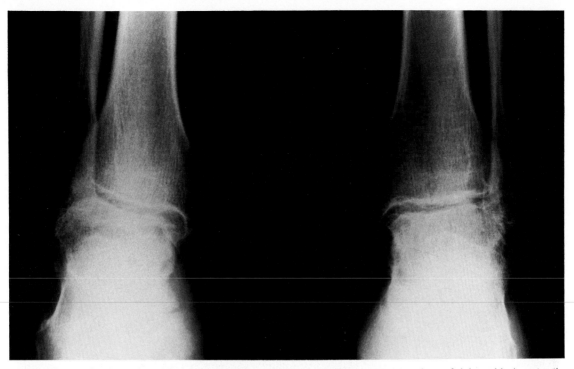

Figure 13.58. Hemophilia: bilateral AP ankle examination. Observe tibiotalar slant of right ankle (see text).

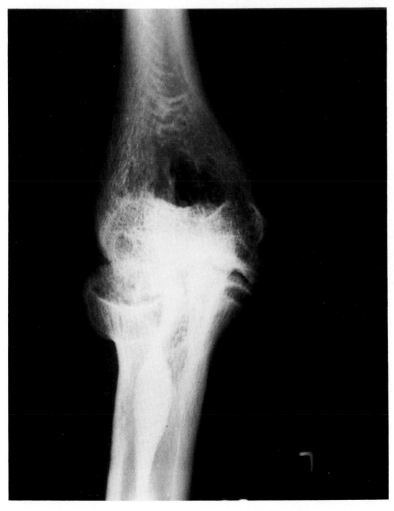

Figure 13.59. Hemophilia: AP elbow examination. Observe enlargement of the radial head (representing a growth disturbance) in this patient with hemophilia.

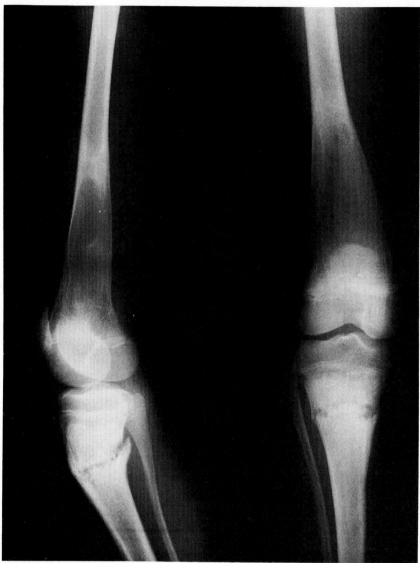

Figure 13.60. Gaucher's disease: AP and lateral lower extremity examination. The distal femur is widened and flared (as well as osteoporotic), reflecting marrow expansion due to marrow packing with Gaucher cells. This deformity is known as an "Erlenmeyer flask" configuration. Observe the pathologic transverse fracture through the proximal tibial metaphysis.

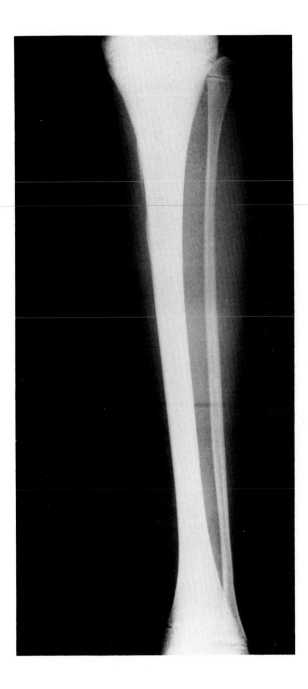

Figure 13.61.   Gaucher's disease: AP lower extremity examination. A fine periosteal layer of new bone is noted along the upper inner aspect of the tibial shaft in this patient with Gaucher's disease. This represents a somewhat unusual x-ray feature seen in this disorder.

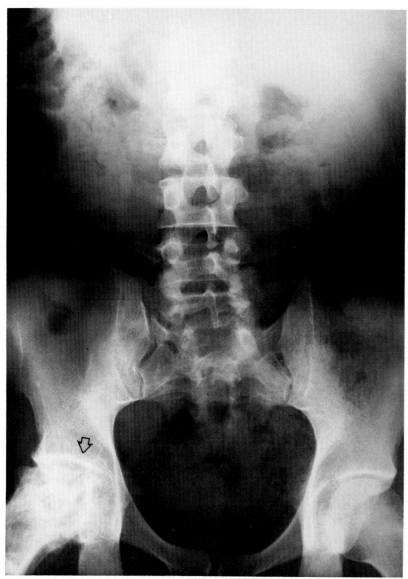

Figure 13.62. Gaucher's disease: abdominal radiograph. The osseous structures of the spine demonstrate trabecular prominence and osteoporosis. The right hip (*arrow*) demonstrates fragmentation, flattening, and sclerosis of the femoral head due to osteonecrosis, a complication of this disorder.

IV. DYSPLASTIC DISORDERS

(*Figures appear on pages 384–414.*)

Paget's Disease

Paget's disease of bone (also known as osteitis deformans) represents a condition of unknown etiology in which there is accelerated osteoclasis of bone accompanied by concomitant osteogenesis of poorly mineralized and poorly organized new bone. The disorder is thought to actually consist of two phases, active and inactive. During the active phase of Paget's disease, there is uncontrolled bone resorption (osteolysis) and bone formation, while in the inactive phase there is a decreased rate of bone turnover. A third stage, that of malignant degeneration of pagetic bone, is also recognized. Each of these phases is associated with rather specific radiographic findings.

Paget's disease, a disorder of middle and older aged groups, is frequently encountered on radiographs of patients being studied for other reasons unrelated to the bone disorder. Symptomatology directly related to the bone abnormality is varied and is probably more common in patients with widespread, multifocal disease (polyostotic Paget's disease) than in those with solitary bone involvement (monostotic). Patients may experience pain localized to pagetic bone or symptoms may occur secondary to bony deformity which is common in this disorder. Kyphosis of the spine, bowing of the long bones, protrusio acetabuli deformity of the hips, and enlargement of the cranial vault with basilar invagination all result from the attendant enlargement and softening of pagetic bone. Pathologic fractures through abnormal bone represent a relatively common complication. Spontaneous avulsion-type fractures at sites of muscular attachment are also noted. Neurologic abnormality and deficits can occur secondary to spinal involvement with pathologic fractures and secondary to basilar impression of the skull. Deafness can result from involvement of the temporal bone with compression of the VIII cranial nerve within the narrowed internal auditory canal. There appears to be an associated increased incidence of arteriosclerosis, hypertension, and congestive heart failure in patients with this disorder.

Laboratory values will characteristically demonstrate a normal serum calcium and phosphorus level, while demonstrating an elevated serum alkaline phosphatase level. Rarely, hypercalcemia is present.

RADIOLOGY

Paget's disease most commonly involves the bones of the axial skeleton and proximal appendicular skeleton, especially the skull, spine, pelvis, and femora. The bones of the more distal skeleton are also the sites of occasional involvement with only infrequent involvement of the small bones of the hands and feet being seen. As eluded to above, the radiographic appearance varies with the stage of the disease. The early active osteolytic phase of Paget's yields lytic bone lesions on radiography, the best example of which is seen in the skull as the entity *osteoporosis circumscripta* (Fig. 13.63). Usually seen in the frontal or occipital area as large geographic areas of bone destruction with relatively sharp margins, the process may on occasion extend throughout the cranium to involve the entire skull. This osteolytic process is sometimes encountered in the long bones of the extremities where a characteristic "blade" of radiolucency is identified extending into the shaft of the bone from a subarticular location; this abnormality is sometimes known as the "blade of grass" or "bayonet" sign.

Most commonly, the process is detected radiographically in its later stages when bone lysis is admixed with bone sclerosis or when there is complete bony sclerosis. The finding of bone sclerosis indicates attempts at repair with recalcification and is responsible for the classic x-ray appearance of Paget's disease. In the skull, there is evidence of calvarial thickening with mottled areas of radiodensity giving the skull a "cotton-wool" appearance (Fig. 13.64). Long bones also may appear larger and thicker than their normal size due to irregular cortical thickening, an important radiographic feature of Paget's disease. Internal trabeculations of these bones may appear prominent and thickened, giving the bone a coarsened texture, and a clear-cut corticomedullary junction is frequently lost (Fig. 13.65). The long bones also may be bowed owing to the softness of the new, pagetic bone. Incomplete or incremental pseudofractures are common, being characteristically found along the convex border of bowed bones; these may progress to frank and complete pathologic fractures (Figs. 13.66 and 13.67).

The pelvis probably represents the most common site of involvement (Fig. 13.68). Usually identified along the ilio-pectineal inner aspect of the pelvis, the process is characteristically blastic here with the x-ray features of cortical thickening and trabecular prominence.

Involvement of the spine may be limited to one vertebral body (producing the so-called "ivory" vertebral body (Fig. 13.69)) or may involve multiple vertebral segments (Fig. 13.70). An important point of differential in distinguishing a pagetic vertebral body from other causes of dense sclerotic vertebral bodies (notably blastic metastases) is the characteristic enlargement of the bone seen in the former. Vertebral compression fractures (and resultant neurologic sequelae) may occur due to the abnormal softness of involved bones.

Involvement of the small tubular bones of the hands and feet is infrequent, but does occur (Fig. 13.72). Most commonly when small bone involvement is encountered, a pattern of homogeneous sclerosis with some bone enlargement is seen. In the foot, the calcaneus is probably the most commonly involved bone, showing cortical thickening and trabecular coarsening (Fig. 13.71).

The complication of malignant degeneration may complicate the radiologic picture of Paget's disease. Degeneration into osteosarcoma, fibrosarcoma, chondrosarcoma, and giant cell tumor of bone have all been described. The radiologic features of Paget's disease become distorted with the additional superimposed findings of malignancy, including frank bony destruction, periosteal reactive change, malignant calcifications, and soft tissue mass. A changing x-ray picture on sequential radiographs should arouse suspicion of this complication.

When Paget's disease is extensively polyostotic, it must be differentiated from other causes of diffuse bony sclerosis (Table 13.5). There is usually no problem in differentiation if the salient features of cortical thickening, trabecular prominence, and bone enlargement are looked for.

It should also be noted that pagetic bone is characteristically responsible for reproducing very "hot" radionuclide bone scans, probably resulting from new bone formation and a high rate of bone metabolism, as well as from the increased regional blood flow to the pagetic bone (Fig. 13.73). The bone scan will accurately determine the distribution and extent of the process throughout the skeleton.

Fibrous Dysplasia

Fibrous dysplasia represents an interesting dysplasia of the skeleton characterized by replacement of medullary bone with fibrous tissue containing varying amounts of osteoid. Often discovered during the first two decades of life, the condition is important due to its ability to produce bony deformity and pathologic fracture. The process, like Paget's disease, may be monostotic or polyostotic in its distribution. Occasionally, the polyostotic variety is associated with sexual precocity and café-au-lait spots of the skin, a disorder known as the McCune-Albright syndrome (seen almost exclusively in females). A variety of other endocrinologic abnormalities have also infrequently been described in association with polyostotic fibrous dysplasia, including hyperthyroidism, acromegaly, and Cushing's disease.

The process is occasionally noted incidentally in patients being studied for other reasons, particularly with involvement of the ribs and small bones.

Distinctly unusual and uncommon, degeneration into fibrosarcoma has been described as an unfortunate complication.

RADIOLOGY

Classically, fibrous dysplasia will lead to osteolytic bone lesions of varying sizes localized to the medullary spaces of bone, and exhibiting a so-called "ground-glass" appearance radiographically. This "ground-glass" appearance refers to a smudgy gray or smokey appearance on x-ray thought to be due to the admixture of fibrous tissue and variably mineralized osteoid. It should be noted, however, that in actuality, all degrees of radiodensity are noted within these lesions ranging from frank lucency to dense sclerosis, reflecting the degree of osteoid mineralization.

The femur represents a common site of involvement, and with extensive involvement of the proximal portion of this bone, a characteristic "shepard's crook" deformity results (Fig. 13.74). The weakened bone becomes bowed, expanded, and radiolucent, and may show evidence of stress fractures or complete pathologic fractures. The entire shaft of any long bone may be involved, or involvement may be localized to a small focus with medullary rarefaction and relatively non-distinct radiographic features. Large masses of fibrous tissue within the medullary canal will lead to endosteal scalloping that thins the surrounding cortical bone. There is an absence of periosteal proliferative change (Figs. 13.75 to 13.77).

Skull involvement is relatively common and may involve both the calvarium and facial bones. Involvement of the calvarium is characteristically lytic, while involvement of the skull base and cranial floors may be densely sclerotic. With extensive involvement of the facial bones, marked facial deformity can result with the patient assuming a lion-like facies (leontiasis ossea deformity). Spinal involvement is relatively uncommon but will be seen with extensive polyostotic disease.

Lesions of the small bones of the hands and feet are occasionally noted, often incidentally (Fig. 13.77). The radiographic features are similar to findings identified in larger bones with medullary lysis, endosteal scalloping, and absence of internal calcification and periosteal reaction. Occasionally, these small bone lesions are sclerotic and blastic in appearance.

Osteopoikilosis

Osteopoikilosis, also known as spotted bone disease, represents an osteosclerotic bone dysplasia characterized by multiple small dense condensations of medullary bone, which is usually unassociated with clinical symptoms. When symptoms are present, symptomatology is classically mild. Minimal joint pain is occasionally present (approximately 20% of patients), as are various skin abnormalities such as a propensity toward keloid formation. The condition is most commonly discovered incidentally in patients over 3 years of age being studied for unrelated reasons. The disorder may be genetically transmitted as an autosomal dominant trait, or cases may appear sporatically.

RADIOLOGY

X-rays demonstrate a classic appearance with multiple small, oval sclerotic foci measuring a few millimeters in diameter. The lesions resemble the small, solitary medullary hamartomatous "bone islands" so commonly noted as incidental findings on bone x-rays (Figs. 13.78, 13.79, and 13.81). The lesions vary in number and are most commonly congregated around joints, particularly around the wrist, ankle, hip, and shoulder. Involvement of the spine and skull is less common. Although a patient with both osteopoikilosis and osteosarcoma has been described, the lesion is best thought of as a benign dysplastic entity without malignant potential. The lesions must be differentiated, however, from osteoblastic metastases and the bony lesions of two uncommon disorders, mastocytosis and tuberous sclerosis.

A related disorder of bone, osteopathia striata, represents a similar dysplastic condition characterized by radiating streaks of increased radiodensity, also characteristically localized around joints.

Achondroplasia

Achondroplasia, representing the most common form of dwarfism, results from a defect in enchondral bone formation. The condition is he-reditary, being transmitted as an autosomal dominant trait; spontaneous mutations probably result in a large number of cases. Bony abnormalities are present at birth in those cases that survive intrauterine life. Many cases do not survive the first year of life, but in those patients who survive this period, life span is good.

Physically, achondroplasts average a height of 50 inches and demonstrate very short limbs, a lordotic spinal curvature with a protuberant abdomen and a shallow thorax, and an enlarged head with a prominent forehead and jaw. There is no mental retardation.

RADIOLOGY

Radiographs display symmetric shortening of all tubular bones with a disproportionate shortening of the proximal segments of the extremities in relation to the distal segments (rhizomelic dwarfism) (Figs. 13.82 to 13.84). The long bones may appear rectangular and broadened and may be bowed with cortical thickening at the sites of muscular insertion. In the lower extremities, the femoral necks are characteristically shortened and the fibula is often longer than the tibia resulting in inversion of the foot. In the upper extremity, the ulna is characteristically shorter than the radius.

The tubular bones of the hands and feet are also shortened and broad, and in the hand a characteristic separation of the third and fourth digits is present, leading to the so-called "trident" hand.

Due to communicating hydrocephalus seen in these persons, the skull is enlarged with a small foramen magnum. The frontal bone is particularly prominent, as is the mandible.

The spine demonstrates flattened vertebral bodies at birth with widening of the intervertebral disc spaces. This widening of the disc spaces often persists into adult life when the vertebral bodies will also characteristically demonstrate concave scalloping of their posterior margins and a decreased interpediculate distance in the lumbar area, resulting in a narrowed spinal canal (spinal stenosis) with frequent neurologic complaints in adulthood. A lumbar lordosis is usual with an abnormal horizontal orientation of the sacrum which is characteristically narrowed. The iliac bones may appear squared and the pelvis small; the superior borders of the acetabula appear horizontal in orientation with flattening of the acetabular angle.

Although the degree of severity of the osseous abnormalities as enumerated above may vary from case to case, these findings in the skull, spine, and extremities are characteristic and are usually diagnostic (Fig. 13.80).

Enchondromatosis (Ollier's Disease)

Enchondromas, representing benign cartilaginous tumors, most commonly exist as solitary lesions of the small bones of the hands and feet. Multiple and disseminated lesions are sometimes encountered, the syndrome of multiple enchondromas being known as Ollier's syndrome or enchondromatosis. The cartilaginous lesions of enchondromatosis are felt to be due to an aberration of enchondral bone growth with resultant involvement of cylindrical bones where masses of abnormal, hamartomatous cartilage proliferate within the metaphyseal areas of the bone. These cartilaginous masses result in distortion of normal architecture and a disturbance in the normal growth pattern of the affected bone. The small bones of the hands and feet are often completely replaced with bulbous masses or cartilage which may grossly deform the bone. There is a high incidence of unilateral involvement of the skeleton in this disorder which is usually recognized in childhood due to the disturbances of skeletal growth inherent to the condition. Unilateral limb shortening involving the lower or upper extremity may result due to impairment of normal epiphyseal growth, usually at the knee and wrist. Occasionally, the first symptoms are related to pathologic fractures occurring in childhood, adolescence, or adulthood. The condition gains further clinical significance due to the complication of malignant degeneration into chondrosarcoma which is occasionally noted.

There is no genetic transmission of the disorder nor is there any sex predilection. When this condition is associated with multiple soft tissue hemangiomas, the resulting disorder is known as Mafucci's syndrome.

RADIOLOGY

The degree of bony involvement in this condition varies greatly with the important radiographic features being those of abnormal and irregular areas of radiolucency at bone ends, often longitudinally oriented, representing the masses of abnormal cartilage extending into the metaphyseal and diaphyseal areas of long bones from epiphyseal locations. The affected areas of the bone will often appear widened and bulbous (reflecting abnormal enchondral ossification), with endosteal scalloping and cortical thinning (Fig. 13.85).

Spotty, amorphous deposits of calcification, the x-ray hallmark of cartilaginous bone lesions, are usually present within these radiolucent areas (Fig. 13.86). The small bones of the hands and feet represent the most common site of involvement where multiple radiolucent lytic lesions are seen which are often expansile and contain spotty calcific deposits (Fig. 13.87).

The lesions of enchondromatosis usually cease growth following puberty. Malignant degeneration into chondrosarcoma, however, may occur, resulting in regrowth of the lesions following this period, a complication which may occur in 5–20% of cases.

Multiple Hereditary Exostoses (Diaphyseal Aclasis)

This condition represents a dysplasia of bone characterized by the presence of multiple osteochondromas of bone (exostoses), usually arising from the ends of tubular bones and in other bones which are preformed in cartilage. It is an autosomal dominant disorder usually leading to clinical abnormality within the first two decades of life. Palpable bony masses are discovered around joints, these masses representing the abnormal osteochondromas which are most frequently noted at sites of greatest skeletal growth, including the knee, shoulder, and wrist. Osteochondromas may be less frequently found in the ribs, pelvis, scapulae, and spine. The lesions grow during childhood, characteristically ceasing their growth upon closure of the neighboring growth plate, and their presence in long bones is capable of causing an abnormality of bone growth with occasional shortening of the involved bone. Compression of adjacent blood vessels and nerves can lead to a variety of symptoms. Just as in the syndrome of enchondromatosis, a malignant potential exists, with malignant degeneration into chondrosarcoma being reported in anywhere from 5–20% of cases. The greatest risk area for this development is in the axial skeleton, notably the pelvis. Skeletal pain in the adult may herald the onset of this complication.

RADIOLOGY

The bony lesion of this disorder, the osteochondroma (Fig. 13.88), represents a benign cartilaginous neoplasm of bone seen radiographically as a bony projection originating from the metaphyseal area of a host bone which has been preformed in cartilage (Fig. 13.89). These neoplasms represent defects in cortical bone formation allowing for enchondral bone growth in a direction perpendicular to the shaft of the host bone. The existence of such multiple lesions will interfere with normal growth and modeling of the shaft (Figs. 13.90 to 13.92). The lesions of multiple exostoses are similar in appearance to solitary osteochondromas but are often smaller in size. Arising most commonly from the metaphyseal area of the bone, they may appear as broad-based, sessile bony projections blending with the underlying shaft cortex of the host bone or they may also produce pedunculated bony excrescences showing a narrow base and a bulbous bony cap. The lesions characteristically grow in a direction away from the nearest joint, producing the so-called "coat hanger exostoses." Osteochondromas also contain a cartilaginous cap which may calcify, sometimes with spotty, amorphous calcification or sometimes with very dense flocculent calcification. The number of lesions varies in the condition from several lesions to hundreds of lesions. They are most commonly clustered around the knees, but lesions can be found in all of the long bones, the scapulae, the pelvis (Fig. 13.93), ribs, clavicles and rarely the spine. There is often resultant shortening of the fibula and ulna (Fig. 13.94). In the forearm, the ulnar shortening results in curvature of the radius and ulnar deviation of the carpus with a subluxed distal radius ("bayonet hand"). Occasionally, shortening of the metacarpals, metatarsals, and phalanges is seen.

Osteopetrosis

Also known as "marble bone" disease or Albers-Schonberg disease, osteopetrosis represents an uncommon bone dysplasia characterized by a failure of osteoclasis. The deficit of endosteal osteoclasis in developing bone leads to a failure of development of a normal medullary cavity, and a deficiency of periosteal osteoclasis leads to a lack of normal bone modeling. The disorder is important due to the failure in producing normal marrow bone and a resultant lack of formation of the normal bone marrow elements. Anemia, thrombocytopenia, and a decreased white cell count can result. Resulting extramedullary hematopoiesis,

in an attempt to correct the deficiency of blood elements, may result in hepatosplenomegaly. It should also be mentioned that although the bones are dense radiographically, they are actually brittle and prone to the development of fracture.

Varying degrees of clinical severity exist. The disorder may be discovered at birth (osteopetrosis congenita) or shortly thereafter, or may be detected in adulthood (osteopetrosis tarda). The congenita form results in the most severe clinical abnormalities with the affected infant showing hepatosplenomegaly, jaundice, adenopathy, pathologic fractures, cranial nerve deficits, and a failure to thrive. Death often occurs in the first year of life. In older individuals affected by the tarda form of the disease, symptoms may be related to fractures occurring through the brittle, dense bones, or may be related to anemia or thrombocytopenia. These patients also demonstrate poor dentition, carious teeth, and osteomyelitis of the jaw.

RADIOLOGY

Three important x-ray characteristics are noted in this disease: increased skeletal radiodensity, modeling defects of bone, and a characteristic "bone-within-a-bone" appearance. The increased bony density, most severe in the congenita variety, is widespread and is associated with a loss of demarcation between cortical and medullary bone.

The abnormality of osteoclastic activity will result in modeling defects of bone, particularly the tubular bones, which will show flaring and underconstriction of their metaphyseal ends. This produces the "Erlenmeyer flask" deformity of the large tubular bones.

The "bone-within-a-bone" appearance refers to alternating bands of radiodensity within bones paralleling the outer bony contours of tubular bones, pelvis, and vertebrae. These linear zones of condensed bone are felt to reflect the intermittent nature of the process responsible for the disorder, and help allow for differentiation of this sclerotic bone dysplasia from other sclerotic bone disorders (Figs. 13.95 to 13.102).

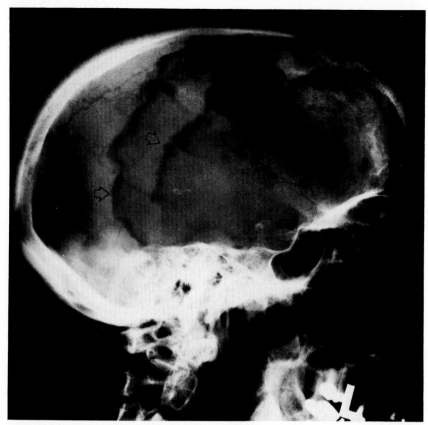

Figure 13.63. Paget's disease: lateral skull examination. A large focus of geographic osteolysis extends posteriorly into the parietal areas of the skull from the frontal region. This represents the lesion osteoporosis circumscripta, the lytic stage of Paget's disease (two advancing edges of osteolysis are noted (*arrows*) reflecting bilateral cranial involvement).

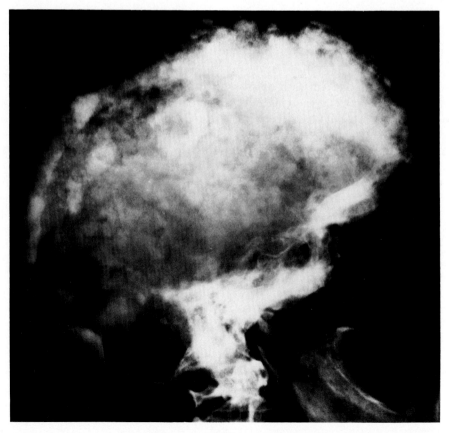

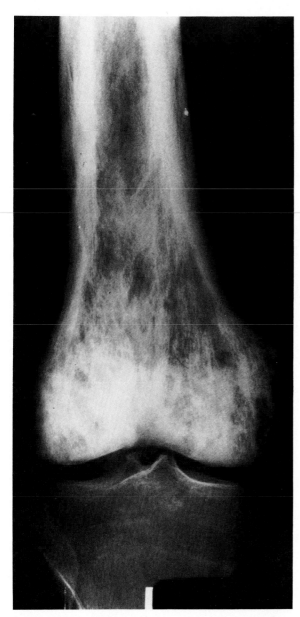

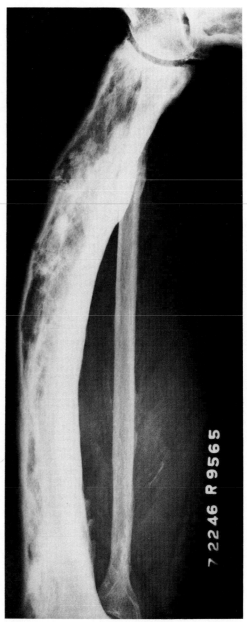

Figure 13.65. Paget's disease: AP knee examination. Pagetic involvement of the distal femur is identified. Observe the increase in bone density, the cortical thickening, and the trabecular prominence. The x-ray appearance is pathognomonic of this entity.

Figure 13.66. Paget's disease: lateral examination lower extremity. The tibia is markedly bowed owing to the softness of the pagetic bone. Small pseudofractures are identified along the anterior border of the distal tibia.

Figure 13.64. Paget's disease: lateral skull examination. Blotchy appearing patches of osteosclerotic new bone and a thickened calvarium give a "cotton-wool" appearance to the skull in this patient with extensive calvarial involvement.

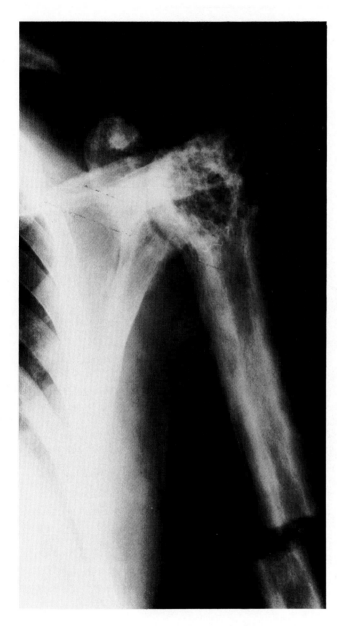

Figure 13.67. Paget's disease: left humerus examination. Extensive pagetic bone change is noted involving the humerus. A transverse pathologic fracture is seen.

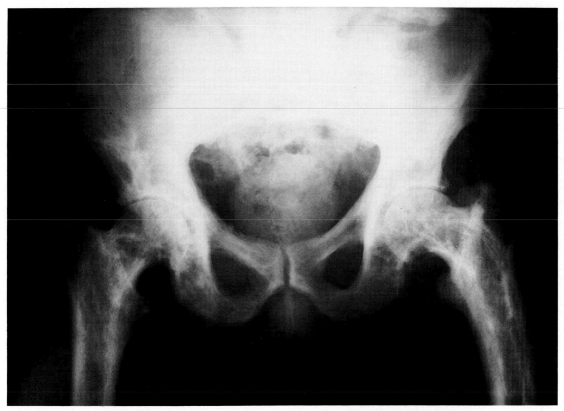

Figure 13.68. Paget's disease: AP pelvis examination. The bones of the pelvis are sclerotic and dense in appearance with a coarsened, mottled trabecular pattern. Involvement extends into both femora.

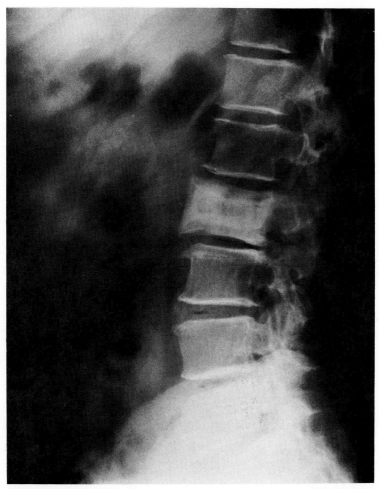

Figure 13.69. Paget's disease: lateral lumbar spine. Vertebral body L₂ is noted to be sclerotic ("ivory" vertebral body); it is also enlarged in comparison to the other lumbar spinal segments, this feature helping to distinguish this condition from other causes of dense vertebral bodies (e.g., metastases, lymphoma, chronic infection, etc.).

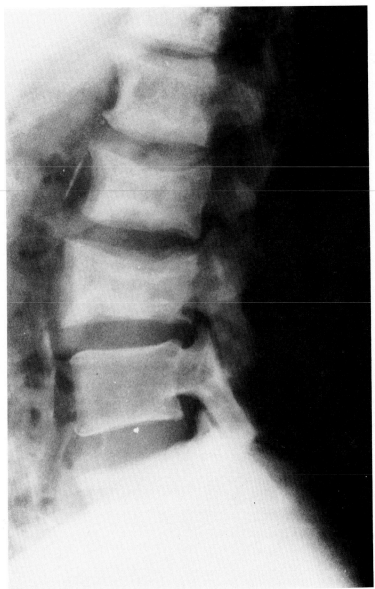

Figure 13.70. Paget's disease: lateral lumbar spine. Involvement of vertebral bodies L_1, L_2, and L_3 is noted with particular enlargement of L_3. Linear calcification anterior to the spine represents calcific atherosclerotic plaques within the abdominal aorta.

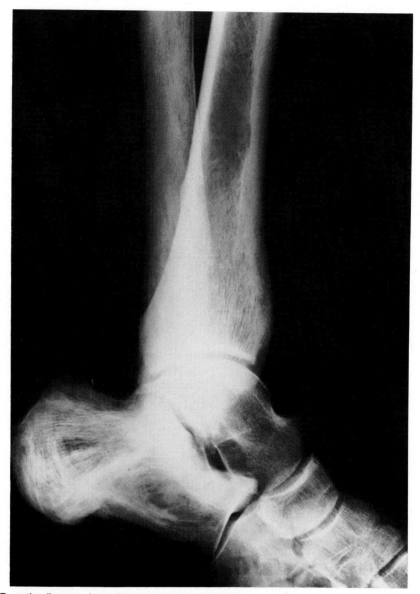

Figure 13.71.   Paget's disease: lateral lower extremity. There is particular involvement of the os calcis which is dense with marked thickening of internal trabeculation. This distal tibia and fibula are also involved.

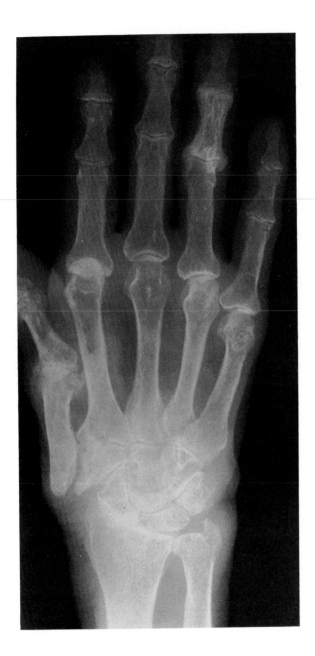

Figure 13.72. Paget's disease: hand examination. Sixty-eight-year-old female with advanced rheumatoid arthritis (note destructive changes and joint space loss, particularly at the wrist) whose hand and wrist study incidentally showed changes of Paget's disease involving the middle phalanx of the fourth digit. Involvement of the small tubular bones of the hands and feet is relatively unusual.

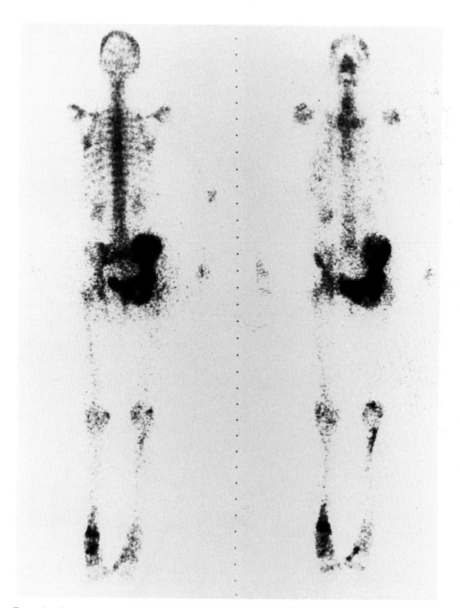

Figure 13.73.   Paget's disease: radionuclide bone scan (Tc-99m MDP). Dense accumulation of the radioisotope in the hemipelvis is observed. This represents a common site of involvement with Paget's disease. (Increased uptake in the right ankle was attributed to degenerative change.)

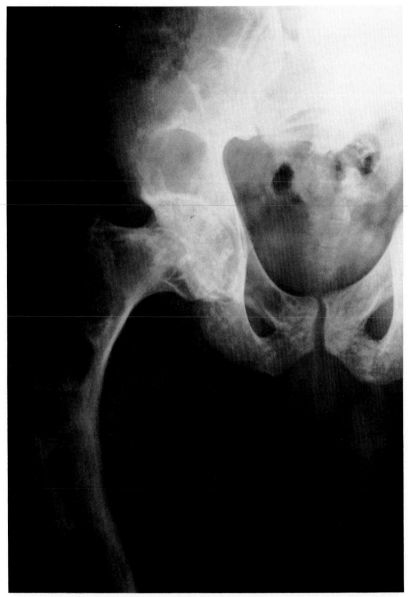

Figure 13.74. Fibrous dysplasia: AP pelvis and right hip examination. The proximal femur is bowed ("shepard's crook deformity") and demonstrates medullary lucency and endosteal scalloping due to replacement of marrow bone with fibrous tissue. A pathologic fracture of the proximal femur is noted. Also, observe the multiple small blastic bone lesions involving the pubic bones, ischiae, and right femoral head in this interesting patient with two dysplasias of bone, fibrous dysplasia, and osteopoikilosis (see text).

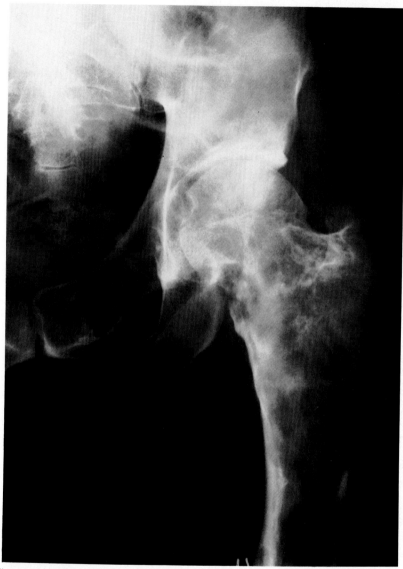

Figure 13.75.   Fibrous dysplasia: AP hip examination. Involvement of the femoral head, neck, and shaft is identified. Notice the deformity in structure of the involved hip.

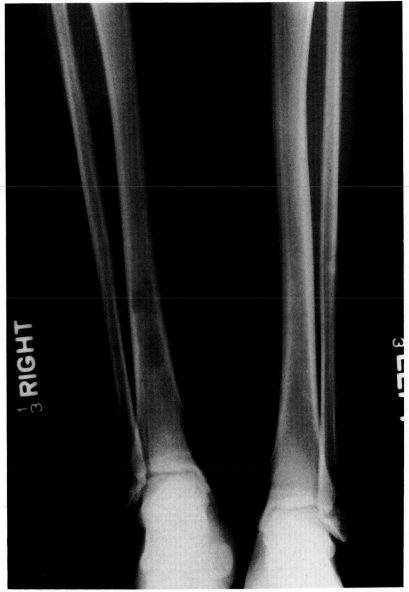

Figure 13.76. Fibrous dysplasia: AP examination of the lower extremities. A well-defined medullary osteolytic lesion of the distal right tibia is noted. It is unassociated with calcification, periosteal reactive new bone, or cortical breakthrough. Endosteal scalloping can be seen. Biopsy demonstrated fibrous dysplasia.

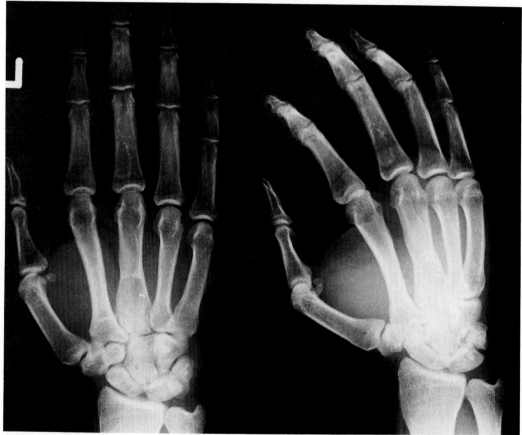

Figure 13.77.   Fibrous dysplasia: oblique and PA views of the left hand. As an incidental finding in a patient having sustained trauma to the hand, fibrous dysplasia involving the third metacarpal, is noted. The bone is expanded with a ''ground-glass'' appearance of the matrix.

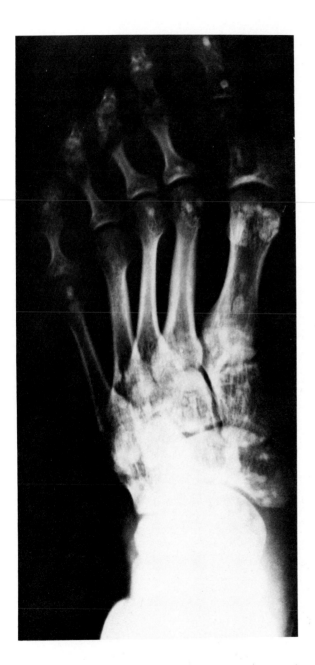

Figure 13.78. Osteopoikilosis: foot examination. Multiple small ovoid densities are identified in the mid-foot and tubular bones of the forefoot. These represent multiple benign hamartomatous ''bone islands'' (see text).

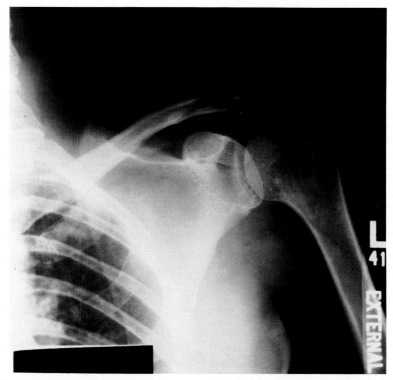

Figure 13.79. Osteopoikilosis: AP shoulder. Small sclerotic lesions of the humeral head are noted.

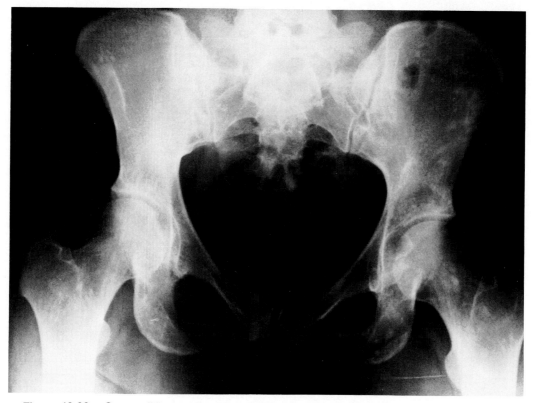

Figure 13.80. Osteopoikilosis: AP pelvis. Multiple desseminated lesions are noted bilaterally.

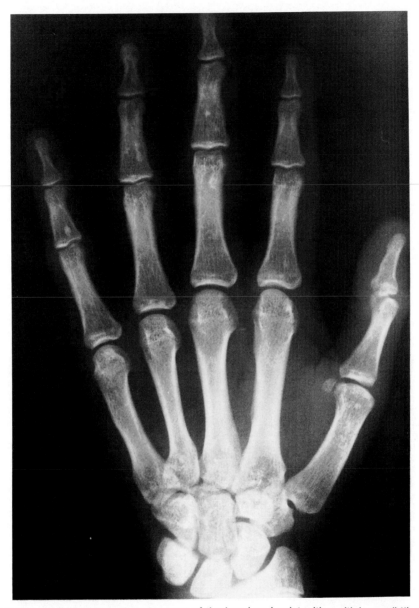

Figure 13.81.   Osteopoikilosis. Involvement of the hand and wrist with multiple small "bone islands."

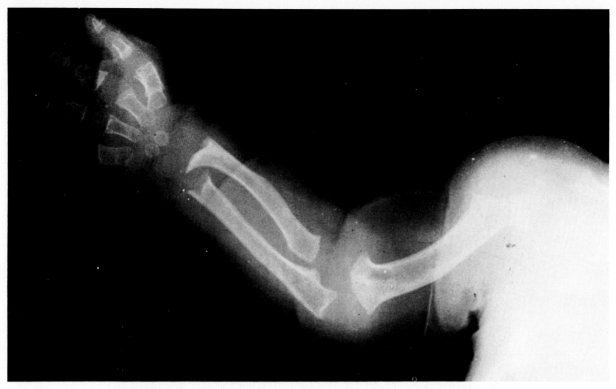

Figure 13.82. Achondroplasia: forearm examination. Shortening of the tubular bones of the arm and hand is evident. The bones also appear somewhat broad and rectangular in appearance.

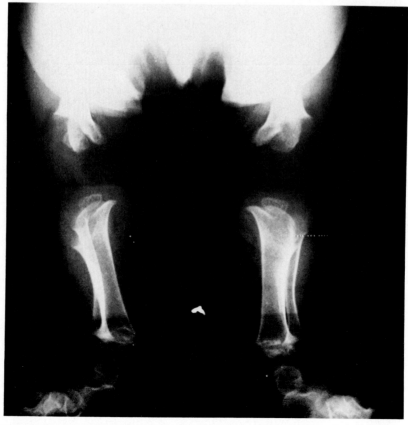

Figure 13.83. Achondroplasia: lower extremities. The long bones are shortened and demonstrate splaying and sloping of the metaphyses.

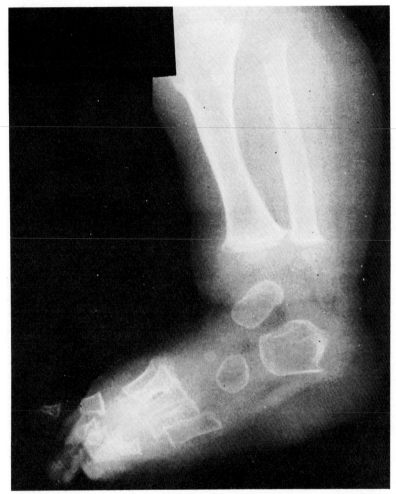

Figure 13.84.   Achondroplasia: lateral lower extremity. Shortening of the long and short tubular bones is evident.

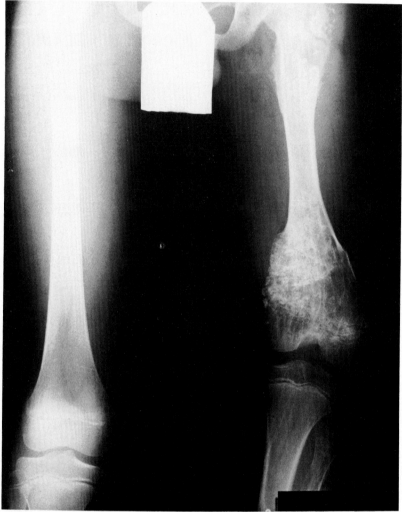

Figure 13.85.   Enchondromatosis: AP examination of the femora. Marked abnormality in bone development of the left femur has resulted in bulbous widening and expansion of the distal femur which is radiolucent and contains stippled cartilaginous calcifications. Proximal femoral involvement is also evident. The involved femur is distinctly shortened (see text).

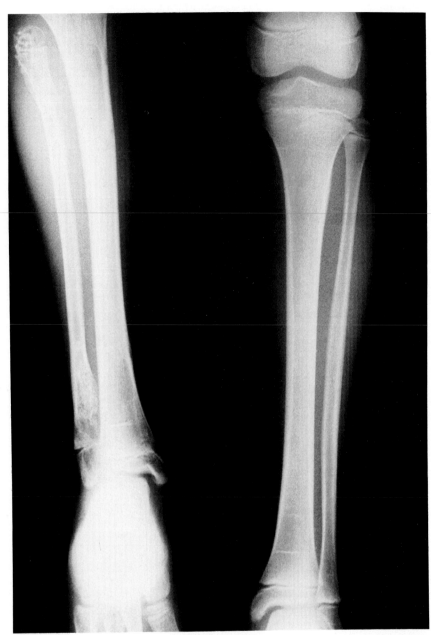

Figure 13.86.   Enchondromatosis: AP examination of the lower extremities. The right leg shows modeling deformities of the proximal and distal tibiae. A few speckled calcifications (particularly in the proximal fibula) indicate the cartilaginous nature of the process.

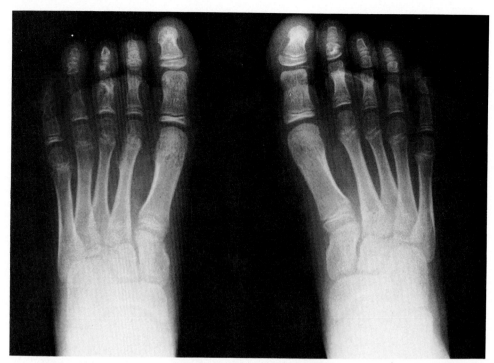

Figure 13.87. Enchondromatosis: bilateral foot examination. Relatively subtle change is noted involving the right third, fourth, and fifth proximal phalanges which are involved with enchondromata. Occasionally, involvement of the small bones of the hands and feet with large, grossly expansile and deforming cartilaginous masses is encountered.

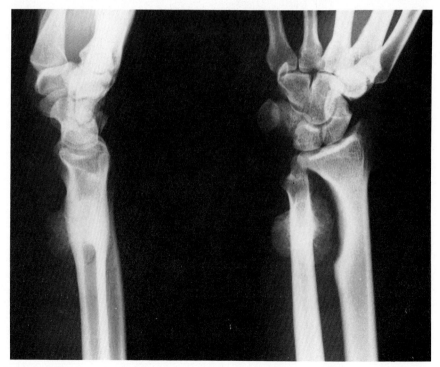

Figure 13.88. Solitary osteochondroma of bone. A solitary lesion of the distal ulna is identified which has caused pressure erosion on the adjacent radius. When such bony lesions are multiple, the syndrome of multiple cartilaginous exostoses results.

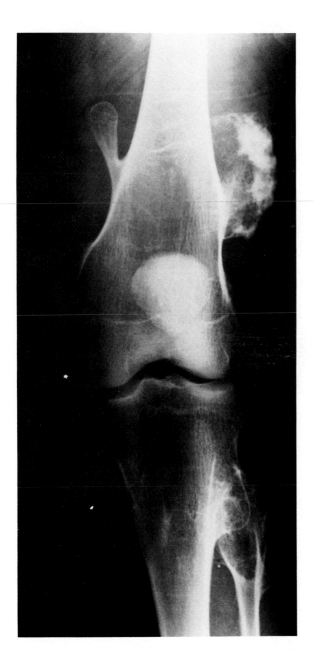

Figure 13.89.   Multiple hereditary exostoses: multiple exostoses are centered around the knee. Pedunculated lesions arise from the distal femur, the largest of which demonstrates amorphous ("snow-cap") calcification on its cartilaginous surface. The pedunculated lesions characteristically grow away from the nearest joint.

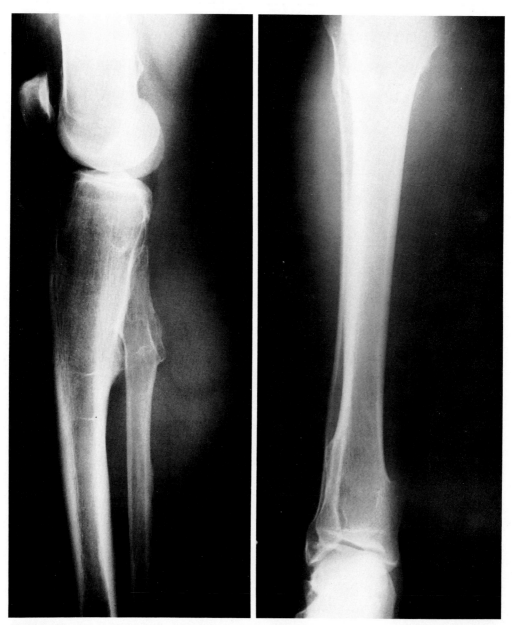

Figures 13.90 (*left*) and 13.91 (*right*).   Multiple hereditary exostoses: lateral examination of the lower extremity. Observe the lack of normal development of the proximal and distal tibia and fibula with abnormal bony protuberances representing exostosis formation.

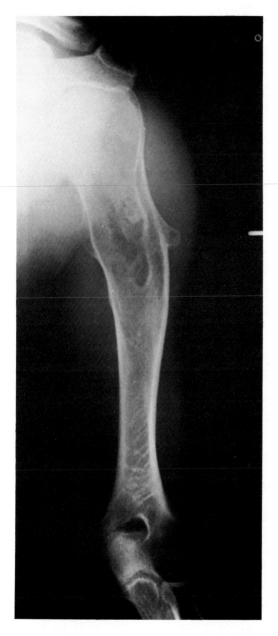

Figure 13.92.   Multiple hereditary exostoses: humerus examination. The humerous displays abnormal modeling with proximal exostosis formation.

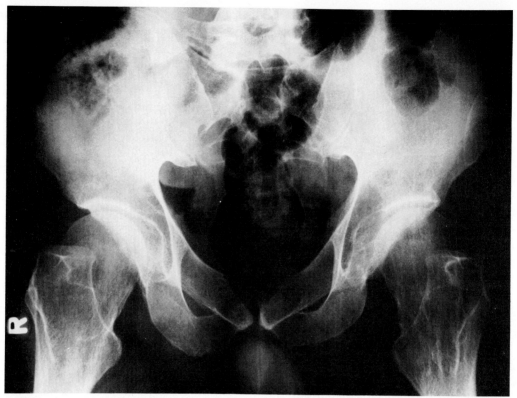

Figure 13.93. Multiple hereditary exostosis: AP pelvis examination. Growth abnormality of the proximal femora bilaterally has resulted in broad and thickened femoral necks.

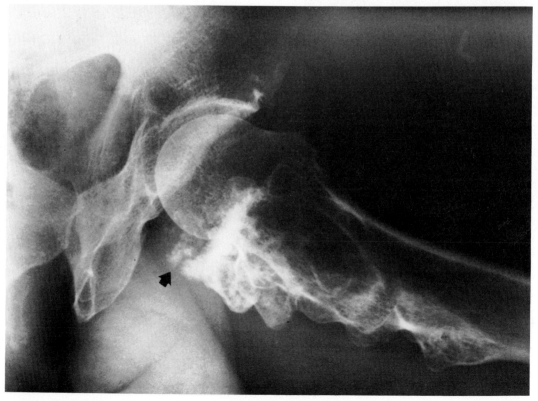

Figure 13.94. Multiple hereditary exostoses: lateral hip examination. The proximal femur is deformed by multiple bony exostoses. Flocculent calcifications cap the most proximal lesions (*arrow*).

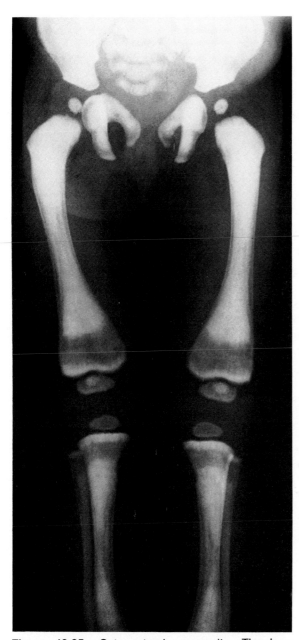

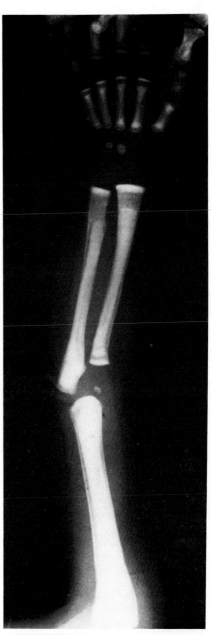

Figure 13.95. Osteopetrosis congenita. The long bones of the lower extremity are dense with the characteristic "bone-within-a-bone" appearance. Observe the flaring of the distal femora ("Erlenmeyer flask deformity"), representing an abnormality in normal bone development inherent to this entity. The bones of this pelvis are also osteosclerotic.

Figure 13.96. Osteopetrosis congenita: involvement of the upper extremity. Observe osteosclerosis of the bones, "bone-within-a-bone" appearance, and the rectangular shape of the tubular bones.

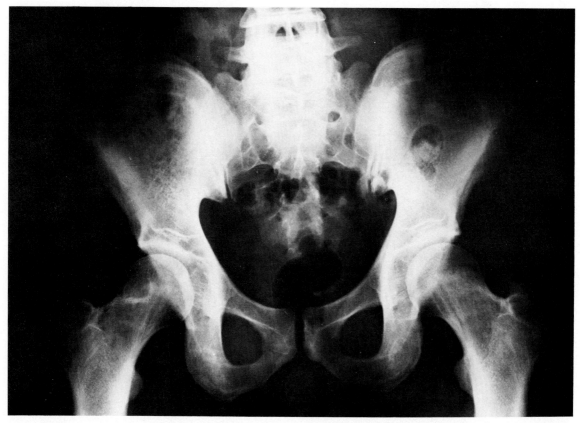

Figure 13.97. Osteopetrosis tarda: AP pelvis. Alternating parallel bands of osteosclerosis are evident in the pelvis.

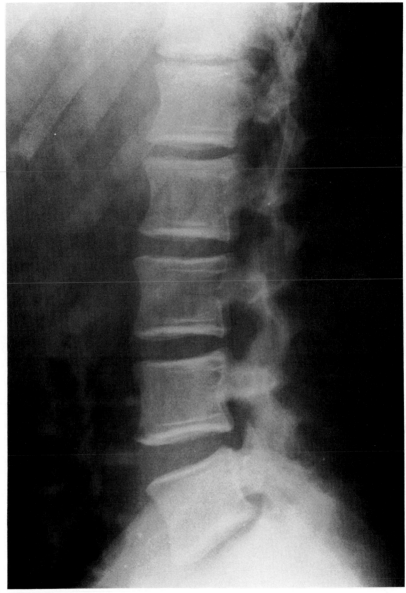

Figure 13.98.   Osteopetrosis tarda: lateral lumbar spine. A "bone-within-a-bone" appearance involving the vertebral bodies is noted.

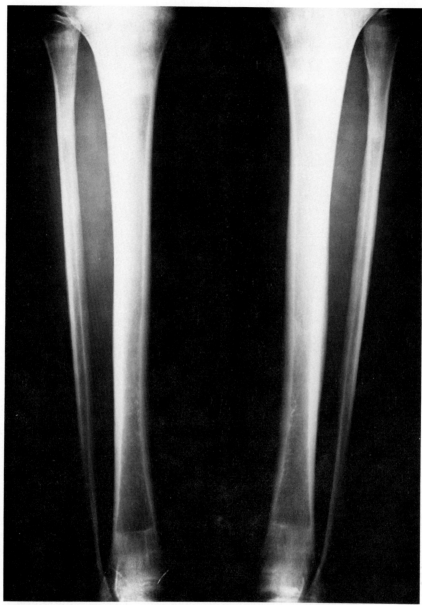

Figure 13.99. Osteopetrosis tarda: lower extremity examination. Bands of increased density are seen in the proximal and distal metaphyses of the tibia and fibula.

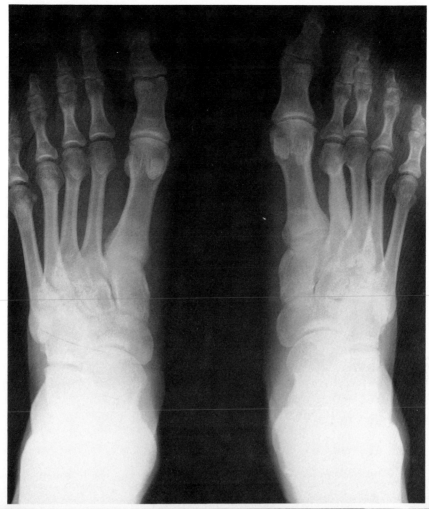

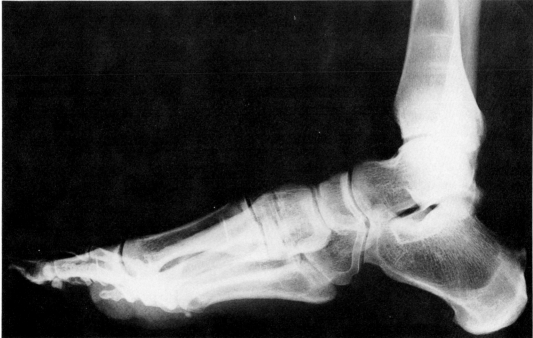

Figures 13.100 (*top*) and 13.101 (*bottom*).   Osteopetrosis tarda. Foot examination shows paralleling bands of osteosclerosis involving the bones of the midfoot and forefoot, os calcis, and distal tibia.

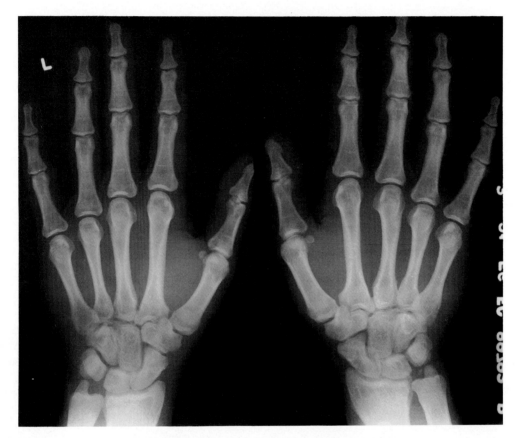

Figure 13.102.   Osteopetrosis tarda: hand involvement.

V. NEOPLASTIC AND PARANEOPLASTIC

(Figures appear on pages 418–431.)

Metastases

Obviously, metastases can produce a myriad of various systemic abnormalities, depending on their site of deposition within the body, with the osseous skeleton representing one of the most common sites of hematogenous spread of tumor; therefore, bone pain represents a common complaint. In childhood, skeletal metastases most frequently result from neuroblastomas, and in adulthood, carcinoma of the lung in males and carcinoma of the breast in women account for the largest number of metastatic cases. By a great margin, metastases represent the most common tumor of bone.

RADIOLOGY

Bony metastases are characteristically divided into blastic and lytic varieties. Although there is considerable overlap, with certain tumors capable of producing both osteolytic and osteoblastic metastases, such a classification can be useful, however, in differential diagnosis (Table 13.6). Mixed osteolytic and osteoblastic lesions are also encountered characterized by both bony lysis and bony sclerosis. Diffuse lytic metastases must be differentiated from other conditions also capable of producing multiple sites of bone destruction (Table 13.7).

Although metastatic disease is more common to the axial skeleton, skull, and large tubular bones, involvement may on occasion be seen in the small bones of the hands and feet. The terminal phalanges seem to be most commonly involved in the hand, with bronchogenic carcinoma being a particularly frequent site of the primary neoplasm. In the foot, involvement is primarily noted in the calcaneus with lesions having also been noted in the talus, metatarsals, and phalanges. Foot involvement with metastases is frequently due to renal neoplasms with tumors of the lung, breast, and colon occasionally responsible.

Lytic metastases most commonly present with relatively well-circumscribed areas of bone lysis involving medullary bone, cortical bone, or both, most frequently without any evidence of concomitant bony sclerosis or periosteal reactive change. Lytic metastases may, however, be very ill-defined, sometimes permeative in character, and if not destroying a significant amount of bone,

Table 13.6.
Metastatic Disease: Osteolytic versus Osteoblastic

Osteolytic Metastases	Osteoblastic Metastases
1. Bronchogeneic carcinoma	1. Prostate carcinoma
2. Breast carcinoma	2. Breast carcinoma
3. Renal cell carcinoma	3. Lymphoma
4. Gastrointestinal malignancies	4. Carcinoid tumor
5. Thyroid carcinoma	5. Medulloblastoma
6. Neuroblastoma	6. Bladder carcinoma
7. Melanoma	7. Pancreatic carcinoma

Table 13.7.
Multiple Lytic Lesions of Bone

1. Lytic metastases
2. Multiple brown tumors of hyperparathyroidism
3. Histiocytosis X
4. Multiple myeloma
5. Lymphangiomatosis and angiomatosis of bone
6. Lymphoma
7. Sarcoidosis
8. Tuberculous osteomyelitis (cystic variety)

can be difficult to detect radiographically. On occasion, lytic metastases may assume a "bubbly," aneurysmal appearance with bone expansion and thinned, eggshell-like cortical margins. Metastases from carcinoma of the kidney and thyroid characteristically are associated with this unusual x-ray picture. Metastatic disease to the spine may involve the vertebral body or posterior elements of a vertebra. Involvement of the pedicle of a vertebral body is characteristic of metastatic disease, and destruction of the pedicle helps differentiate lytic metastatic disease of the spine from multiple myeloma (where the pedicles are commonly spared destructive change). Pathologic fracture through metastatic bone is a common complication occurring in long bones, as well as in the spine where compression fractures and flattened vertebral bodies (vertebra plana deformity) may be noted (Figs. 13.103 to 13.109).

Radionuclide bone scanning is characteristically more sensitive at detecting osseous metastatic disease than conventional radiography (Fig. 13.115). Bone scans may be positive even in the absence of radiographically detectable lesions, reflecting the sensitivity of this modality at detecting skeletal disease before it can be picked up on conventional x-rays. In the patient with known malignancy, the radionuclide bone scan can be helpful in detecting the presence of bony metastases, the extent of such metastatic disease, and the response of disease to therapy (Figs. 13.110 to 13.114).

Multiple Myeloma

Multiple myeloma represents a relatively common bone malignancy, usually seen in patients over the age of 40 years, which is characterized by the proliferation of malignant plasma cells within bone marrow. It represents a condition that is capable of producing protean systemic manifestations. Many patients initially present with bone pain, particularly back pain which is caused by spontaneous compression fractures of involved vertebral bodies. Anemia, which may be severe, is almost always present and may be responsible for the patient seeking medical help. The various sequelae of hypercalcemia, which is common in this disorder, may also be responsible for the discovery of underlying myeloma, such complications including nephrolithiasis, nausea and vomiting, and CNS problems. The malignancy may be associated with amyloidosis (in approximately 15% of cases), amyloid deposits being occasionally discovered in and around joints giving rise to various rheumatologic complaints. Multiple myeloma may also be associated with gout. Susceptibility to bacterial infections reflects the altered immunologic status of these patients with impairment in the production of normal gamma-globulins. Impairment of renal function can be secondary to infiltration of the kidney with malignant plasma cells or amyloid, nephrolithiasis and nephrocalcinosis, renal infection, and tubular injury created by the intratubular precipitation of immunoproteins (myeloma kidney). Death may be the result of renal failure, uncontrollable infection, hemorrhage, or cachexia.

RADIOLOGY

The radiographic findings in multiple myeloma are variable. The appearance of the skeleton may be normal radiographically or the radiographs may merely demonstrate a pattern of diffuse osteoporosis mimicking the changes of senile osteoporosis. This form of the disorder characterizes the myelomatosis form of the disease where plasma cells diffusely permeate the bone without the tendency of forming discrete tumor-like masses. The characteristic and best-known changes of multiple myeloma are the typical diffuse lytic lesions bearing a resemblance to osteo-

lytic bone metastases. The most common sites of this form of involvement are areas of red bone marrow, including the calvarium, ribs, vertebral bodies, pelvis, and proximal long bones. Less commonly will there be detectable lytic lesions in the more distal appendicular skeleton and only relatively rarely will lesions be seen in the small bones of the hands and feet. When lesions of the hand and feet are seen, there will invariably be involvement of other bones. The lytic lesions of multiple myeloma are characteristically well circumscribed, rounded or oval in shape, and are of relatively uniform size, particularly in the skull. The lesions may be associated with adjacent soft tissue masses, a feature which is relatively common in multiple myeloma and less frequent in lytic bone metastases. Spinal involvement may lead to vertebral body collapse (Fig. 13.116) and pathologic fractures through osteolytic lesions of the extremities are relatively common. Occasional lesions are expansile and "bubbly" in appearance, resembling aneurysmal bone cysts. This form is characteristically seen in solitary plasmacytoma of bone (Figs. 13.119 and 13.120), a precursor form of the disease which antedates the occurrence of multiple myeloma as a single focus of disease. Usually, within months or years, other skeletal lesions occur (multiple myeloma).

Probably the most unusual radiographic appearance of multiple myeloma is bone sclerosis, either focal or diffuse. When focal, the condition will resemble osteoblastic metastatic disease, and when diffuse, it must be differentiated from the many causes of diffuse dense bones. It should be noted that osteosclerotic lesions of multiple myeloma may result following irradiation or chemotherapy of the more characteristic lytic lesions.

It should also be mentioned that bone scanning with radionuclides characteristically yields a negative bone scan, even with evidence of widespread bony involvement. This is felt to reflect the purely osteolytic character of the osteolytic bone lesions of multiple myeloma which demonstrate no concomitant osteogenesis and bone repair, factors felt to be necessary in the production of positive nuclear scans.

In summary, the plain film findings in multiple myeloma vary, with several different x-ray patterns possible, including (Figs. 13.117, 13.118, and 13.121):

1. Normal appearance of the osseous structures
2. Generalized bone demineralization
3. Multiple "punched-out" lesions

4. Expansile "bubbly" lesions
5. Widespread bone destruction
6. Osteosclerosis (very rare)

Hypertrophic Pulmonary Osteoarthropathy (HPO)

An intriguing disorder of unclear etiology, HPO represents a triad of abnormality consisting of clubbing of the digits of the hands and feet, periostitis of bone, and synovitis. It is occasionally encountered in patients with bronchogenic carcinoma, thus representing one of the various paraneoplastic syndromes of this group of neoplasms. The condition may also be seen secondary to a variety of other chest and lung disorders, as well as secondary to conditions occurring outside the chest (hence, some prefer the term secondary hypertrophic osteoarthropathy to hypertrophic pulmonary osteoarthropathy). Mesotheliomas, bronchiectasis, cystic fibrosis, empyema, lung metastases, cyanotic congenital heart disease, inflammatory bowel disease, biliary cirrhosis, and nasopharyngeal carcinoma are all conditions that can lead to the development of this entity. Occasionally, the symptoms of HPO are responsible for a patient's initial clinical presentation, the underlying abnormality being discovered after x-rays demonstrate the characteristic periostitis of the extremities. Patients may experience joint pain involving the knees, ankles, elbows, wrists, or metacarpophalangeal joints, and synovial effusion may be present. The periostitis may on occasion be painful. Clubbing of the digits may be accompanied by skin thickening and swelling of the extremities, hands, and feet. The clubbing is often painful with an erythematous rim surrounding the bases of the nails of affected digits.

RADIOLOGY

The finding of disseminated periosteal reactive change in the long bones of the extremities and in the short tubular bones of the hands and feet should arouse suspicion of this entity. Characteristically, the periostitis involves the tibiae and fibulae, radii and ulnae, the femora, and occasionally the metatarsals, metacarpals, and phalanges. The periostitis affects the diaphyses and metaphyses while sparing the epiphyses. Various radiographic patterns of periostitis may be noted, including a simple linear form, a lamellated, onion-skin type, or a thickened, undulating variety. The periosteal new bone may eventually merge with the underlying bony cortex resulting in cortical thickening. Juxtaarticular osteoporosis, particularly around small joints, is usually noted. Digital clubbing may be recognized radiographically with acral soft-tissue prominence and occasional resorption of the osseous tufts.

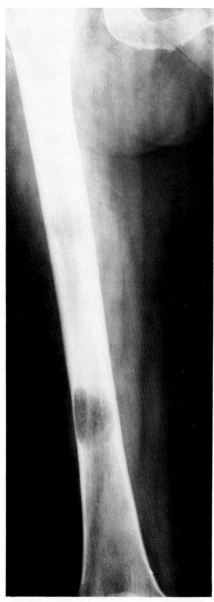

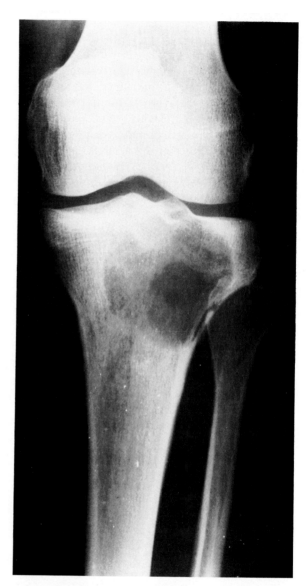

Figure 13.103. Metastases. Two large osteolytic metastatic deposits are identified in the femur in this 42-year-old woman with breast carcinoma. Notice the medullary location of the lesions with endosteal scalloping. Breast carcinoma represents a common neoplasm responsible for bony metastatic disease.

Figure 13.104. Metastases. A large lytic lesion of the proximal tibia is noted representing a metastasis from primary renal cell carcinoma. This represented the only focus of metastatic bone disease in this middle-aged male patient who presented with hematuria.

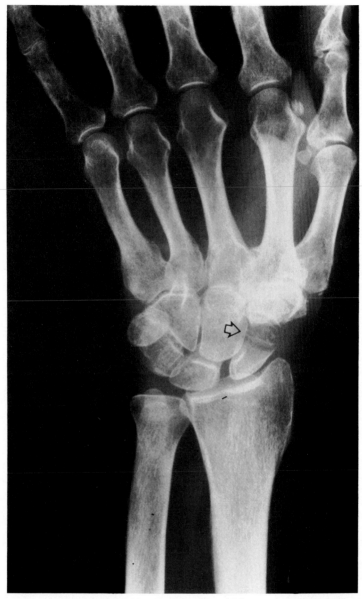

Figure 13.105.   Metastases. Hand and wrist examination of a middle-aged male patient who presented with pain in the wrist demonstrates destruction of the distal half of the navicular bone due to metastatic involvement (*arrow*). The primary neoplasm was a bronchogenic carcinoma. Small-bone involvement with metastases is occasionally encountered, with bronchogenic lung tumors commonly responsible.

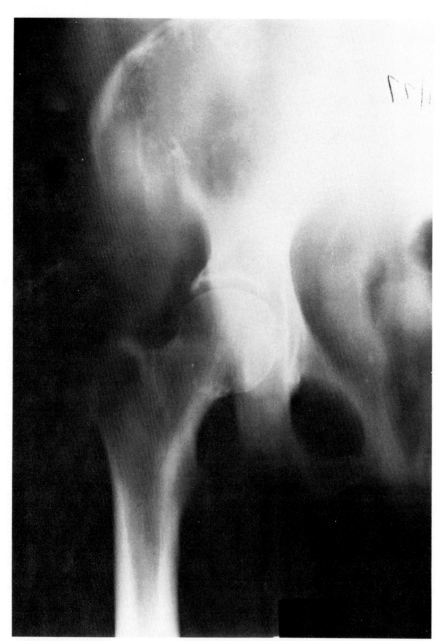

Figure 13.106. Metastases. Tomogram of the right hemipelvis and femur demonstrates a large lytic lesion of the right pelvis proven to be an expansile metastatic deposit from a renal cell carcinoma.

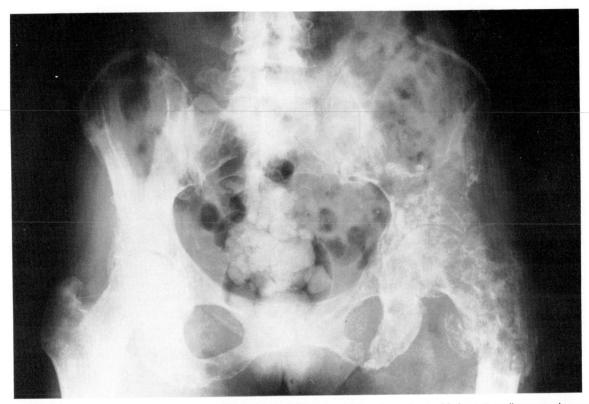

Figure 13.107.   Metastases: AP pelvis examination. A 57-year-old female patient with breast malignancy demonstrates extensive osteolytic metastatic disease, particularly of the left hemipelvis and proximal femur. Notice the pathologic fracture of the left femur.

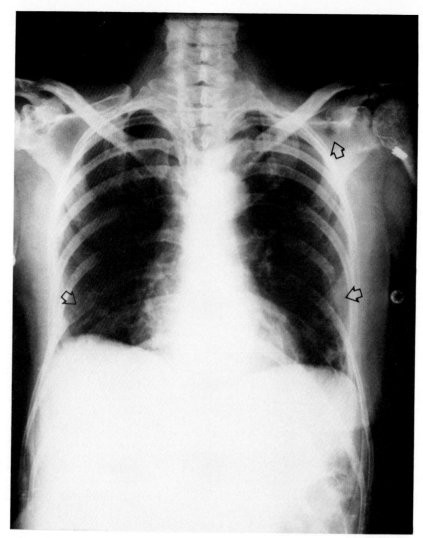

Figure 13.108. Metastases: PA chest examination. Multiple lytic bone lesions are identified (*arrows*), particularly involving the ribs. Primary neoplasm was breast carcinoma.

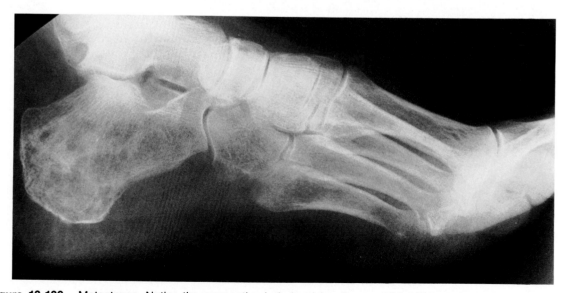

Figure 13.109. Metastases. Notice the permeative lysis involving the os calcis. This patient with bronchogenic carcinoma presented clinically with heel pain.

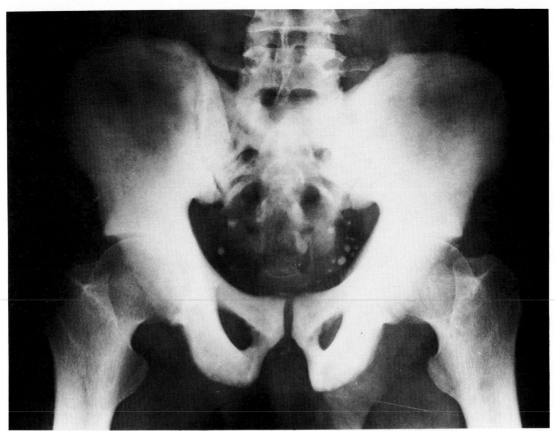

Figure 13.110. Metastases: AP pelvis examination. The pelvis is homogeneously osteosclerotic due to osteoblastic metastatic bone involvement secondary to adenocarcinoma of the prostate.

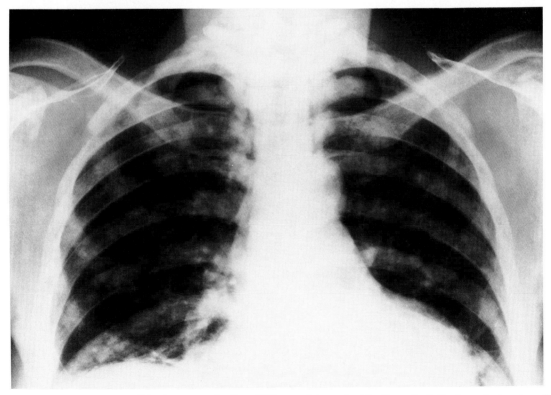

Figure 13.111. Metastases: PA chest examination. Diffuse patchy osteoblastic metastatic deposits involve all the osseous structures in this patient with prostate carcinoma.

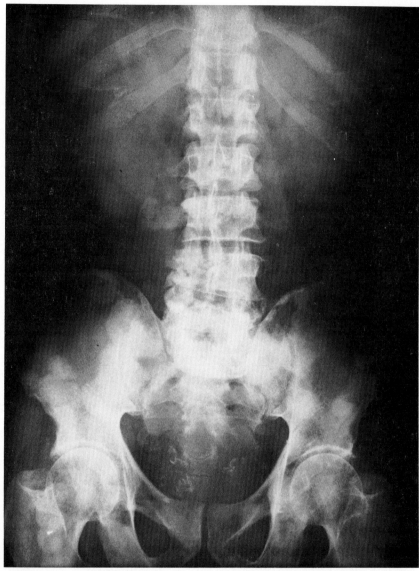

Figure 13.112. Metastases. Rounded osteoblastic metastatic disease to the pelvis is evident. Calcifications incidentally noted in the pelvis have been deposited in the seminal vesicles and vascular structures in this patient with prostate carcinoma and hypercalcemia.

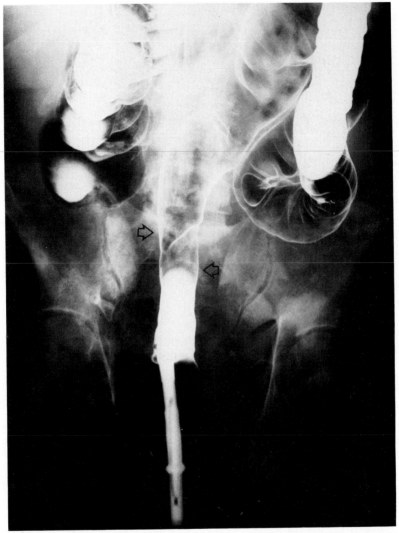

Figure 13.113. Metastases: barium enema examination. Patchy osteoblastic metastases involve the pelvis. The rectum and rectosigmoid colon (*arrows*) are circumferentially compressed within the pelvis by prostate carcinoma and carcinomatous involvement of pelvis lymph nodes.

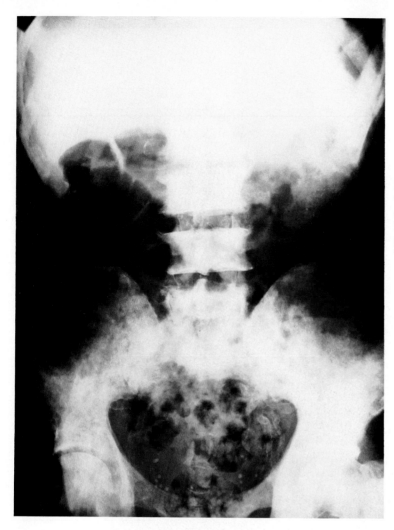

Figure 13.114. Metastases. Widespread osteosclerotic bone change is identified secondary to osteoblastic metastases. The primary lesion was a malignant carcinoid tumor of the gastrointestinal tract. Notice the extensive vascular calcification in the pelvis.

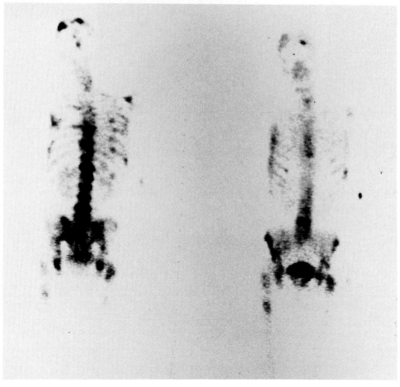

Figure 13.115. Metastases: radionuclide bone scan (TC-99m MDP). Posterior and anterior images demonstrate multiple "hot" foci of activity in a patient with disseminated metastases from carcinoma of the thyroid.

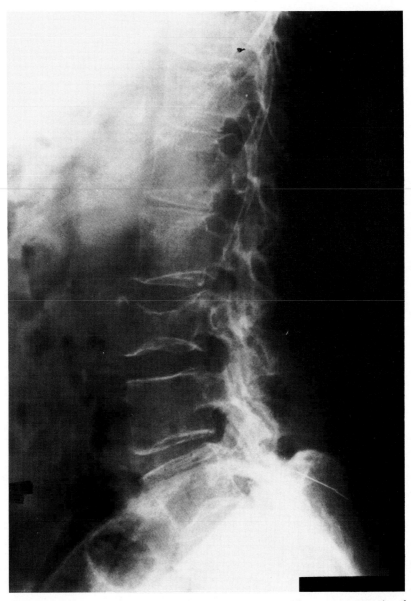

Figure 13.116.   Multiple myeloma: lateral lumbar spine examination. Diffuse osteoporosis of the spine with a "washed-out" appearance of the vertebral bodies is seen. A compression fracture of L_3 has resulted secondary to the weakened vertebral bodies in this 71-year-old patient with multiple myeloma who presented with back pain.

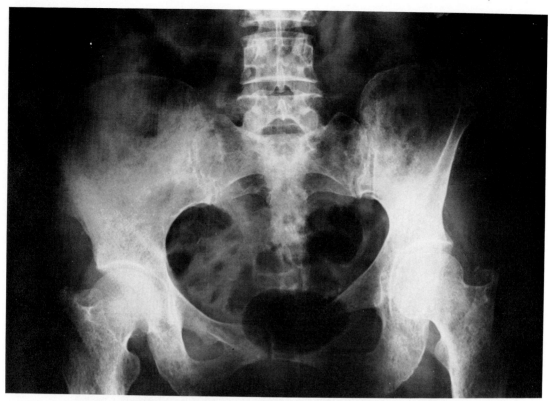

Figure 13.117. Multiple myeloma: AP pelvis examination. The only radiographic feature is osteoporosis of the osseous structures, a finding which may be the only indicator of the underlying disease process.

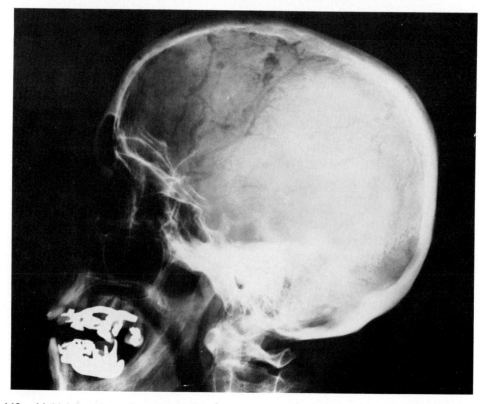

Figure 13.118. Multiple myeloma: lateral skull examination. Multiple small punched-out lesions along the convexity of the skull represent a "classic" x-ray pattern encountered in multiple myeloma. These are sometimes extremely widespread and extensive, involving the entire calvarium.

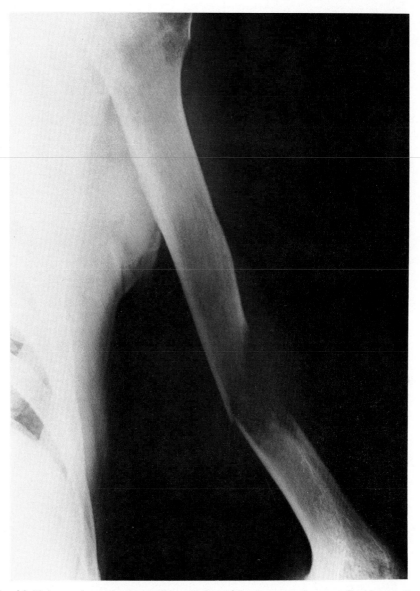

Figure 13.119.   Multiple myeloma. Lytic myeloma lesion of the humerus has resulted in a pathologic fracture.

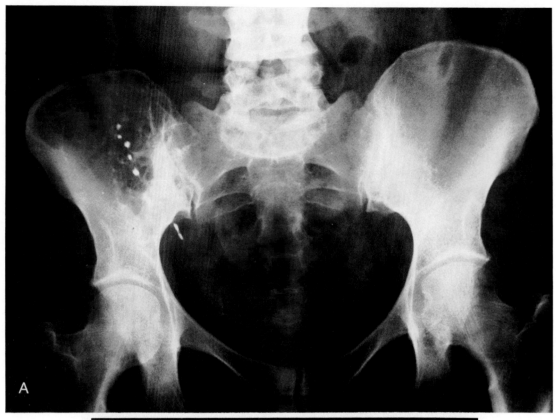

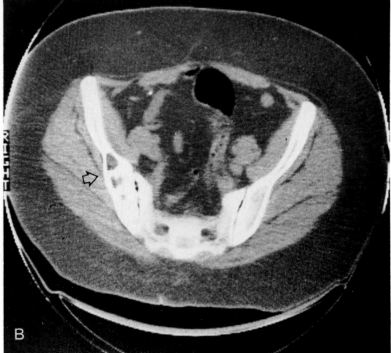

Figure 13.120. *A* and *B*, multiple myeloma. A 52-year-old patient presented with ill-defined right hip pain. Conventional AP radiograph of the pelvis demonstrates a multi-septated lytic lesion of the right innominate bone (barium in the appendix from barium enema exam overlies the bone lesion). Computerized axial tomography through the pelvis demonstrates the same lesion (*arrow*) which was unassociated with any cortical breakthrough or pelvis soft-tissue mass. No other skeletal lesions were found. Diagnosis: solitary plasmacytoma of bone.

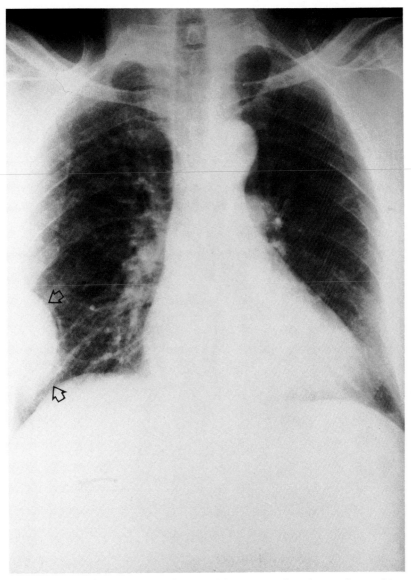

Figure 13.121.   Multiple myeloma: PA chest examination. A large extrapleural mass (*arrows*) is seen along the right lateral chest wall representing a tumor mass of myelomatous tissue extending into the chest from adjacent rib involvement.

VI. MISCELLANEOUS

(Figures appear on pages 433–440.)

Sarcoidosis

Sarcoidosis represents a granulomatous disease (with non-caseating granulomas representing the pathologic hallmark) capable of affecting multiple organ systems in the body, including the lungs, liver, lymph nodes, eyes, skin, and salivary glands. Pulmonary involvement most frequently dominates the clinical picture. Involvement of bones and joints also occurs, but is usually not an important part of the patients' clinical picture. Bone involvement is felt to be most common in the small bones of the hands and feet, but x-ray abnormalities have been described throughout the skeleton. The hands are probably somewhat more commonly involved than the feet. The exact incidence of skeletal involvement in sarcoidosis is actually unknown with undoubtedly a large percentage of cases going unrecognized due to a lack of symptoms and x-ray investigation. Involvement of the small bones of the hands and feet may result in minimal arthritic symptomatology.

RADIOLOGY

The osseous changes of sarcoidosis are most characteristically observed in the small bones of the feet and hands, and vary in severity from minimal, almost imperceptible change to gross destructive change. Probably the most common pattern of abnormality is a reticulated, lace-like appearance of the spongiosa of the short tubular bones, particularly the middle and distal phalanges, owing to granulomatous infiltration of the medullary cavities. Larger, cystic-appearing lesions can occur in more severe cases, and a mutilating variety with larger areas of bone and joint destruction can be identified in the most severe cases. When multiple lytic lesions of the hands and feet are noted, sarcoidosis must be differentiated from gout, metastatic disease, fibrous dysplasia, the bone lesions of tuberous sclerosis, tuberculous dactylitis, and enchondromatosis. Characteristically, the bony lesions of sarcoidosis are unassociated with any periosteal reactive change (which is only very rarely seen) or soft-tissue abnormality (soft tissue nodularity is a very unusual feature). Endosteal sclerosis of small tubular bones may be noted. Acroosteosclerosis represents another occasional radiographic characteristic seen in the hands and feet. The bones are characteristically normally mineralized with no evidence of osteoporosis.

Involvement of the skull, spine, and long bones with lytic lesions is less common. A very rare manifestation of skeletal sarcoidosis is diffuse bony sclerosis (Figs. 13.122 to 13.129).

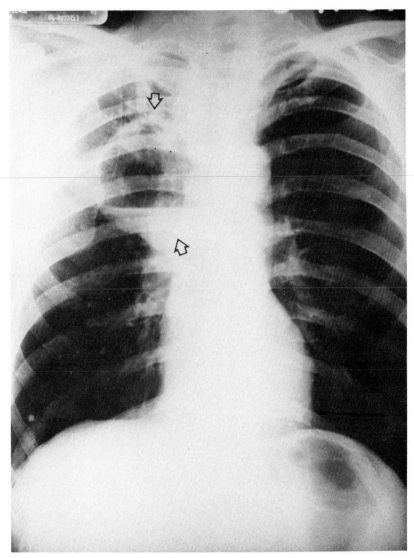

Figure 13.122.   Hypertrophic pulmonary osteoarthropathy: PA chest examination. A large cavitating right upperlobe mass (which contains an air-fluid level) (*arrows*) representing a cavitating squamous cell bronchogenic carcinoma was responsible for the development of HPO in this patient.

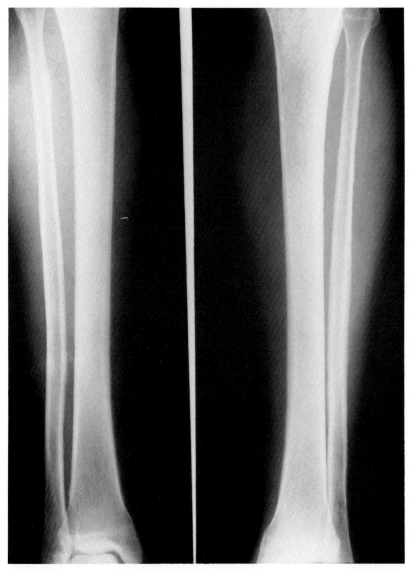

Figure 13.123.   Hypertrophic pulmonary osteoarthropathy. The tibia and fibula bilaterally demonstrate fine periosteal new-bone formation in the same patient whose chest exam is shown in Figure 13.122.

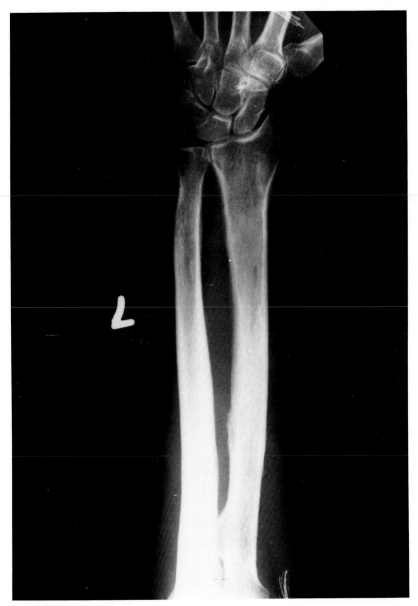

Figure 13.124. Hypertrophic pulmonary osteoarthropathy. Another patient with the entity of HPO demonstrating fine periosteal proliferation along the distal shafts of the radius and ulna. The change was due to a malignant mesothelial tumor of the pleura.

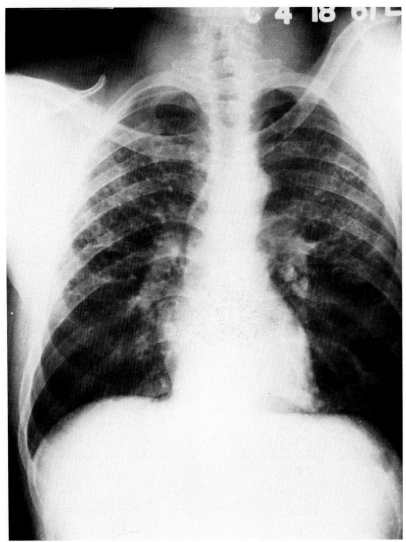

Figure 13.125. Sarcoidosis: PA chest examination. Upper lobe fibrosis bilaterally represents change commonly seen in sarcoidosis. Pulmonary involvement commonly dominates the clinical picture in patients with sarcoid and can progress to respiratory failure.

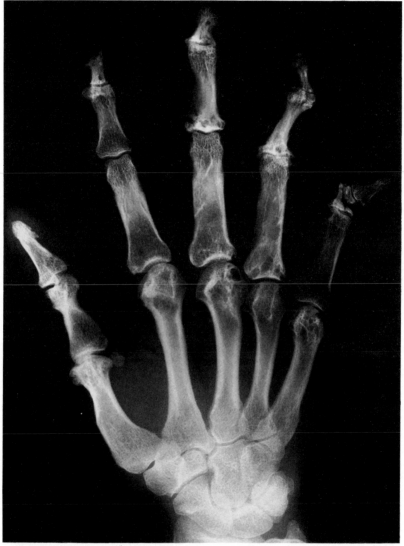

Figure 13.126.   Sarcoidosis. Hand examination demonstrates multiple cystic lesions primarily centered around joint articulations. Such a distribution is unusual with small cystic lesions seen more characteristically within the medullary spaces of the small tubular bones.

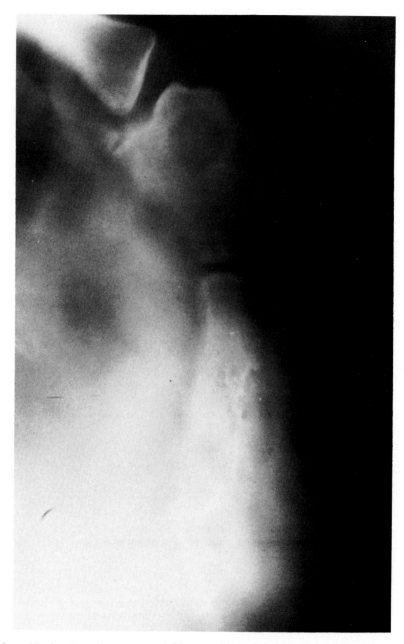

Figure 13.127.   Sarcoidosis: sternal tomogram. A 30-year-old black female presented with anterior chest wall pain. Tomography of the sternum demonstrates a large lytic lesion of the manubrium and destructive change involving the body of the sternum in this unusual example of sarcoid bone involvement.

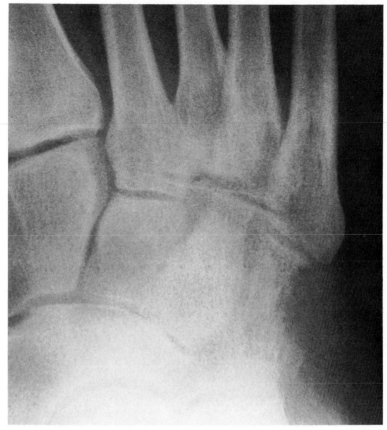

Figure 13.128. Sarcoid arthritis. Sarcoidosis frequently erodes bone and has been known to completely destroy joints.

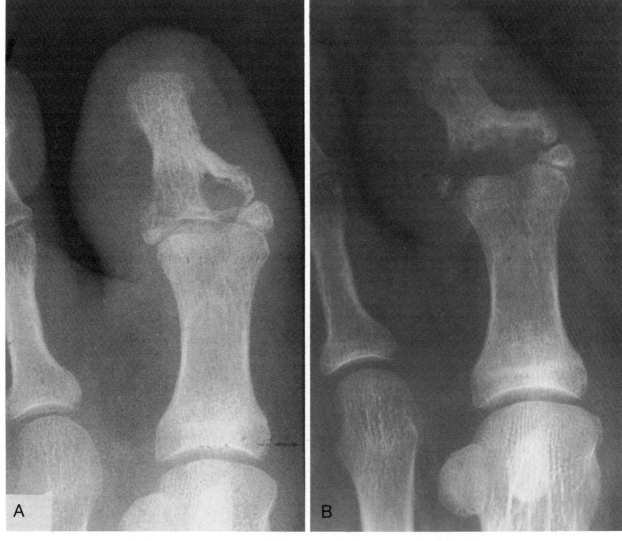

Figure 13.129. Sarcoidosis of bone. *A*, sarcoidosis affecting the proximal interphalangeal joint of the hallux. *B*, progressed to completely destroy the interphalangeal joint. Radiographs compliments of Dr. Vincent Mandracchia.

REFERENCES

1. AEGERTER, E., AND KIRKPATRICK, J. A., JR.: *Orthopedic Diseases,* 4th Ed, Saunders, Philadelphia, 1975.
2. AGUS, Z. S., AND GOLDBERG, M.: Pathogenesis of uremic osteodystrophy. Radiol. Clin. North Am., **10:** 545, 1972.
3. BJARNASON, D. F., FORRESTER, D. M., AND SWEZEY, R. L.: Destructive arthritis of the large joints. A rare manifestation of sarcoidosis. J. Bone Jt. Surg., **55-A:** 618, 1973.
4. DELETED IN PROOF.
5. CARACHE, S., AND PAGE, D. L.: Infarctions of bone marrow in sickle cell disorders. Ann. Intern. Med., **67:** 1195, 1967.
6. CURRANINO, G., AND ERLANDSON, M. E.: Premature fusion of epiphyses in Cooley's anemia. Radiology, **83:** 656, 1964.
7. DIGGS, L. W.: Bone and joint lesions in sickle cell disease. Clin. Orthop. Rel. Res., **52:** 119, 1967.
8. DODDS, W. J., AND STEINBACH, H. L.: Primary hyperparathyroidism and articular calcification. Am. J. Roentgenol., **104:** 884, 1968.
9. DOYLE, F. H.: Radiologic assessment of endocrine effects on bone. Radiol. Clin. North Am., **5:** 289, 1967.
10. EDEIKEN, J.: *Roentgen Diagnosis of Diseases of Bone,* 3rd Ed, Williams & Wilkins, Baltimore, 1981.
11. EDEIKEN, J., DEPALMA, A. F., AND HODES, P. J.: Paget's disease: Osteitis deformans. Clin. Orthop. Rel. Res., **146:** 141, 1966.
12. EHRENPREIS, B., AND SCHWINGER, H. N.: Sickle cell anemia. Am. J. Roentgenol. Radium Ther. Nucl. Med., **68:** 28, 1952.
13. FORBES, G. S., MCLEOD, R. A., AND HATTERY, R. R.: Radiographic manifestations of bone metastases from renal carcinoma. Am. J. Roentgenol., **129:** 61, 1977.
14. FORNASIER, V. L., AND HORNE, J. G.: Metastases to the vertebral column. Cancer, **36:** 590, 1975.
15. FRASER, S. A., SMITH, D. A., ANDERSON, J. B., AND WILSON, G. M.: Osteoporosis and fractures following thyrotoxicosis. Lancet, **1:** 981, 1971.
16. FRIEDMAN, A., ORCUTT, J., AND MADEWELL, J.: Paget's disease of the hand: Radiographic spectrum. Am. J. Roentgenol., **138:** 691, 1982.
17. GALL, R. J., SIM, F. H., AND PRITCHARD, D. J.: Metastatic tumors to the bones of the foot. Cancer, **37:** 1492, 1976.
18. GIBSON, M. J., AND MIDDLEMISS, J. H.: Fibrous dysplasia of bone. Br. J. Radiol., **44:** 1, 1971.

19. GLEASON, D. G., AND POTCHEN, E. J.: The diagnosis of hyperparathyroidism. Radiol. Clin. North Am., **5:** 277, 1967.

20. GONTICAS, S. K., IKKOS, D. G., AND STERIGIOU, L. H.: Evaluation of the diagnostic value of heel-pad thickness in acromegaly. Radiology, 92: 304, 1969.

21. GRABIAS, S. L., AND CAMPBELL, C. J.: Fibrous dysplasia. Orthop. Clin. North Am., **8:** 771, 1977.

22. GREENFIELD, G. B.: Bone changes in chronic adult Gaucher's disease. Am. J. Roentgenol., **110:** 800, 1970.

23. GREENFIELD, G. B.: *Radiology of Bone Diseases,* 2nd Ed, J. B. Lippincott, Philadelphia, 1975.

24. GREENFIELD, G. B.: Roentgen appearance of bone and soft tissue changes in chronic renal disease. Am. J. Roentgenol., **116:** 749, 1972.

25. GRIFFITHS, H. J.: *Basic Bone Radiology,* Appleton-Century-Crofts, New York, 1981.

26. HELMS, C. A., O'BRIEN, E. T., AND KATZBERG, R. W.: Segmental reflex sympathetic dystrophy syndrome. Radiology, **135:** 67, 1980.

27. HOLLING, H. E.: Pulmonary hypertrophic osteoarthropathy. Ann. Intern. Med., **66:** 232, 1967.

28. HOLMAN, C. B.: Roentgenologic manifestations of vitamin D intoxication. Radiology, 59: 805, 1952.

29. HOWLAND, W. J., JR., PUGH, D. G., AND SPRAGUE, R. G.: Roentgenologic changes of the skeletal system in Cushing's syndrome. Radiology, **71:** 69, 1958.

30. HYDE, S.: Acromegalic arthropathy. Ann. Rheum. Dis. **30:** 243, 1971.

31. JENSEN, P. S., AND KLIGER, A. S.: Early radiographic manifestations of secondary hyperparathyroidism associated with chronic renal disease. Radiology, **125:** 645, 1977.

32. LANG, E. K., AND BESSLER, W. T.: The roentgenologic features of acromegaly. Am. J. Roentgenol., **86:** 321, 1961.

33. LEVIN, B.: Gaucher's disease: Clinical and roentgenologic manifestations. Am. J. Roentgenol., **85:** 685, 1961.

34. MASSRY, S. G., COBURN, J. W., POPORTZER, M. M., SHINABERGER, J. H., MAXWELL, M. H., AND KLEEMAN, C. R.: Secondary hyperparathyroidism in chronic renal failure. Arch. Intern. Med., **124:** 431, 1969.

35. MEUNIER, P. J., S-BIANCHI, G. G., EDOUARD, C. M., BERNARD, J. C., COURPRON, P., AND VIGNON, G. E.: Bony manifestations of thyrotoxicosis. Orthop. Clin. North Am., **3:** 745, 1972.

36. MINDELL, E. R., NORTHUP, C. S., AND DOUGLASS, H. O., JR.: Osteosarcoma associated with osteopoikilosis, Case report. J. Bone Jt. Surg., **60-A:** 406, 1978.

37. MOULE, B., GRANT, M. D., BOYLE, I. T., MAY, H.: Thyroid acropachy. Clin. Radiol., **21:** 329, 1970.

38. MULVEY, R. B.: Peripheral bone metastases. Am. J. Roentgenol., **91:** 155, 1964.

39. MURRAY, R. O.: Radiological bone changes in Cushing's syndrome and steroid therapy. Br. J. Radiol., **33:** 1, 1960.

40. PRICE, C. H. G., AND GOLDIE, W.: Paget's sarcoma of bone. J. Bone Jt. Surg., **51-B:** 205, 1969.

41. PUGH, D. G.: Subperiosteal resorption of bone. A roentgenologic manifestation of primary hyperparathyroidism and renal osteodystrophy. Am. J. Roentgenol. Radium Ther. Nucl. Med., **66:** 577, 1951.

42. REISS, E., AND CANTERBURY, J. M.: Spectrum of hyperparathyroidism. Am. J. Med., **56:** 794, 1974.

43. RESNICK, D., AND NIWAYAMA, G.: *Diagnosis of bone and joint disorders,* W. B. Saunders, Philadelphia, 1981.

44. RESNICK, D., AND NIWAYAMA, G.: Subchondral resorption of bone in renal osteodystrophy. Radiology, **118:** 315, 1976.

45. ROBBINS, S. L., AND ANGELL, M.: *Basic Pathology,* W. B. Saunders, Philadelphia, 1971.

46. SCANLON, G. T., AND CLEMETT, A. R.: Thyroid acropachy. Radiology, **83:** 1039, 1964.

47. SCHREIBER, M. H., AND RICHARDSON, G. A.: Paget's disease confined to one lumbar vertebra. Am. J. Roentgenol., **90:** 1271, 1963.

48. SHAPIRO, R.: Radiologic aspects of renal osteodystrophy. Radiol. Clin. North Am., **10:** 557, 1972.

49. SHAUB, M. S., ROSEN, R., BOSWELL, W., GORDONSON, J.: Tibiotalar slant: A new observation in sickle cell anemia. Radiology, **117:** 551, 1975.

50. SIMPSON, W., KERR, D. N. S., HILL, A. V. L., AND SIDDIQUI, J. Y.: Skeletal changes in patients on regular hemodialysis. Radiology, **109:** 313, 1971.

51. SOLOMON, L.: Hereditary multiple exostoses. J. Bone Jt. Surg., **45-B:** 292, 1963.

52. SPANGER, J. W., LANGER, L. O., JR., AND WIEDEMANN, H.-R.: Bone dysplasias—An atlas of constitutional disorders of skeletal development. W. B. Saunders, Philadelphia, 1974.

53. STEIN, G. N., ISRAEL, H. L., AND SONES, M.: A roentgenographic study of skeletal lesions in sarcoidosis. Arch. Intern. Med., **97:** 532, 1956.

54. STEINBACH, H. L., AND NOETZLI, M.: Roentgen appearance of the skeleton in osteomalacia and rickets. Am. J. Roentgenol., **91:** 955, 1964.

55. STEINBACH, H. L.: Some roentgen features of Paget's disease. Am. J. Roentgenol., **86:** 950, 1961.

56. STEINBACH, H. L.: The roentgen appearance of osteoporosis. Radiol. Clin. North Am., **2:** 191, 1964.

57. TENG, C. T., AND NATHAN, M. H.: Primary hyperparathyroidism. Am. J. Roentgenol., **83:** 716, 1960.

58. WELLER, M., EDEIKEN, J., AND HODES, P. J.: Renal osteodystrophy. Am. J. Roentgenol., **104:** 354, 1968.

59. WIETERSEN, F. K., AND BALOW, R. M.: The radiologic aspects of thyroid disease. Radiol. Clin. North Am., **5:** 255, 1967.

60. WOOD, K., ET AL.: Hemophilic arthropathy: A combined radiologic and clinical study. Br. J. Radiol., **42:** 498, 1969.

CHAPTER 14

Special Studies: Bone Scans and Computerized Axial Tomography

VINCENT J. HETHERINGTON, D.P.M., M.S.

BONE SCANNING

Oftentimes, in managing podiatric complaints, clinical and conventional radiographic techniques are insufficient in determining a patient's problem. This is especially true in the early stages of bone infection. Bone scanning or imaging can provide additional information in the diagnosis of the disorder. However, bone scans are not specific and must be correlated with clinical, radiographic, and laboratory evaluation. In other words, bone scanning does not provide the diagnosis, but is an important bit of information aiding in the process of diagnosis.

How Bone Scans Are Performed

The more useful radionuclides in skeletal imaging are technetium phosphate complexes and gallium citrate. These compounds are administered intravenously and are detected at specific time intervals postinjection by a rectilinear scan-

ner or gamma camera. A rectilinear scanner with minification is used and the entire skeleton can be imaged from head to toe. Minification allows visualization of the entire skeleton in a single image. A gamma camera can concentrate on an isolated area. However, it requires multiple views to complete the whole skeletal image.

Magnification of certain areas can also be obtained with a pinhole columnator (Fig. 14.1). Recent advances have allowed computer augmentation of the data received from radionucleotide imaging. The purpose of this chapter is to present the current radionuclides clinically useful in podiatric patients and not a review of instrumentation and the history of radiopharmaceuticals.

Mechanisms of Radionuclide Uptake

TECHNETIUM PHOSPHATE COMPOUNDS

Technetium phosphate compounds are deposited in bone by a proposed two-phase mechanism.[1] The first phase is a vascular phase, depend-

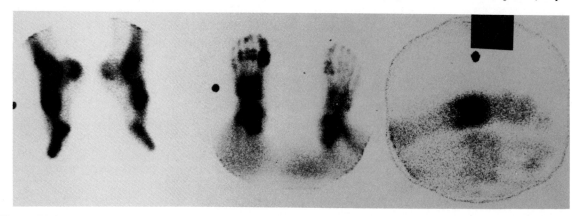

Figure 14.1. Technetium bone scan with a pinhole image for magnification of the right first metatarsophalangeal joint. Localized increased uptake of the radionuclide is well demonstrated in the head of the first metatarsal.

ent upon increased blood flow to bone. The second phase is termed the bone phase, dependent upon the bone radionuclide interaction. Technetium in the vascular phase is a reflection of increased blood flow to an area of bone.[2,3] Reactive bone formation, whether it be due to metastasis of a malignant lesion, infection, fracture, or the reparative process of infarction, all present with increased blood flow to bone. The initial increase in vascularity is due to hyperemia with vessel dilation and recruitment of adjacent vessels. Neovascularization may occur with time, increasing blood flow. In the microcirculation of bone, capillaries contained in the haversian system carry the radioisotope to the extravascular and extracellular space of bone. The second phase of the mechanism requires healthy, vital bone. By the process of passive diffusion, the radionuclide enters the bone fluid space and eventually can come in contact with the bone. The exact mechanism of uptake, binding, or exchange with the hydroxyapatite crystals of bone is not completely understood. Therefore, the initial phases in the technetium scan are dependent upon increased vascularity to an area of bone. This increased vascularity brings greater concentration of the radionuclide in contact with the injured or diseased segment. This increase in radionuclide to the localized area is what is commonly referred to as a "hot spot" on the technetium scan.

There are, however, various factors which can affect the uptake of the radionuclide in bone, e.g., changes in blood flow to bone. Decreased uptake of the radionuclide may occur in cases of infarction (sickle cell infarct), aseptic necrosis, or congestive heart failure. Areas of diminished uptake are referred to as photopenic, or photon-deficient.

Increased uptake is seen with increased bone blood flow. Such conditions that may be associated with increased bone blood flow are those in which sympathetic control is eliminated and recruitment of existing vessels, usually under sympathetic control, deliver increased amounts of radionuclide.[4,5] This can be seen after stroke, sympathectomy, and in certain cases of neuropathy. Focal abnormalities in bone that destroy or functionally impair the interosseous sympathetics can also produce this hyperemic effect. This may be seen in fractures, osteomyelitis, infarction, or new growths. Clarke[5] described these scan appearances as a hot focus and diffusely increased tracer activity within the bone.

Technetium scans can be static or dynamic.

After IV administration of the radionuclide, flow studies can be performed immediately after injection at 2- or 3-second intervals (Fig. 14.2). This allows the radioisotope to be monitored in its relationship to blood flow to the segment. Areas of photopenic activity may be detected initially at this time by lack or delay of uptake of the radioisotope. Five minutes after injection, a blood pool image can be performed (Fig. 14.3). The scan is usually completed 2–4 hours after injection of the radionuclide.

Technetium phosphate compounds have been used predominately in the diagnosis of hematogenous osteomyelitis. Gilday et al.,[6] in 1975, using technetium phosphate compounds, defined osteomyelitis as a well-defined focus of increased radioactivity in the bone image with an identical area on the blood pool images. Cellulitis was a diffuse increase in radioactivity involving the soft tissues with no focal bone component; in other words, soft tissue hyperemia secondary to the infection with no focal bone component. Septic arthritis was defined as a diffuse uptake in the blood pool images with a diffuse increase periarticularly. Duszynski[7] found that the suspected diagnosis can be confirmed as early as 48 hours after the onset of clinical symptoms. Localization of the site of infection is obtained and it can help in the planning of surgical drainage. They also noted that uptake may be present for as long as 6 months after treatment of the infection (Fig. 14.11).

Not all bone scans associated with osteomyelitis may initially present with an area of hot uptake. In certain cases, a normal bone scan or photon-deficient area may be seen.[8,9] It is believed that this is probably secondary to local ischemia produced by vessel tamponade or compromise of the microcirculation from subperiosteal or intraosseous pus.

Extended patterns of radionuclide uptake may also be seen secondary to a hyperemia in response to inflammatory and reparative processes due to infection and trauma. Thrall[10] found that this extended pattern is non-specific tracer accumulation and is more likely to occur in the extremities. The uptake of technetium compounds have also been found associated with an abdominal scar that was 5 weeks postoperative,[11] and in growing bone islands.[12] Christensen[13] studied the distribution of 99 technetium phosphate compounds in osteoarthritic femoral heads. His findings revealed that the technetium became localized in areas of new bone formation, particularly in chondral ossification, and felt that it reflected

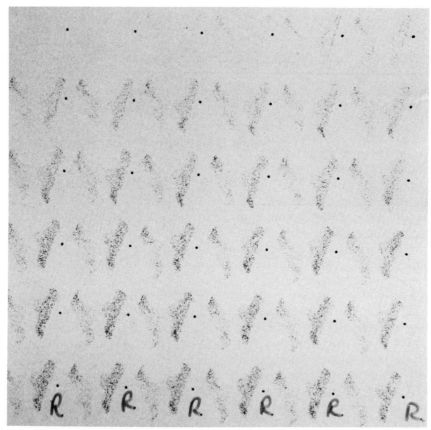

Figure 14.2.   A dynamic flow study at 2-second intervals using technetium which reveals increased uptake of the tracer in the right foot.

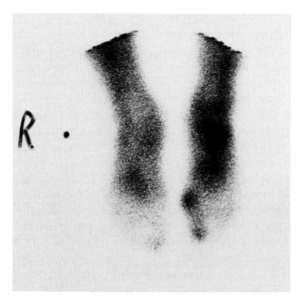

Figure 14.3.   This is illustrative of a 5-minute blood pool image revealing increased uptake (hyperemia) of the left foot. There is noticeably increased uptake in the first metatarsophalangeal joint and great toe.

primarily the rate of osteogenesis in the subchondral bones and osteophytes.

Technetium has also been shown to be accurate in defining the extent of non-viable bone sequestrum (photon-deficient) and viable bone involucrum, which showed increased uptake due to new bone formation.[14] Technetium compounds have also been used in detection of benign bone tumors, malignant tumors, metastatic tumors of the bone, and bone disease associated with systemic disease and various rheumatoid variants.

One must remember, however, that technetium uptake is not specific, and a focus of uptake may be associated with osteomyelitis, fracture, degenerative arthritis, or trauma. It is therefore imperative to correlate the clinical and laboratory finding with the technetium scan.

Gallium—67 Citrate

A second useful isotope is gallium. Gallium may be considered an inflammatory imaging agent. As with technetium, gallium is initially localized in the tissues via blood flow. Hoffer[15] postulated three mechanisms for gallium-67 localization at the site of infection. These are: 1) leukocyte localization or incorporation (leukocytes are rich in lactoferrin and gallium is taken up by the leukocytes and is primarily bound to the lactoferrin); 2) direct lactoferrin binding at the site of infection (lactoferrin is released from the leukocytes or may be present by leakage of the protein through the permeable vessel endothelium); and 3) direct bacterial uptake by siderophores. Yuan Tzen et al.[16] also felt that gallium-67 accumulation is caused by increased capillary permeability and iron-binding proteins, such as transferrin or lactoferrin. Weiner et al.[17] also felt that lactoferrin appears to be the major binding protein for gallium present in the neutrophil.

Gallium, similar to technetium, causes an increased focal uptake at the area of infection. Gallium is less dependent on blood flow than technetium and it seems capable of localizing in lesions despite ischemia caused by tamponade. Hoffer[18] also pointed out that, when osteomyelitis is suspected as a result of spread from adjacent areas of cellulitis, the gallium-67 scan may be difficult to interpret due to the inability to distinguish which activity is in bone and which is soft tissue. He also noted that recent surgical wounds are positive on gallium scans for an excess of 2 weeks.

Teates,[19] using gallium scanning as a screening test for inflammatory lesions, found that a normal scan did not rule out inflammatory lesions, but no significant pyogenic lesions were missed. Deysine et al.[20] demonstrated that gallium-67 can be used in the early detection of acute exacerbations of chronic osteomyelitis and postoperative bone infection. Early diagnosis is important in these cases to prevent the sequelae due to an untreated infection. Abdominal abscesses secondary to anerobic infections, however, can interfere with the uptake of ferric ions and, therefore, presumably gallium-67 citrate by anerobic organisms.[21] Gallium binds to at least four of the iron binding molecules: transferrin, lactoferrin, ferritin, and siderphores. Gallium citrate is injected intravenously and the scan is usually completed 24–72 hours postinjection with sequential images (Fig. 14.4).

The combined use of gallium and technetium scans has been helpful in the evaluation of osteomyelitis. This is based on the assumption that technetium is a bone imaging radionuclide and gallium would be an inflammatory imaging nuclide. On the basis of their findings, Lisboma and Rosenthall[22] used combined scanning with the following results. A positive technetium and negative gallium scan was indicative of chronic osteomyelitis (Fig. 14.5). A negative technetium scan and positive gallium scan represented cellulitis. A positive technetium scan and a positive gallium scan revealed active osteomyelitis or septic arthritis (Fig. 14.6). They also felt that cellulitis is generally defined more clearly by gallium than by technetium blood pool images and also felt that gallium was more accurate in the pediatric group due to the concentration of technetium at the epiphyseal plates. Combined scans have also been used in the evaluation of painful total hip joint replacements.[23]

Technetium is a bone imaging nuclide dependent on blood flow and incorporation into vital bone. It is also non-specific and, therefore, one cannot count on it to make the diagnosis. Gallium is an inflammatory imaging agent which relies on its incorporation into iron-binding proteins and white blood cells for its localization. In combination, radionuclides can distinguish acute from chronic osteomyelitis and cellulitis in certain instances (e.g., hematogenous osteomyelitis).

Neurotrophic Foot

The neurotrophic foot, especially one which is ulcerated and infected, can present a dilemma in the diagnosis of osteomyelitis of the underlying bone. In these patients, oftentimes an ulceration is present, which may give rise to a positive gallium scan and also increased technetium uptake in the hyperemic soft tissues. Whether the bone is truly infected or increased uptake is present due to the bone being previously diseased secondary to the neurotrophic destructive processes cannot always be differentiated (Fig. 14.7).[24]

One must also remember that in neuropathy, increased radionuclide is delivered to the extremity due to the recruitment of vessels caused by the autosympathectomy that often occurs. Gallium uptake can also be observed in non-infected areas. This may be due primarily to the fact that gallium also accumulates from increased vessel permeability in areas undergoing repair and also from the presence of an increased number of white blood cells due to both the repair of the neurotrophic bone process and soft tissue infection.[24]

Park et al.[25] performed a three-phase scan in the diabetic foot. His three-phase scan included a first phase dynamic flow study at 3 seconds per frame for 12 frames, a blood pool image, and a 2-hour image. Scan abnormalities were graded to the background activity. Scans scored in all three phases were significantly higher in proven sites of osteomyelitis than in areas with degenerative disease. Ischemic ulcers scored lower in phases 1 and 2 than in phase 3. Cellulitis without osteomyelitis was high in phase 1 and 2, but low in phase 3.

Bone scanning in the neurotrophic foot for the detection of osteomyelitis does not appear to offer any advantages. In these cases, bone biopsy and bone culture must still be relied upon (Fig. 14.8).

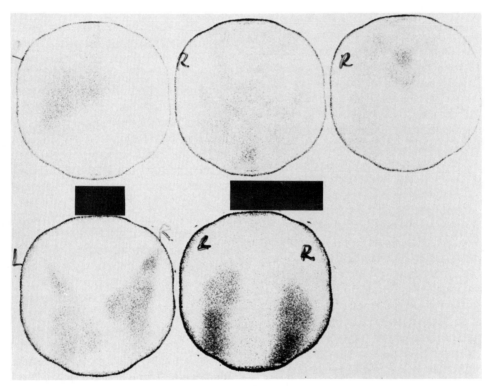

Figure 14.4. Normal gallium scan at 24 hours (anterior and lateral views).

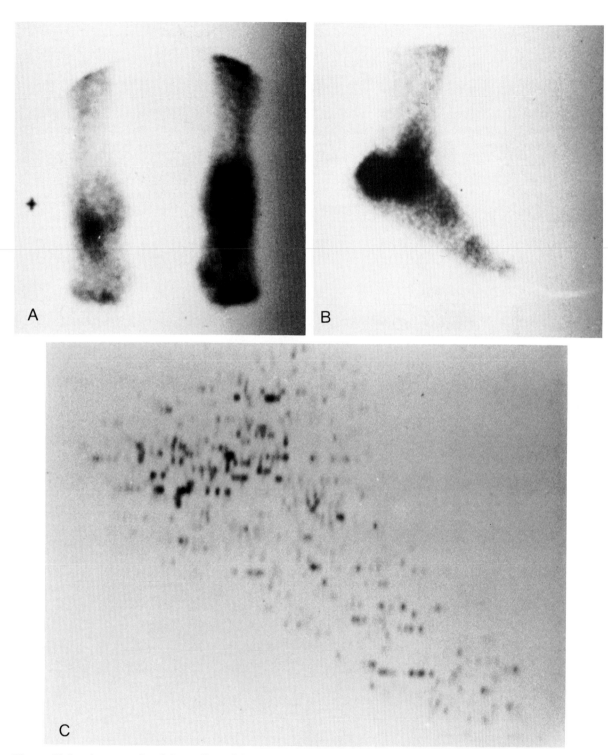

Figure 14.5. An example of the radionuclide pattern seen in chronic osteomyelitis. *A,* 5-minute blood pool image demonstrating increased uptake in the left rear foot using technetium. *B,* technetium bone scan showing focal uptake isolated to the left calcaneus. *C,* normal gallium scan. Although this is consistent with chronic osteomyelitis, the diagnoses in this instance was the sclerosing non-suppurative osteomyelitis of Garré.

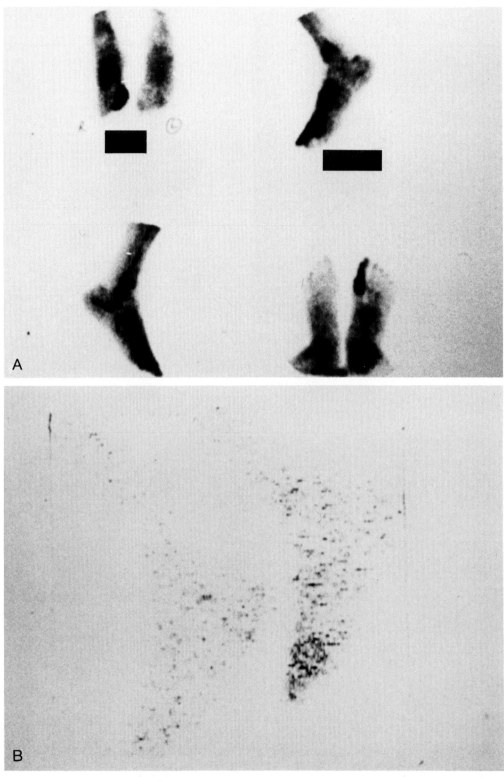

Figure 14.6.   An illustration of acute osteomyelitis of the right great toe which was confirmed by biopsy. *A,* technetium bone scan showing focal uptake to the right great toe. *B,* gallium scan showing the focal uptake involving the right great toe.

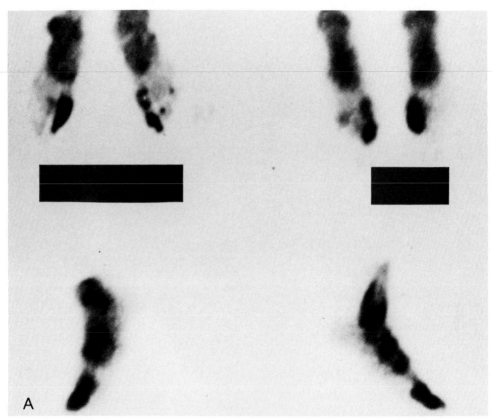

Figure 14.7.   A patient with peripheral neuropathy secondary to ethanol abuse. Focal uptake was seen in the areas of the great toes of both feet and the second and fourth digits of the right foot using the technetium bone scan. Radiographically, the patient had osteomyelitis of the left great toe. There did not appear to be any destructive changes involving the right great toe, and that also went on to heal uneventfully. However, radiographically, in *B* one can see the destructive changes that have occurred in the second and fourth digits of the right foot secondary to the patient's neuropathy. There is a mortar and pestle appearance to the joint.

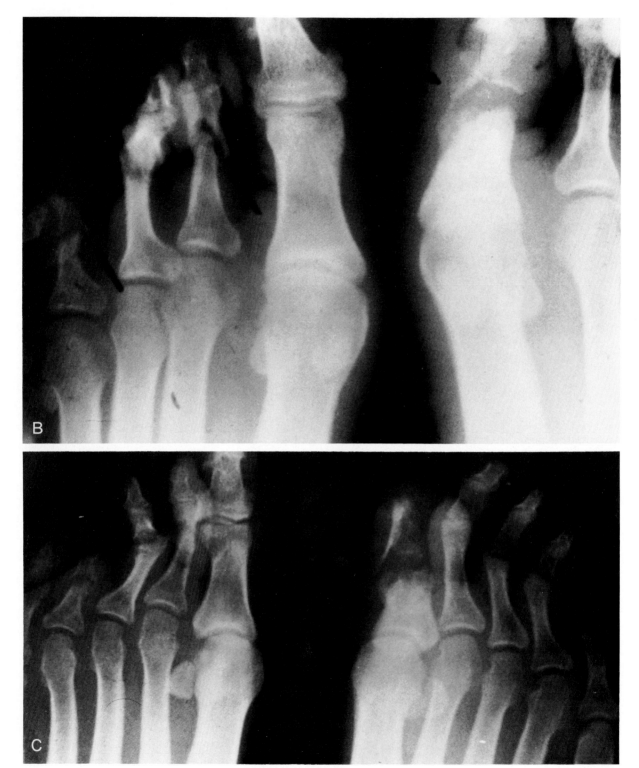

Figure 14.7. (*B* and *C*)

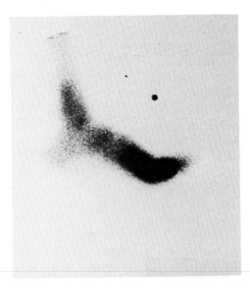

Figure 14.8. A technetium bone scan showing focal uptake of the first metatarsal of the right foot in a diabetic patient. Clinically, the patient presented with ulceration on the plantar and medial aspects of the head of the first metatarsal secondary to diabetic neuropathy. There was an abscess involving the first intermetatarsal space. Osteomyelitis could not be confirmed in this patient by biopsy. The patient's biopsy was consistent with a phase of bone healing with callus formation. This patient healed uneventfully after debridement of the ulcers and incision and drainage of the abscess. Approximately 6 months postoperatively, neurotrophic bone changes of the mortar and pestle variety were seen to involve the first metatarsal phalangeal joint of the right foot.

Trauma

Fractures can be revealed within 7 hours after injury.[26] Radionuclide imaging of fractures is indicated only when the radiograph is not definitive or is normal, but with a strong suspicion of fracture remaining. Transient traumatic synovitis or hyperemia may produce a generalized increase in concentration, which may obscure focal uptake. Patients fitting this description should be restudied in 3 days to a week after initial scanning. Failure to reveal a focal lesion excludes fracture. If the scan is negative, the cast may be removed to prevent unnecessary immobilization and its consequences. However, one must keep in mind that focal concentration does not represent a gross fracture. Ligamentous avulsion or periosteal injury could yield similar pictures.

Martin,[27] in 1979, described the appearance of bone scan following fractures. Three phases were presented. One, the acute phase for the first 3 or 4 weeks post-injury. It is characterized by diffuse area of increased activity surrounding the fracture site. A distinct fracture was frequently seen during this stage. Phase 2, the subacute phase, was a well-defined linear abnormality showing the most intense uptake; this stage lasted approximately 8–12 weeks. The third phase, or healing phase, showed a gradual diminution in intensity of the abnormality until the scan returned to normal. A return to normal scan varied on the area of the body injured. Also, patients over the age of 65 showed a greater delay in the return to normal after fracture, and a delay in onset of a normal scan was also noted. O'Reilly et al.[28] found that, with technetium phosphate compounds, one could not detect any early pattern of change between normal healing and delay or non-union. In the study of non-united fractures undergoing percutaneous, low-grade, direct current stimulation,[29] the response was correlated with three distinct patterns of osseous activity. Group 1 revealed an intense activity at the fracture line, of which 95% went on to heal. Group 2 showed a line of decreased tracer uptake surrounded by increased uptake on both sides. This may be possibly representative of a non-union or pseudarthrosis, and none of the patients went on to heal. In the third group were placed patients who did not fit either pattern and 50% healing occurred. It was their feeling that bone scanning is recommended as an important initial examination for proper selection of patients for percutaneous electrical stimulation.

One can see that in evaluation of osteotomies and/or fracture sites with questionable healing potential, radionuclide imaging may be of value.

Stress Fractures

Bone scanning may be used in the differential diagnosis of shin splints or exercise-induced lower extremity discomfort.[30] Geslein[31] found that stress fractures could be detected before radiographic evidence by radionuclide imaging to allow early treatment. Spencer[32] and others found a diverse appearance of bone scan abnormalities in shin splints. Four variants were described in four different patients. One was focal tibial uptake; the second was diffuse tibial uptake; the third was combined tibial and fibular uptake; and the last was fibular uptake. In their findings, fibular abnormal uptake are of particular interest since such lesions make it particularly difficult for the patient to locate the source of the trouble. Lieberman and Hemmingway[33] found that the double-strip sign, which was previously described as specific for hypertrophic pulmonary osteoarthropathy, was also found in patients with shin splints.

Inflammatory Arthritis and Bone Disease

Increased uptake at joint sites related to inflammatory joint disease is most likely related to increased blood flow to bone secondary to inflammatory synovitis.[34, 35] Hyperemia surrounding an inflamed joint includes the periarticular bone. This hyperemia to bone, with or without pannus erosion of the subchondral bone, leads to increased bone turnover and, therefore, increased deposition of technetium phosphate compounds. Continued uptake of radionuclides in clinically asymptomatic joints may be related to continued osseous activity secondary to pannus erosion, low-grade hyperemia, and inflammation or healing of the articular bone. Desaulneirs et al.[34] pointed out 99 technetium phosphate compounds are useful and recommended as radiopharmaceuticals of choice in screening patients with arthralgias for the presence of inflammatory articular disease, disclosing affected joints not clinically suspected, and in detecting extensions of disease during follow-up.

Miscellaneous Entities

Tracer uptake may be detected in cases of plantar fasciitis[36] (Fig. 14.9) and in various types of rheumatoid variants, such as Reiter's syndrome.[37] Reflex sympathetic dystrophy shows a characteristic pattern of increased periarticular uptake that can be useful in excluding the diagnosis in suspected cases (Fig. 14.10).[38] Bone scans may also be useful in the detection of benign bone tumors, such as the osteoid osteoma. There are two basic indications for scanning patients with suspected benign bone tumors.[39] These are: 1) to locate the lesion causing the pain; and 2) to determine if the lesion is benign or malignant. Blood pool images with malignant lesions tend to be more hyperemic than the benign lesions. Gallium-67 appears superior when distinguishing malignant from benign lesions and are more accurate in delinating the local extent of primary bone tumors.[40]

Radionuclides are also further entering the field of podiatric surgery with the prospective use of

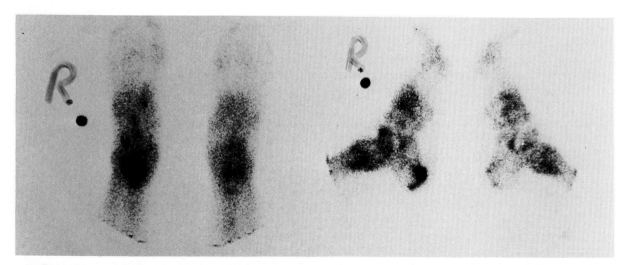

Figure 14.9.   A technetium bone scan of a patient who was complaining of chronic heel pain and had not responded to conservative treatment over an extended period. The technetium bone scan of the right foot reveals increased uptake of the radionuclide in the inferior portion of the calcaneus. A relatively normal technetium scan is demonstrated on the left foot.

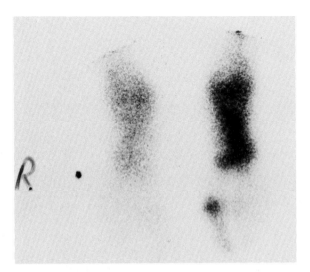

Figure 14.10. A patient who exhibited reflex sympathetic dystrophy showing increased periarticular uptake unilaterally. The involvement shows the first metatarsal phalangeal joint and the tarsal articulations.

xenon-133 for establishing amputation level selection in patients, with ischemic vascular disease.[41] Thallium[42] has also been used in a ratio to determine the healing ability of ischemic ulcers. The ratio is obtained by point counting directly over the ulcer and at three points (2.5 cm) from the edge of the ulcer over relatively normal tissue. Counting was performed for 60 seconds over each site. A 2.54 × 1.27 cm pinhole-columnated scintillation detector was used. The ratio for healing was determined as the activity per unit area of the ulcer over the activity per unit area of the surrounding tissue. Minimum hyperemic response for healing was 1.5. It was found that "healing" was not related to the presence or absence of diabetes, and was not dependent upon a palpable arterial pulse. It is obviously related to the adequacy of the microcirculation and its capacity to produce a hyperemic, inflammatory response.[42] In seven of seven patients with a ratio in excess or equal to 1.5, 100% healing occurred. In those patients with a ratio of less than 1.5, five of six of the patients, or 83%, went on to amputation.

Indium[43] may also be used in the future for detection of infectious lesions as it is perhaps more specific than gallium in detection of infectious process.

Conclusions

Radionuclide imaging can add valuable information in evaluation of the podiatric patient. However, one must be aware of the limitations of the individual scans and interpret their findings judiciously.

COMPUTERIZED AXIAL TOMOGRAPHY

Computerized axial tomography is a radiographic scanning technique which allows the visualization of a cross-sectional plane of the body.[44-47] A CT scanner consists of an X-ray generator, scanning gantry, data processing and storage system, and a viewing component, usually a video monitor. Each cross-sectional slice is divided into numerous small units of volume. An x-ray attenuation value is determined for each unit in the cross-section. Attenuation values are expressed as a computed tomography number. CT numbers range from −1000 to +1000 and are expressed as houdsfield units. The range is −1000 for air with +1000 for compact bone. The small units called pixels are displayed on a video monitor using a gray scale where varying shades of gray represent differences in density of the tissue contained in the small unit. CT data may also be displayed on a color scale or as numerical values. In the computer-reconstructed image, the denser tissues appear white, whereas tissues of less density appear black. The resolution power ranges from 1.5–2.0 mm.

Computerized tomography has multiple applications in orthopaedic and podiatric pathology. Weis et al.[48] found computerized tomography to be particularly useful in examining tumors of the lower extremity. The advantages of CT in tumor evaluation are: 1) precise mass size determination; 2) localization of the mass in relationship to muscle bundles and fascial planes; 3) marginal definition of the mass; 4) relationship of neurovascular structures to the mass; and 5) relation of masses to osseous structures. CT is useful in both osseous and soft tissue tumors.[49-51] Osteomyelitis may also be evaluated for progression and/or regression by recording changes in the attenuation coefficient of the medullary canal. In acute and subacute osteomyelitis, the attenuation coefficient is high. Involucrum in chronic stages is reported to be well defined on CT scans.[52] CT was found to be useful in the follow-up of bone infection to differentiate healing from progression when obvious changes were not apparent with conventional radiology.

CT has also been advocated for use in the evaluation and diagnosis of muscular atrophy and hypertrophy.[53] CT may also be used in the evaluation of unilateral extremity swelling. Comput-

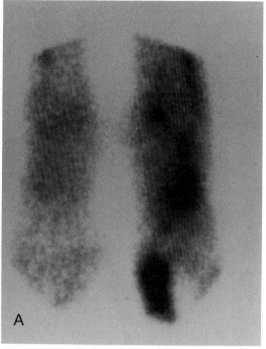
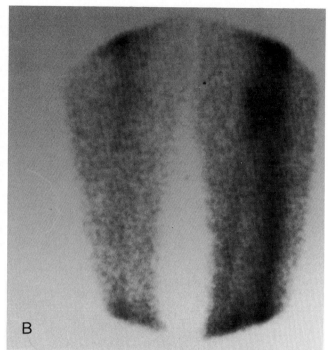

Figure 14.11. *A* and *B*, this patient had a clinical diagnosis of osteomyelitis of the left great toe. He had edema extending throughout the left foot and up to the left knee. The technetium bone scan shows an increase of uptake of the entire left leg; left foot with a focal uptake of the left great toe.

erized tomographic angiography is also available in evaluation of arterial disease and in arterial bypass grafts,[54] as well as diagnosis of caval thrombosis.[55]

Evaluation of lower extremity fractures may be aided by CT. Better visualization of the relationship of the fracture fragments, as well as intraarticular involvement,[56] will be attainable. CT may also be helpful in establishing the diagnosis of tarsal coalition and degenerative change of the tarsus and lesser tarsus, which are not readily available with conventional techniques. High-resolution computed tomography will make the small joints of the foot accessible.[57] Atlases of normally and pathologically computed axial tomographic anatomies have been published.[58, 59]

Congenital deformities, as well as the relationship of structures in pathologic conditions, will be better visualized, allowing better understanding of their processes and anatomy.

REFERENCES

1. HUGHES, S.: Radionuclides in orthopedic surgery. J. Bone Jt. Surg., **62B:** 141, 1980.
2. SIEGEL, B. A., DONOVAN, R. L., ANDERSON, P. O., AND MACK, G. R.: Skeletal uptake of 99ᵐ Tc-diphosphate in relation to local bone blood flow. Radiology, **120:** 121, 1976.
3. CHARKES, N. D.: Mechanisms of skeletal tracer uptake. J. Nucl. Med., **20:** 794, 1979.
4. SAGER, V. V., PICCONE, J. M., AND CHARKES, N. D.: Studies on skeletal tracer kinetics: III. Tᶜ-99 m (Sn) methylenediphosphonate uptake in the canine tibia as a function of blood flow. J. Nucl. Med., **20:** 1257, 1979.
5. CHARKES, N. D.: Skeletal blood flow: Implications for bone scan interpretation. J. Nucl. Med., **21:** 91, 1980.
6. GILDAY, D. L., PAUL, D. J., AND PATERSON, J.: Diagnosis of osteomyelitis in children by combined blood pool and bone imaging. Radiology, **117:** 331, 1975.
7. DUSZYNSKI, D. O., KUHN, J. P., AFSHANI, E., AND RIDDIESBURGER, M. M.: Early radionuclide diagnosis of acute osteomyelitis. Radiology, **117:** 337, 1975.
8. TEATES, C. D., AND WILLIAMSON, B. R. J.: "Hot and cold" bone lesions in acute osteomyelitis. Am. J. Roentgenol., **129:** 517, 1977.
9. JONES, D. C., AND CADY, R. B.: "Cold" bone scans in acute osteomyelitis. J. Bone Jt. Surg., **63B:** 376, 1981.
10. THRALL, J. H., GESLIEN, G. E., CORCORON, R. J., AND JOHNSON, M. C.: Abnormal radionuclide deposition patterns adjacent to focal skeletal lesions. Radiology, **115:** 659, 1975.
11. SIDDIQUI, A. R., AND STOKKA, C. L.: Uptake of Tc-99m-methylene diphosphate in a surgical scar. Clin. Nucl. Med., **5:** 274, 1980.
12. ROBACK, D. L.: Tᶜ-99m-MDP bone scintigraphy and "growing" bone islands: A report of two cases. Clin. Nucl. Med., **5:** 98, 1980.
13. CHRISTENSEN, S. B., AND ARNOLDI, C. C.: Distribution of ⁹⁹ᵐTc-phosphate compounds in osteoarthritic femoral heads. J. Bone Jt. Surg., **62A:** 90, 1980.
14. HEMINGWAY, D. L., AND LIEBERMAN, C. M.: Bone scan findings with radiographic, clinical and surgical correlation in extensive osteomyelitis: A case report. Clin. Nucl. Med., **5:** 29, 1980.
15. HOFFER, P.: Gallium mechanisms. J. Nucl. Med., **29:** 282, 1980.
16. YUAN TZEN, K., OSTER, Z. H., WAGNER, H. H., AND TSAN, M.: Role of iron binding proteins and enhanced

capillary permeability in the accumulation of gallium-67. J. Nucl. Med., **21**: 31, 1980.

17. WEINER, R., HOFFER, P. B., AND THAKUR, M. L.: Lactoferrin: It's role as a GA-67 binding protein in polymorphonuclear leukocytes. J. Nucl. Med., **22**: 32, 1981.

18. HOFFER, P.: Gallium and infection. J. Nucl. Med., **21**: 484, 1980.

19. TEATES, C. D., AND HUNTER, J. G.: Gallium scanning as a screening test for inflammatory lesions. Radiology, **116**: 383, 1975.

20. DEYSINE, M., RAFKIN, H., TEICHER, SILVER, L., ROBINSON, R., MANLY, J., AND AUFSES, A. H.: Diagnosis of chronic and postoperative osteomyelitis with gallium 67 citrate scans. Am. J. Surg., **129**: 632, 1975.

21. HOLLAND, R. D., GOONRATNE, H. S., WEST, T. E., AND SELBY, J. B.: Gallium-67 scintigraphy in abdominal anaerobic abcesses. Clin. Nucl. Med., **5**: 393, 1980.

22. LISBOMA, R., AND ROSENTHALL, L.: Observations on the sequential use of ^{99m}-Tc-phosphate complex and ^{67}-GA imaging in ostomyelitis, cellulitis and septic arthritis. Radiology, **123**: 123, 1977.

23. REING, C. M., RICHIN, P. F., AND KENMORE, P. J.: Differential bone scanning in the evaluation of a painful total joint replacement. J. Bone Jt. Surg., **61A**: 933, 1979.

24. HETHERINTON, V. J.: Technetium and combined technetium and gallium scans in the neurothrophic foot. J.A.P.A., **72**: 459, 1982.

25. PARKS, N., WHEAT, J., SIDDIQUI, A., BURT, R., ROBB, J., AND WELLMAN, H. H.: Three-phase bone scan in diabetic foot. J. Nucl. Med., **20**: 602, 1979 (abstract).

26. ROSENTHALL, L., HILL, R. O., AND CHUANG, S.: Observations on the use of ^{99m}Tc-phosphate imaging in peripheral bone trauma. Radiology **119**: 637, 1976.

27. MARTIN, P.: The appearance of bone scans following fractures including immediate and long-term studies. J. Nucl. Med., **20**: 1227, 1979.

28. O'REILLY, R. J., COOK, D. J., GAFFNEY, R. D., ANGEL, K. R., AND PATERSON, D. C.: Can serial scintigraphic studies detect delayed fracture union in man? Clin. Orthop. Relat. Res. **160**: 227, 1981.

29. DESAI, A., ALAVI, A., DALINKA, M., BRIGHTON, C., AND ESTERHAI, J.: Role of scintigraphy in the evaluation and treatment of non-united fractures: Concise communications. J. Nucl. Med., **21**: 931, 1980.

30. MILLS, G. Q., MARYMONT, J. H., AND MURPHY, D. A.: Bone scan utilization in differential diagnosis of exercise-induced lower limb pain. Clin. Orthop. Relat. Res. **149**: 207, 1980.

31. GESLEIN, G. E., THRALL, J. H., ESPINOSA, J. L., AND OLDER, R. A.: Early detection of stress fracture using ^{99m}Tc-Polyphosphate. Radiology, **121**: 683, 1976.

32. SPENCER, R. P., LEVINSON, E. D., BALDWIN, R. D., SZIKLAS, J. J., WITEK, J. T., AND ROSENBERG, R.: Diverse bone scan abnormalities in "shin splints." J. Nucl. Med., **21**: 1271, 1979.

33. LIEBERMAN, C. M., AND HEMMINGWAY, D. L.: Scintigraphy of shin splints. Clin. Nucl. Med., **5**: 31, 1980.

34. DESAULNIER, M., FUKS, A., HAWKINS, D., LACOURCIERE, Y., AND ROSENTHALL, L.: Radiotechnetium polyphosphate joint imaging. J. Nucl. Med., **15**: 417, 1974.

35. HANDMAKER, H., AND LONEARDS, R.: The bone scan in inflamatory osseous disease. Semin. Nucl. Med., **6**: 95, 1976.

36. SEWELL, J. R., BLACK, C. M., CHAPMAN, A. H., STATHAM, J., HUGHES, G. R. V., AND LAVENDER, J. P.: Quantitative scintigraphy in diagnosis and management of plantar fascitis (calceaneal periostitis): Concise communication. J. Nucl. Med., **21**: 633, 1980.

37. KHALKHALI, I., STADALNIK, R. C., WEISNER, K. B., AND SHIAPIRO, R. F.: Bone imaging of the heel in Reiter's syndrome. Am. J. Roentgenol., **132**: 110, 1979.

38. SIMON, H., AND CARLSON, D. H.: The use of bone scanning in the diagnosis of reflex sympathetic dystrophy. Clin. Nucl. Med., **5**: 116, 1980.

39. GILDAY, D. O., AND ASH, J. M.: Benign bone tumors. Semin. Nucl. Med., **6**: 33, 1976.

40. SIMON, M. A., AND KIRCHNER, P. J.: Scintigraphic evaluation of primary bone tumors: Comparison of techetium-99m phosphonate and gallium citrate imaging. J. Bone Jt. Surg., **62A**: 758, 1980.

41. MOORE, W. S., HENRY, R. E., MALONE, J. M., DALY, M. J., PATTON, D., AND CHILDERS, S. J.: Prospective use of xenon XE-133 clearance for amputation level selection. Arch. Surg., **116**: 86, 1981.

42. SIEGEL, M. E., STEWART, C. A., WAGNER, W., AND SAKIMURA, I.: A new objective criterion for determining noninvasively healing potential of ischemic ulcers. J. Nucl. Med., **22**: 187, 1981.

43. LANTIERI, R. L., FAWCETT, H. D., MCKILLOP, J. H., AND MCDOUGALL, I. R.: GA-67 or In-111 white blood cell scans for abscess detection. Clin. Nucl. Med., **5**: 185, 1980.

44. MELINCOFF, R. N.: Computed tomography: The CT scanner. A new diagnostic and research potential for podiatric medicine. J.A.P.A., **70**: 161, 1980.

45. SCHUMACHER, T. M., GENANT, H. K., KOROBKIN, M., AND BOVILL, E. C.: Computed tomography. J. Bone Jt. Surg., **60A**: 600, 1978.

46. O'CONNOR, J. F., AND COHEN, J.: Computerized tomography (CAT scan, CT scan) in orthopedic surgery. J. Bone Jt. Surg., **60A**: 1096, 1978.

47. GENANT, H. K., WILSON, J., BOVILL, E. G., BRUNELLE, F. O., MURRY, W. R., AND RODRIGO, J. J.: Computed tomography of the musculo skeletal system. J. Bone Jt. Surg., **62A**: 108, 1980.

48. WEIS, L., HEELAN, R. T., AND WATSON, R. C.: Computed tomography of orthopedic tumors of the pelvis and lower extremities. Clin. Orthop. Relat. Res. **130**: 254, 1978.

49. HEELMAN, R. T., WATSON, R. C., AND SMITH, J.: Computed tomography of the lower extremities. Am. J. Roentgenol., **132**: 933, 1979.

50. LAURSEN, K., AND REITER, S.: Computed tomography in soft tissue disorders of the lower extremities. Acta Orthop. Scand., **51**: 881, 1980.

51. MCLEOD, R. A., STEPHENS, D. H., BEABOUT, J. W., SHEEDY, P. F., AND HATTERY, R. R.: Computed tomography of the skeletal system. Semin. Roentgenol., **13**: 235, 1978.

52. HERMAN, G., AND ROSE, J.: Computed tomography in bone and soft tissue pathology of the extremities. J. Comput. Assist. Tomogr. **3**: 58, 1979.

53. TERMOTE, J., BERT, A., CROLLA, D., PALMERS, Y., AND BULCKE, J. A.: Computed tomography of the normal and pathologic muscular system. Radiology, **137**: 439, 1980.

54. LEVINSONN, E. M., AND BRYAN, P. J.: Computed tomography in unilateral extremity swelling of unusual cause. J. Comput. Assist. Tomogr. **3**: 67, 1979.

55. JOHNSON, W. C., PALEY, R. H., CASTROUOVO, J. J., ET AL.: Computed tomographic angiology. Am. J. Surg., **141**: 434, 1981.

56. VUJIC, I., STANLEY, J., AND TYMINSKI, L. J.: Computed tomography of suspected caval thrombosis secondary to proximal extension of phlebitis from the leg. Radiology, **140**: 437, 1981.

57. REIS, N. D., ZINMAN, C., BESSLER, M. I. D., ET AL.: High resolution computerized tomography in clinical orthopedics. J. Bone Jt. Surg., **64B**: 20, 1982.

58. CHIU, L. C., AND SCHAPIRO, R. L.: A primer in computed axial tomographic anatomy: VI. The lower extremities. J. Comput. Tomogr. **2**: 349, 1978.

59. CHIU, L. C., YIU, V. S., AND SCHAPIRO, R. L.: An introduction to abnormal computed tomographic anatomy: VI. The lower extremities. J. Comput. Tomogr. **2**: 367, 1978.

Index

Page numbers in italics denote figures; those followed by t or f denote tables and footnotes, respectively.

Accessory bones, 243
Achilles tendon
  shortened, 171
  thickened, 219
Achondroplasia, 381–382, *400–401*
  hydrocephalus in, 381
  trident hand in, 381
Acid neutralizer, x-ray processing and, 16
Acromegaly, 139–140, 320–321, *325–331*
  diabetes mellitus in, 320
  dorsal kyphosis in, 320
  fibrous dysplasia and, 380
  heel pad sign and, 139
  hyperthyroidism in, 320
  joint space and, 202
  osteophytes and, 204
  radiologic findings
    chondrocalcinosis, 321, 321t
    spade-like tufts, 321, *326*
  rheumatologic complaints in, 320
  somatotropin and, 321
Acroosteosclerosis, sarcoidosis and, 432
Acute radiation syndrome, 4
Adamantinoma, anatomic location of, 279
Adduction deformity, of second toe, 123, *124*
Adductus forefoot, 55
Ainhum, 190, *191*
Albers-Schonberg disease (*see* Osteopetrosis)
Albright's syndrome, 282
American College of Podiatric Radiologists, 1, 2
Amyloidosis, multiple myeloma and, 416
Angioma, benign, 281
Ankle
  diastasis of, 40, 236, *258*
  examination of, 40
  fracture of, *274*
  inversion sprain of, 231, *232*, 236
Ankle equinus, 65, 67, *67*
Ankylosing spondylitis, 219, *220–222*
  bamboo spine in, 219, *222*
  bony ankylosis in, 219
  calcaneal erosions and, 219
  Haglund's deformity and, 219
  HLA-B27 antigen and, 219
  paraarticular osteoporosis and, 219
  plantar spur in, 219
  similarity to hyperparathyroidism, 323
  thickening of Achilles tendon in, 219
Anterior drawer view, 31, *31*

Anterior talofibular ligament
  arthrography and, 231
  calcaneofibular ligament and, 231
  Drawer sign x-rays and, 231
  soft tissue injuries and, 231
  stress inversion x-rays and, 231
Apophysis, calcaneal, 77
Arrested epiphyseal growth, fracture healing and, 273
Arteriography, neoplastic evaluation and, 285
Arteriosclerosis obliterans
  differentiated from Mönkeberg's medial sclerosis, *142*
  dystrophic calcification and, 140–141, *142*, *143*
Arteriosclerotic calcification
  Mönkeberg's medial sclerosis and, 145
Arthritis (*see also* specific type), 202–230
  joint space examination, 202
  with acute osteomyelitis, *180*
Arthritis mutilans
  in Reiter's syndrome, 216
Arthritis mutilans
  in rheumatoid arthritis, 215
Arthrography, 231, 236
  anterior talofibular ligament and, 231
  calcaneofibular ligaments and, 231
  diastasis of the ankle and, 236
  inferior tibiofibular syndesmosis and, 236
  inversion sprain of the ankle and, 231, 236
  soft tissue injuries and, 231
Aseptic necrosis
  causal conditions, 322t
  Cushing's disease and, 322, *333*
  decreased uptake of radionuclide and, 443
  fracture healing and, 273
Atom, 6
Atrophic arthropathy, 190–192, *192–194*
  deformities in
    balancing pagoda, 191
    intrusion, 191
    mortar-in-pestle, 191
    pencil-in-cup, 191
    talipes cavus, 191
  osteolysis in, *194*
  similar conditions
    burns, 190
    frostbite, 190
    progressive systemic sclerosis, 190

psoriatic arthritis, 190
Raynaud's disease, 190
rheumatoid arthritis, 190
surgical amputation, 190
trench foot, 190
Atrophy, of soft tissue, 139, *156*
Autosympathectomy
  neuropathy and, 446
  peripheral neuropathy and, 191–192
Avulsion fracture, 243, 245, *250*, 379
Axial calcaneal projection, 24, *25*
Axial sesamoidal projection, 24, *24*, *25*

Balancing pagoda deformity, in atrophic arthropathy, 191
Bamboo spine, in ankylosing spondylitis, 219, *222*
Bayonet hand, in multiple hereditary exostoses, 383
Bayonnet sign (*see* Blade of grass sign)
Benign bone tumor, technetium bone scan and, 445
Bi-malleolar fracture, 261
Bipartite sesamoids, 243
Blade of grass sign, in Paget's disease, 379
Block washer, 3
Blood pool image, in bone scan, 443, *444*
Boehler's angle, fracture of calcaneus and, 276, *277*
Bone cyst, 281, 284–285, *297–298*, *311–313*
  aneurysmal in multiple myeloma, 416
  as differentiated from Brodie's abscess, 187
  of osteoarthritis, 223
Bone healing (*See* Fracture repair)
Bone infarction
  in Gaucher's disease, 361
  in sickle cell anemia, *364*, *365*
Bone islands
  in osteopoikilosis, 381, *397*, *399*
  technetium bone scan and, 443
Bone neoplasms (*See* Neoplastic evaluation and specific disease)
Bone patterns
  neoplastic evaluation and
    moth-eaten, 279
    permeated, 279
Bone scan, 442–443, *444*, 445–446, *446–451*, 451–453
  blood pool image and, 443, *444*
  combined use of gallium, technetium osteomyelitis and, 445, *447*

Bone scan—*continued*
  septic arthritis and, 445
  flow studies and, 443, *444*
  gamma camera in, 442
  in inflammatory arthritis diagnosis, 452
  in multiple myeloma, 416
  in osteoid-osteoma diagnosis, 452
  in plantar fasciitis diagnosis, 452
  in Reiter's syndrome diagnosis, 452
  in stress fracture diagnosis, 452
  in trauma diagnosis
    fracture, 451
    pseudoarthrosis, 451
    synovitis, 451
  indium and, 453
  of metastases, *426*
  of Paget's disease, *392*
  photopenic activity in, 443
  photondeficient area in, 443
  photopenic area in, 443
  pinhole columnator in, 442
  processes
    microcirculation of bone, 443
    neovascularization, 443
    passive diffusion, 443
  rectilinear scanner in, 442
  technetium, 442–443, *442, 444,* 445
  thallium and, 453
  xenon-133 and, 452–453
Bone shortening, fracture healing and, 273
Bone-within-a-bone appearance, in osteopetrosis, 383, *409, 411*
Bony ankylosis, in ankylosing spondylitis, 219
Bony bridging, fracture healing and, *275–276*
Bony deformity, in osteomalacia, 342
Bony destruction, in Paget's disease, 380
Bony equinus (*see* Ankle equinus)
Bony mineralization, abnormalities of, 161, *162,* 163, *163*
  endosteal new bone, 163
  osteomalacia, 163
  osteoporosis, 161, *162*
  Sudek's atrophy, 161, *163*
Bouchard's node, in osteoarthritis, 223
Boutonniere deformity, in rheumatoid arthritis, 205
Bowing deformity, in rickets, 342
Bradymetapody, *127,* 128, *129, 130*
  pseudohypoparathyroidism and, 128
  pseudopseudohypoparathyroidism and, 128
Brodie's abscess, 187, *187, 188*
Bronchiectasis, hypertrophic pulmonary osteoarthropathy and, 417
Bronchogenic carcinoma, hypertrophic pulmonary osteoarthropathy and, 417
Brown tumors
  in hyperparathyroidism, 324, *341*
  in uremic osteopathy, 343
Burns, as similar to atrophic arthropathy, 190

Café-au-lait skin spot, in fibrous dysplasia, 380
Caffey's syndrome, 160
Calcaneal apophysis, 48, *48, 49*
Calcaneal inclination angle, 57, *59*

calcaneovalgus and, *86*
cavus and, *80, 82*
equinus and, *90*
Calcaneal inclination axis, 57, *59*
Calcaneofibular ligament
  anterior talofibular ligament and, 231
  arthrography and, 231
  soft tissue injuries and, 231
  stress inversion x-rays and, 231
Calcaneonavicular bar, 70, 93, *93*
Calcaneovalgus, 84, 87, *89*
  calcaneal inclination angle and, *86*
  factors affecting position, 84–85
  limitation of dorsiflexion, 85
  rigid, *88*
  similarity to vertical talus, 91
  talocalcaneal angle and, *88*
Calcaneus, 17, 20, 38–39, 77
  axis of, 57, *59*
  Boehler's angle and, 276, *277*
  cyma line of, 39
  fracture of, *252–257*
  Haglund's deformity and, 39
  pronation of, 39
  sustentaculum tali and, 39
  talocalcaneal notch and, 39
  tuberosity of, 39, 77
Calcification
  defined, 140
  in Paget's disease, 380
Calcification of Baggenstoss and Keith, etiology of, 145
Calcified thrombae, 147, *147, 148*
Calcifying collagenolysis, 148, *150*
Calcinosis, 140, 147–148, *149–152*
  calcified bursitis, 148, *151, 152*
  secondary hyperparathyroidism and, *153*
  subcutaneous, 148, *149*
  tumoral, 148, *150,* 343
Calcium deposition, in the media, 141
Calcium pyrophosphate, pseudogout and, 230, *230*
Carcinoma, metastasis and, 415
Cartilage formation, neoplastic evaluation and, 279
Cartilaginous matrix
  neoplastic evaluation and, 279
  Ollier's disease and, 279
Cavovarus, tendo-achilles and, *81*
Cavus
  calcaneal inclination and, *80*
  neurological, *82*
  secondary to Charcot Marie Tooth disease, *83*
Cavus deformities, *100*
  rearfoot varus and, 100
  rigid forefoot valgus and, 100
Cavus foot, 64, *68, 69*
Cellulitis, technetium bone scan and, 443
Central ray, 16
Charcot foot, 190, *191*
  penciling in, 190
  peripheral neuropathy and, 191
  sucked-candy deformity in, 190
Charcot joint
  as degenerative osteoarthritis, 192
  diabetic neuropathy and, 191
  neurotrophic arthropathic form, 192
  osteoarthrosis in, 194
  osteophytes in, 194
  syphilitic tabes dorsalis and, 191

zone of subchrondral osteoporosis and, 193
Charcot Marie Tooth disease, cavus deformity and, *83*
Chondroblastoma, anatomic location of, 279
Chondrocalcinosis
  in acromegaly, 321, 321t, *329*
  in primary hyperparathyroidism, 343
Chondroma, 281
Chondrosarcoma
  cartilaginous matrix and, 279
  in enchondromatosis, 382
  in multiple hereditary exostoses, 382
Chopart's joint, 57, *59*
Christmas disease (*see* Hemophilia, B type)
Classic hemophilia (*see* Hemophilia, A type)
Claw foot, *131*
Claw toe, 118, *118,* 206–207
Cleft foot, *131*
Cloaca, as sign of osteomyelitis, 179, *180,* 182
Club foot (*see also* Talipes and specific type), 77–99
Clubbing of digits, in hypertrophic pulmonary osteoarthropathy, 417
Coat hanger exostoses, in diaphyseal aclasis, 383
Coccidioidal granuloma, 190
Codman's triangle, 160, 280
Collimation, of x-ray beam, 3, 7, 16–17
Collum tali axis, *51,* 53, 57, *59*
Comminuted fracture, 245
Complete dislocation, *238*
Compound fracture, 245
Compression fracture, in Paget's disease, 380
Computerized axial tomography, 453–454
  Cushing's disease, *332*
  fracture evaluation and, 454
  involucrum evaluation and, 453
  neoplastic evaluation and, 285
  of multiple myeloma, *430*
  osteomyelitis evaluation and, 453
  tarsal coalition evaluation and, 454
Congenital syphilis, calcification of Baggenstoss and Keith and, 145
Congestive heart failure, decreased uptake of radionuclide and, 443
Congruous joint, 40, 108, *108*
Cooley's anemia, 359, 360, *367*
Cortex, blood sources of, 181
Cottonwool skull, in Paget's disease, 379, *384*
Crescent sign
  Freiberg's infraction and, 167
  in osteonecrosis, 166
Cretinism (*see* Hypothyroidism)
Crew-cut pattern (*see* Hair-on-end pattern)
Crista
  axial sesamoidal view, *106*
  tibial sesamoid and, 106, *107*
Crooke's tube, 1
CRST syndrome, scleroderma and, *155*
Cuboid, 17, 19, 39, 77
Cuboid abduction, *88,* 99
Cuboid abduction angle, *51,* 53
Cuneiforms, 39, 77

Cuneiform split, sign of hypermobility of first ray, 114, *115*
Cushing's disease, 321–322, *332, 333*
  aseptic necrosis in, 322, *333*
  CAT scan, *332*
  features
    buffalo hump, 321
    cutaneous striae, 321
    hirsutism, 321
    moon facies, 321
    osteoporosis, 321, 322
  fibrous dysplasia and, 380
  glucocorticoids and, 321
  osteoporosis and, 343
  radiologic findings
    demineralization, 321–322
    osteoporosis, 321–322
  similarity to hyperparathyroidism, 323
Cutaneous gangrene, hyperparathyroidism and, 152
Cutaneous induration, *138*
Cutaneous striae, Cushing's disease and, 321
Cyma line, 57, *59,* 67
Cystic fibrosis, hypertrophic pulmonary osteoarthropathy and, 417
Cystic lesion, *313*

Dactylitis, in sickle cell anemia, 359
Darkroom processing technique, of x-ray, 8
Degenerative arthritis (*see* Osteoarthritis)
Delayed union of fracture, 273–274
Dermatomyositis, 156, *156*
Developer, 16
Deviated joint, 40
  defined, 108
  increased proximal articular set angle, *109*
Diabetes mellitus, in acromegaly, 320
Diabetic foot, 190
Diabetic neuropathy
  as basis for Charcot joint disease, 191
  bone scan, *451*
Diabetic osteopathy, 190
  osteosclerosis in, 190
  sequestration in, 190
Diaphyseal aclasis (*see* Multiple hereditary exostoses)
Diastasis
  arthrography and, 236
Diastasis
  of ankle, 40, 236, *258–259*
Digital deformity, 118–130
Digital excrescence, 119
Digiti quinti varus, hallux-abducto-valgus in, 125, *125*
Digit, longitudinal axis of, *52, 53*
Direct extension osteomyelitis, 179, 182, *182*
Dislocation, 236, *238–242*
  defined, 236
  Lisfranc's, *240–241*
  peritalar, *242*
Displaced fracture, *243*
Disseminated periostitis, in thyroid acropachy, 322–323, *334*
Distal articular set angle, *56,* 57, 103–104
Dorsal kyphosis, in acromegaly, 320
Dorsoplantar projection
  calcaneus, 17
  cuboid and, 17

interphalangeal joint and, 17
Lis Franc's joint and, 17
medial cuneiform and, 17
metatarsophalangeal joints and, 17
navicular and, 17
talus and, 17
Double-strip sign
  hypertrophic pulmonary osteoarthropathy and, 452
  shin splints and, 452
Drawer sign x-rays, 231
  anterior talofibular ligament and, 231
  inversion sprain of the ankle and, 231
  soft tissue injuries and, 231
Dwarfism (*see* Achondroplasia)
Dysplastic disorder, 379–414
  achondroplasia, 381–382, *400–401*
  enchondromatosis, 382, *402–404*
  fibrous dysplasia, 380–381, *393–396*
  multiple hereditary exostoses, 382, *405–408*
  osteopetrosis, 383, *409–414*
  osteopoikilosis, 381, *393, 397–399*
  Paget's disease, 379–380, *384–392*
Dystrophic calcification, 140–146
  arteriosclerosis obliterans, 140–141, *142, 143*
  Mönkeberg's medial sclerosis and, 144–145, *144–146*

Ebuneration, in osteoarthritis, 223
Edema
  infectious, 132, *133, 134, 184*
  traumatic, 132, *133*
Emphysema, of soft tissue, 139, *141*
Enchondroma, 281, 284–285, *296*
  cartilaginous matrix and, 279
  Ollier's disease and, 279
Enchondromatosis, 382, *402–404*
  chondrosarcoma in, 382
  hamartomatous cartilage and, 382
  Mafucci's syndrome and, 382
  multiple hereditary exostoses and, 382
  pathologic fracture in, 382
  sarcoidosis and, 432
Endocrinologic disease, 320–341
  acromegaly, 320–321, *325–331*
  Cushing's, 321–322, *332, 333*
  hyperparathyroidism, 323–324, *337–341*
  hyperthyroidism, 322
  hypothyroidism, 323, *334–336*
  thyroid acropachy, 322–323, *334*
Endosteal new bone, osteopetrosis and, 163
Endosteal osteoclasis, deficit in osteopetrosis, 383
Endothelial myeloma (*See* Ewing's sarcoma)
Energy transfer, types, 6–7
Eosinophilic granuloma, periosteal reaction and, 158, 279–280
Epiphyseal fracture, 260, *260–261*
Epiphysiolysis, in hemophilia, 360
Epiphysis, 77
Equino varus, 77, 79–80
Equinus, 62
  ankle, 65, 67, *67*
  calcaneal inclination angle and, *90*
  compensated, *63*
  defined, 90
  genu recurvatum and, 62f

hallux abducto valgus and, 62
microtrauma and, 62
midtarsal joint in, 90
navicular cuneiform fault and, 62
partially compensated, 62
retrocalcaneal spur and, 62
subtalar joint in, 90
wedged-shaped navicular and, 62, *90*
Erlenmeyer flask deformity
  in Gaucher's disease, 361, *376*
  in osteopetrosis, 383, *409*
  in thalassemia, 360
Erosion
  in ankylosing spondylitis, 219
  in gouty arthritis, 225
  in hemophilia, 360
  in psoriatic arthritis, 215
  of gouty arthritis, 202, *204*
  of inflammatory arthritis, 202
  of psoriatic arthritis, 202, *203*
  of rheumatoid arthritis, 202, *203,* 205, *212, 213*
Ewing's sarcoma, 282, 285, *300, 305*
  anatomic location of, 278
  bone patterns and, 279
  periosteal reactions and, 280
Exostoses, 280–281, 285, 382, *404*
Exposure time, x-rays and, 8
Extramedullary hematopoiesis, in osteopetrosis, 383

Fairbank's disease, *177,* 178
Fanconi's syndrome, osteomalacia and, 342
Fatigue fracture, 264
Fibrosarcoma of bone, 284, *284, 291, 295*
Fibrous dysplasia, 380–381, *393–396*
  acromegaly and, 380
  café-au-lait skin spots and, 380
  Cushing's disease and, 380
  hyperthyroidism and, 380
  of bone, 282
  radiologic findings
    leontiasis ossea deformity, 380
    osteolytic bone lesion, 380
    pathologic fracture, 380
    shepard's crook deformity, 380, *393*
    stress fracture, 380
  sarcoidosis and, 432
  sexual precocity and, 380
Fibula, fracture of, *258–259*
Film speed, x-ray exposure and, 8
Filtration, of x-ray beam, 7
First metatarsal declination angle, in first ray evaluation, 113
First metatarsal declination axis, 57, *59*
First metatarsal first cuneiform angle, 105
First metatarsophalangeal joint
  alignment of, 108
  result of microtrauma to, 113
First ray, hypermobility of, 114
First ray deformity
  bunion, 102
  hallus-abducto-valgus, 102
Fixer, 16
Flow study, bone scan and, 443, *444*
Foot
  biomechanics of, 50–76
  bones of, 38–40
    calcaneus, 38–39
    cuboid, 39
    cuneiforms, 39

first metatarsal, 39
navicular, 38
second through fifth metatarsals, 39–40
supernumerary, 40–45, *41–45*
talus, 38
normal, 38–49
Forefoot adductus angle, *54*, 55, 102
Forefoot supinatus, *63*, 64
Forefoot valgus, 64, *65–67*, 67, 100–101
flexible cavus foot, 101
flexible plantarflexed first ray, 64, 101
rigid, 64, *66*, 67, 100–101
semi-rigid, 64, *65*, 67
Forefoot varus
compensated, 58, *61*, 62
Forefoot varus
naviculocuneiform fault and, 62
wedge-shaped navicular and, 58, *61*
Foreign bodies, x-ray evaluation of, *233–235*
Fracture, 243–277, *243–277*
avulsion, 243, 245, *250*
bi-malleolar, 261
Boehler's angle and, 276, *277*
bone scan diagnosis, 451
comminuted, 245
compound, 245
computerized axial tomography and, 454
defined, 243
dislocation and, 236, *238, 240, 244, 261*
displaced, *243*
epiphyseal, 260, *260–261*
Gosselin's, 261
greenstick, 245
impaction, *246–247*, 261
incomplete, 245
increased uptake of radionuclide and, 443, 445
Jones, 261
microfracture, 265
of calcaneous, *252–257*, 276, *277*
of fibula, *258–259*
of navicular, *248–249*
of talus, *251*
pathologic, 271, *271*
physiological anesthesia and, 271
Potts, 261
repair, 271–274, *273–276*
spiral, 245
stress, 264–266, *264–270*
fatigue, 264
insufficiency, 264–265, 271
osteonal remodeling and, 265
systemic diseases and, 265
technecium bone scan and, 266
tibial sesamoid, *244*
transverse, *243*, 245
tri-malleolar or cotton, 261
Fracture repair, 271–274, *273–276*
arrested epiphyseal growth and, 273
aseptic necrosis and, 273
bone shortening and, 273
bony bridging and, *275–276*
complications of, 273–274
delayed union and, 273–274
infection and, 273
inflammatory stage of healing, 271
mal-union of bone and, 273
non-union of bone and, 273–274, *273*

physiological anesthesia and, 271
primary, 272–273
primary cellular callus, 271–272
pseudoarthrosis and, 274
reorganization and remodeling of primary bone, 272
reparative phase of healing, 271
secondary, 273
systemic factors and, 273
Free radicals, 4
Freiberg's disease, etiology of, 165
Freiberg's infraction, 166–168, *168–172*
crescent sign in, 167
hypermobile first metatarsals and, 166
metatarsalgia and, 166
subchondral bone fracture and, 167
Frontal plane evaluation, of first ray deformities, 114
Frostbite, as similar to atrophic arthropathy, 190
Functional coalition, 70, *71, 73*
Fungal infection
ainhum, 190, *191*
Coccidioidal granuloma, 190

Gait
normal foot
gastrocnemius muscle, 80
triceps surae, 80
spastic equinus foot, 80
Gallium bone scan, 445, *446, 447*
lactoferrin and, 445
siderophores and, 445
Gamma camera, in bone scanning, 442
Ganglion, *136*
Garrè's non-suppurative osteitis, 189–190
Gastrocnemius equinus, 90
Gaucher's disease, 361, *376–378*
bone infarction, 361
Erlenmeyer flask deformity, 361, *376*
Genu recurvatum, 62f
Giant cell sarcoma, 279, 281, 284–285, *290, 301–302, 314–315*
Gigantism (*see* Acromegaly)
Glucocorticoids, Cushing's disease and, 321
Goiter (*see* Grave's disease)
Gosselin's fracture, 261
Gout
multiple myeloma and, 416
sarcoidosis and, 432
Gouty arthritis, 225, *225–229*
erosion in, 202, *204*, 225
hyperuricemia and, 225
martel sign and, 202, *204*, 225
tophi in, 225, *229*
Graves' disease, in hyperthyroidism, 322
Greenstick fracture, 245, 342
Growth hormone (*see* Somatotropin)
Gummatus destruction, luetic osteomyelitis and, 188

Haglund's deformity, 39, 219
Hair-on-end pattern
in sickle cell anemia, 358, *361*
in thalassemia, 360, *370*
Hallux
os interphalangeum of, 43, *43*
subungual exostosis of, *121, 122*
valgus rotation of, *116*
Hallux abducto valgus
absence of, 62

in digiti quinti varus, *125*
second toe overlap, 123, *123*
Hallux-abducto valgus deformity
development of, 206
first metatarsal cuneiform angle and, 103
forefoot adductus angle and, 103
frontal plane evaluation, 114
hallux abductus angle and, *103*
in rheumatoid arthritis, 205, 206, *207, 209*
intermetatarsal angle and, 103
sesamoid position and, 103
Hallux abductus angle, *52*, 55
ideal, 102
in first ray evaluation, 102
Hallux abductus varus, *104*
Hallux-adducto varus, *104*
Hallux interphalangeal angle, *52*, 55, 102, 112, *112*
Hallux limitus, *114*
first metatarsal declination angle, 113
structural, 113
Hallux rigidus, 113, *113*
Hallux varus
iatrogenically caused, 103
metatarsus adductus and, 103
Hamartomatous cartilage, enchondromatosis and, 382
Hammer toe, 118, *118*
Hand-foot syndrome, in sickle cell anemia, *363*
Hansen's disease, 190
Harris and Beath angle, 53
Harris and Beath projection, 26, *26*, 70–73
demonstrating talocalcaneal coalition, 94, *95*
subtalar joints and, 26
sustentaculum tali and, 26
Heberden's node, in osteoarthritis, 223
Hemangioendothelioma, 283
Hemarthrosis, hemophilia and, 360
Hematogenous osteomyelitis, 179, 180–182
in infants and children, 180
technetium bone scan and, 443
Hematologic and reticuloendothelial disease, 358–378
Hematoma, ossifying, 281, 284–285
Hemophilia, 360–361, *372–375*
A type, 360
B type, 360–361
epiphysiolysis in, 360
hemarthrosis and, 360
leg length discrepancy in, 360
radiologic findings
blow-out lesion of bone, 361
erosion, 360
osteoporosis, 360
pseudotumors, 361
subchondral cyst, 360
Hirsutism, Cushing's disease and, 321
HLA antigen
ankylosing spondylitis and, 219
association with inflammatory arthritis, 207
Hodgkin's disease, 284
Hydrocephalus, in achondroplasia, 381
Hypercalcemia, multiple myeloma and, 416
Hyperemia, osteomyelitis and, 186

Hypermobility
  defined, 62
  of first ray, 62
Hypernephroma, 284
Hyperostosis head, of proximal phalanx of fifth toe, *120*
Hyperparathyroidism, 152, *153,* 323–324, *337–341*
  brown tumors in, 324, *341*
  calcification of Baggenstoss and Keith and, 145
  compression fracture in, 324
  cutaneous gangrene and, 152
  elevated serum calcium in, 323
  hypervitaminosis D and, 344
  nephrocalcinosis in, 324, *337*
  osteoporosis in, 324
  pathologic fracture in, 324
  radiologic findings
    acroosteolysis, 323, 324t
    periosteal resorption of bone, 323
    similarities to inflammatory conditions, 323
  resorption of bone in, 204
  salt and pepper skull in, *341*
  secondary (*see also* Renal osteodystrophy), 152, *153,* 342–343, *349–352*
  soft tissue calcification in, 324
  subcutaneous calcinosis and, 148
Hyperthyroidism
  fibrous dysplasia and, 380
  goiter and, 322
  in acromegaly, 320
  osteoporosis in, 322
  primary, 323–324, *337–341*
  radiologic findings
    compression fractures, 322
    pathologic fractures, 322
Hypertrophic arthropathy, distinguished from peripheral neuropathy, 192
Hypertrophic osteoarthropathy, 192–194, *195–201*
Hypertrophic pulmonary osteoarthropathy, 417, *433–435*
  bronchiectasis and, 417
  bronchogenic carcinoma and, 417
  clubbing of digits and, 417
  cystic fibrosis and, 417
  double-strip sign in, 452
  mesotheliomas and, 417
  periostitis of bone and, 417
  solid periosteal reaction and, 158
  synovitis and, 417
Hyperuricemia, gouty arthritis and, 225
Hypervitaminosis A, 160, 344
Hypervitaminosis D, 344
  calcification of Baggenstoss and Keith and, 145
  hyperparathyroidism and, 344
  milk-alkali syndrome and, 344
  multiple myeloma and, 344
  sarcoidosis and, 344
Hypophosphatemia, osteomalacia and, 163
Hypoplastic fibular sesamoid, *117*
Hypothyroidism, 323, *334–336*

Impaction fracture, *246–247,* 261
Incomplete fracture, 245
Indium, detection of infectious lesions and, 453
Infantile cortical hyperostosis, 160

Infarction
  decreased uptake of radionuclide and, 443
  increased uptake of radionuclide and, 443
Infection
  fracture healing and, 273
  periosteal reactions and, 280
Inferior tibiofibular syndesmosis, arthrography and, 236
Inflammatory arthritis
  bone scan diagnosis, 452
  HLA antigens and, 207
  lysosomal enzymes and, 202
Inflammatory stage of fracture healing, 271
Infraction, defined, 166
Insufficiency fracture, 264–265, 271
  osteogenesis imperfecta and, 265
  osteomalacia and, 265
  osteoporosis and, 265
  Paget's disease of bone and, 265
  renal osteodystrophy and, 265
  rheumatoid arthritis and, 265
Intensifying screen, 8, 13–14
  film/screen combinations, 14
  of calcium tungstate, 13
  phosphorescence and, 13
  rare earth type, 14
  speed and, 13–14
Intermetatarsal angle, *52,* 55
  in first ray evaluation, 102
  increased, *123*
Interphalangeal joints, 17
Interstitial polymyositis, in rheumatoid arthritis, 205
Intractable plantar keratosis, plantar-flexed metatarsals and, 116
Intrusion, in atrophic arthropathy, 191
Inversion sprain, of the ankle, 231, *232,* 236
Involucrum
  absence of in tuberculous of bone, *189*
  as sign of osteomyelitis, 179, *180,* 181, 182, *183*
  computerized axial tomography and, 453
  technetium bone scan and, 445
Ionizing radiation, types, 6
Ischemic necrosis, 165–166
  Legg Calvé-Perthes' disease, 166
  of apophysis of calcaneus, 171, *175*
  Osgood-Schlatter's disease, 166, *167*
  radiologic progression
    crescent sign, 166
    snow-cap sign, 166
    step formation, 166
    structural failure, 166
  segmental, 176, *176*
Isherwood views, 69–70, 94
Ivory vertebral body, in Paget's disease, 379, *388*

Jaffe-Lichtenstein syndrome, 282
Joint disease, 202–230
Joint effusion, in peripheral neuropathy, 192
Joint space
  acromegaly and, 202
  in osteoarthritis, 223
  soft tissue effusion and, 202

Joint types
  congruous, 40
  deviated, 40
  subluxed, 40
Jones fracture, 261

Kager's triangle (*see* Toygar's triangle)
Kidney disease, subcutaneous calcinosis and, 148
Kilovoltage, of x-ray beam, 7
Kite's angle, 53
Köhler's disease, 169–171, *173, 174*
  discoid navicular in, 169–170
  etiology of, 165
  ossification of navicular and, 46
  osteochondritis of navicular and, 170
  radionuclide examination in, 170

Lactoferrin binding, gallium-67 localization and, 445
Lamenated periosteal reaction, 158, 159
Lateral ankle projection, 28, *28*
Lateral oblique projection, 22, *22, 23,* 28, *28, 29*
Lateral talocalcaneal angle, 58, *59*
Lead shielding, 15–16
Leg length discrepancy, in hemophilia, 360
Legg Calvé-Perthes' disease, 165, 166
Leontiasis ossea deformity, in fibrous dysplasia, 380
Leprosy, 190, 204
Lesion margin, neoplastic evaluation and, 279
Lesser tarsus
  longitudinal axis of, *52,* 53
  transection of, *52*
Lesser tarsus angle, *54,* 55
Leukemia, 284, 343
Lisfranc's joint, 17
Lisfranc's dislocation, *240–241*
Local cavus (*see* Cavus foot)
Looser's zones, in osteomalacia, 342
Luetic osteomyelitis, 187–188
  gummatus destruction and, 188
  lace-like subperiosteal calcification, 188
  saber shin and, 188
Lytic metastasis, carcinoma of the kidney and, 415

Macrodactyly, 125, *126*
Mafucci's syndrome, enchondromatosis and, 382
Magniposer, *33*
Main-en-lorgnette deformity, in psoriatic arthritis, 215, *216*
Malignant tumor, technetium bone scan and, 445
Mal-union of fracture, 273
Mallet toe, 119, *119*
Marble bone disease (*see* Osteopetrosis)
Martel sign, in gouty arthritis, 202, *204,* 235
Mastocytosis, osteopoikilosis and, 381
Matter, 6
McCune-Albright syndrome, in fibrous dysplasia, 380
Medial cuneiform, 17, 19
Medial oblique projection, 21, *21, 22,* 28, *29*

Mesothelioma, hypertrophic pulmonary osteoarthropathy and, 417
Metabolic disease, 342–358
  hypervitaminosis A, 344
  hypervitaminosis D, 344
  osteomalacia, 342, 346–348
  osteoporosis, 343–344, 353–356
  renal osteodystrophy, 342–343, 349–352
  rickets, 342, 346–348
  scurvy, 344–345, 357, 358
  secondary hyperparathyroidism, 342–343, 349–352
Metaphyseal involvement, in osteomyelitis, 181
Metastasis, 415–416, 418–426
  bone scan, 426
  carcinoma of the breast and, 415
  carcinoma of the lung and, 415
  carcinoma of the kidney and, 415
  lytic type, 415
  neuroblastoma and, 415
  pathologic fracture and, 415
  sarcoidosis and, 432
  tomogram, 420
  vertebra plana deformity and, 415
Metastatic calcification, 140, 152, 152, 153, 154, 154–156
  dermatomyositis, 156, 156
  hyperparathyroidism, 152, 153
  scleroderma, 154, 155
  systemic lupus erythematosus, 154, 154, 155
Metastatic tumor, technetium bone scan and, 445
Metatarsal, 77
  fifth, 19
  first, 19, 39
  second through fifth, 39–40
Metatarsalgia, Freiberg's infraction and, 166
Metatarsophalangeal joints, 17
Metatarsus, longitudinal axis of, 52, 53
Metatarsus adductus, 96, 97–99, 97–99
  talocalcaneal angle and, 78
  types
    Atavistic form of metatarsus primus, 98
    serpentine S-shaped foot, 98
    total, 98
Metatarsus adductus angle, 52, 55, 102
Metatarsus primus adductus angle (see Intermetatarsal angle)
Method of Kho, soft tissue thickness and, 140
Microdactyly, 125
Microfracture, 265
Mid-tarsal joint, 57, 59
Milk-alkali syndrome, hypervitaminosis D in, 344
Mönkeberg's medial sclerosis
  arteriosclerotic calcifications and, 145
  dystrophic calcification and, 144–145, 144–146
  gooseneck lamp sign, 145, 144
Mortar-in-pestle deformity
  in atrophic arthropathy, 191
  in peripheral neuropathy, 192
Mortise projection, 27, 27
Multiple epiphyseal dysplasia, 177, 178
Multiple hereditary exostoses, 382, 405–408

bayonet hand in, 383
chondrosarcoma in, 382
coat hanger lesions in, 383
enchondromatosis and, 382
snow-cap calcification and, 405
Multiple myeloma, 416–417, 427–431
  amyloidosis and, 416
  CAT scan, 430
  gout and, 416
  hypercalcemia and, 416
  hypervitaminosis D in, 344
  negative bone scan and, 416
  radiologic findings
    aneurysmal bone cyst, 416
    diffuse osteoporosis, 416
    solitary plasmacytoma of bone, 416
Muscle myopathy, in acromegaly, 320
Muscular dystrophy, osteoporosis and, 343
Mutation, 2, 4
Myeloma, 283–285
Myositis ossificans
  progressive, 156–157
  traumatic, 156, 157
National Council of Radiation Protection, 2
Navicular, 17, 19, 38, 77
  flattened, 169–170
  fracture of, 248–249
  Köhler's disease and, 169–170
  normal, 173
  pronation of, 38
  wedge-shaped, 58, 61, 62, 88, 90
Naviculocuneiform fault, 62, 114, 115
Necrosis
  aseptic, 165
  avascular, 165
  bone infarction, 165
  ischemic, 165–166
Neoplastic and paraneoplastic disorder, 415–431, 433–435
  hypertrophic pulmonary osteoarthropathy, 417, 433–435
  metastasis, 415–416, 418–426
  multiple myeloma, 416–417, 427–431
Neoplastic evaluation, 278–319 (See also specific disease)
  anatomical location and, 278–279
    adamantinoma, 279
    chondroblastoma, 279
    Ewing's sarcoma, 278
    giant cell sarcoma, 279
  arteriography and, 285
  bone patterns and
    moth-eaten, 279
    permeated, 279
  CAT scan and, 285–286
  lesion margin and, 279
  neoplastic matrix and, 279
    cartilaginous, 279
    osteoid, 279
  of benign tumors, 280–281, 284–285, 293, 296, 308, 318
  of bone cysts, 281, 284, 297–298, 311–313
  of fibrous dysplasia, 282
  of giant cell sarcoma, 281, 284–285, 290, 301–302, 314–315
  of malignant tumors
    metastatic, 283–285, 291, 295, 299, 303, 309
    primary, 282–285, 287–289, 292,

294, 300, 305, 307
  of ossifying hematoma, 281
  of osteoid osteoma, 282, 306, 317
  periosteal calcification and, 280
  periosteal reactions and, 279–280
  tomography and, 285
  xeroradiography and, 285
  cartilaginous, 279
  neoplastic evaluation and, 279
  osteoid, 279
Neovascularization, bone scan and, 443
Nephrocalcinosis, in hyperparathyroidism, 324, 333
Neuroarthropathy, 192, 192–194
Neuroblastoma, 284, 415
Neurological cavus
  calcaneal inclination and, 82
  talocalcaneal angle and, 82
Neuropathy
  autosympathectomy and, 446
  increased uptake of radionuclide and, 443
  peripheral, 449
Neurotrophic arthropathy
  Charcot joint and, 192
  distinguished form hypertrophic osteoarthropathy, 192–193
  osteophytes and, 204
Neurotrophic foot
  autosympathectomy and, 446
  bone scanning in, 445–446, 451
Neurotrophic joint, 193
Non-union of fracture, 273–274, 273
Non-weightbearing lateral view (see Non-weightbearing medial projection)
Non-weightbearing medial projection, 20, 20
  calcaneus and, 20
  talus and, 20
Normal foot, 38–49, 77

Ochronosis, osteophytes and, 204
Ollier's disease (see also Enchondromatosis)
  cartilaginous matrix and, 279
  enchondromas and, 279
Onion skin reaction, 158
Open epiphysis, 243
Orthoposer, 8, 17, 17
Ortho-X-poser (see Orthoposer)
Os calcis (see Calcaneus)
Os intermetatasium, 45, 45
Os interphalangeum, of the hallux, 43, 43
Os peroneum, 43, 43
Os sustentaculi, 45, 45
Os tibiale externum, 40, 41, 45
Os trigonum, 40, 41
Os vesalianum, 44, 44
Osgood-Schlatter's disease, 166, 167
Ossification
  defined, 140
  of primary cellular callus, 272
  of soft tissue, 156–157, 157, 158
Ossification centers, 46, 77
  Köhler's disease and, 46
  normal development, 102
  of thirteen-year-old, 47
  present at birth, 46
  secondary, 48, 48, 49
Osteitis deformans (see Paget's disease)
Osteitis fibrosa cystica, 284–285

Osteoarthritis, 223, *223–224*
  bone cysts of, 223
  Bouchard's nodes in, 223
  Heberden's nodes in, 223
  joint space in, 223
  osteophytes and, 204, *204*
  posttraumatic, *224*
  pseudocysts in, 223
  subchondral sclerosis in, 223
Osteoarthrosis (*see also* Osteoarthritis), 194
Osteoblastic carcinoma, 283, 285, *309*
Osteoblastic metastasis, osteopoikilosis and, 381
Osteoblastoma, periosteal reactions and, 279
Osteochondritis, 165–178
Osteochondritis dissecans, 176, *176*
  crescentic radiolucent zone in, 176
  joint mouse in, 176
Osteochondroma, 279, 281, 285, *293, 308, 318*
Osteochondromatosis, 281
Osteochrondosis
  of femoral head, 166
  of tibial tuberosity, 166
Osteoclastic carcinoma, 283, 324
Osteogenesis imperfecta
  insufficiency fractures and, 265
  osteoporosis and, 343, *353*
Osteogenic sarcoma, 282, 284–285, *307*
Osteoid formation, neoplastic evaluation and, 279
Osteoid matrix, neoplastic evaluation and, 279
Osteoid osteoma, 282, *306, 317*
  bone scan diagnosis, 452
  periosteal reactions and, 279–280,
  solid periosteal reaction and, 158
Osteolysis
  in Paget's disease, 379
  of fifth metatarsal, *123*
Osteolytic bone lesion, in fibrous dysplasia, 380
Osteoma, 281, 284–285
Osteomalacia, 342, *346–348*
  enzyme deficiencies and, 342
  Fanconi's syndrome and, 342
  hypophosphatemia and, 163
  in renal osteodystrophy, 342–343
  insufficiency fractures and, 265
  malabsorption states and, 342
  radiologic findings
    bony deformity, 342
    decreased bony density, 342
    protrusio actabuli deformity, 342
    pseudofractures, 342
  renal tubular acidosis and, 342
  similarity to hyperparathyroidism, 323
  steatorrhea and, 163
  vitamin D deficiency and, 163
  vitamin D-resistant rickets and, 342
Osteomyelitis, 179–190
  acute, *180, 184*
  as distinguished from
    endocrine disorder, 179
    malignant disease, 179
    metabolic disorder, 179
    multiple myeloma, 179
    neurofibromatosis, 179
    Paget's disease, 179
  bone patterns and, 279

bone scan of *447–449, 454*
  chronic, *186*
  combined use of gallium and technetium scans and, 445
  computerized axial tomography and, 453
  demineralization in, 181
  destruction caused by, *181*
  direct extension, 179
  disease progression, *184–185*
  early, *183*
  hematogenous, 179
  in osteopetrosis, 383
  increased uptake of radionuclide and, 443, 445
  metaphyseal involvement in, 181
  signs
    bone destruction, *180, 181, 183*
    cloaca, 179, *180*, 182
    involucrum, 179, *180*, 181, 182, *183*
    radiolucency, 179, *180, 181*
    sclerosis, 179
    sequestration, 179, *180*, 182
    subperiosteal calcification, 180, 181
  Staphylococcus aureus in, 179
  syphilitic, 187–188
  technetium bone scan and, 443, 445
Osteonal remodeling, 265
Osteonecrosis, 165–166
  crescent sign in, 166
  in sickle cell anemia, 359
  snow-cap sign in, 166
  zone of, 165
Osteopathia striata, osteopoikilosis and, 381
Osteopathy
  diabetic, 190
  sensory neuropathic, 190
Osteopetrosis, 383, *409–414*
  congenita, 383, *409*
  endosteal osteoclasis deficit and, 383
  extramedullary hematopoiesis and, 383
  osteomyelitis in, 383
  radiologic findings
    bone-within-a-bone appearance, 383, *409, 411*
    Erlenmeyer flask deformity, 383, *409*
  tarda, 383, *410–414*
Osteophyte, 194, 204, *204*
Osteopoikilosis, 381, *393, 397–399*
  bone islands in, 381, *397, 399*
  keloid formation, 381
  mastocytosis and, 381
  osteoblastic metastases and, 381
  osteopathia striata and, 381
  osteosarcoma and, 381
  tuberous sclerosis and, 381
Osteoporosis, 161, *162*, 343–344, *353–356*
  Charcot joint and, 193
  Cushing's disease and, 321, 322, 343
  forms
    disuse, 344, *355*
    senile, 343, *354*
    spotty, 344
    Sudeck's atrophy, 344, *356*
  in hemophilia, 360
  in hyperparathyroidism, 324
  in hyperthyroidism, 322
  in multiple myeloma, 416
  in peripheral neuropathy, 192
  in Reiter's syndrome, 216

in tuberculous osteomyelitis, 189
  leukemia and, 343
  local, 161
  muscular dystrophy and, 343
  osteogenesis imperfecta and, 343, *353*
  paraarticular, 219
  pathologic fracture and, 344
  radiologic findings, 344
  rheumatoid arthritis and, 343
  subchondral zone, 193
Osteoporosis circumscripta, Paget's disease and, 379
Osteosarcoma, 278–279, 282, 285, *287–289*
  osteoid formation and, 279
  osteopoikilosis and, 381
Osteosclerosis
  associated conditions, 343t
  in diabetic osteopathy, 190
  in renal osteodystrophy, 343

Pachydermoperiostosis
  clubbing of digits and, 160
  osteolysis and, 160
Pad foot syndrome, in sickle cell anemia, 359
Paget's disease, 284, 379–380, *384–392*
  avulsion-type fractures in, 379
  bone scan of, *392*
  insufficiency fractures and, 265
  osteolysis in, 379
  protrusio acetabuli deformity and, 379
  radiologic findings
    blade of grass sign, 379
    compression fracture, 380
    cottonwool appearance of skull, 379, *384*
    ivory vertebral body, 379, *388*
    osteoporosis circumscripta, 379, *384*
    pseudofracture, 379
  similarity to hyperparathyroidism, 323
  superimposed findings
    bony destruction, 380
    malignant calcification, 380
    soft tissue mass, 380
Parathormone, effects of, 323
Parathyroidism, 284
Pathologic fracture, 271, *271*
  in enchondromatosis, 382
  in fibrous dysplasia, 380
  in metastasis, 415
Pediatric radiology, 77–101
Pellegrini-stieda disease, *158*
Pencil-in-cup deformity
  in atrophic arthropathy, 191
  in peripheral neuropathy, 192
Pencil-in-cup deformity in psoriatic arthritis, 192, 215, *215, 216*
Periosteal calcification, neoplasms and, 280
Periosteal chondroma, 279
Periosteal myositis ossificans, *319*
Periosteal new bone, in hypertrophic pulmonary osteoarthropathy, 417
Periosteal reaction
  amorphous, 159
  benign
    Caffey's syndrome, 160
    Codman's triangle, 160
    hypervitaminosis-A, 160
    pachydermoperiostosis, 160
    pseudoperiostitis, 160–161

Periosteal reaction—*continued*
  pulmonary hypertrophic osteoar-
    thropathy, 159–160
  thyroid acropachy, 160
  eosinophilic granuloma and, 279
  interrupted, 158–159
    Codman's triangle, 280
    lamellated, 279
    onion skin type, 158
    spiculated, 280
    sunburst type, 158, 159
  neoplastic evaluation and, 279
  osteoblastoma and, 279
  osteoid osteoma and, 279
  solid, 158, *159*
    eosinophilic granuloma and, 158
    hypertrophic pulmonary osteoar-
      thropathy and, 158
    osteoid osteoma and, 158
  uninterrupted, 279
Periosteum, 157–161
  cambium layer, 157
  new bone formation, *159*
Periostitis, in rheumatoid arthritis, 215
Peripheral neuropathy
  autosympathectomy and, 191–192
  Charcot foot and, 191
  deformities in
    mortar-in-pestle, 192
    pencil-in-cup, 192
  distinguished from hypertrophic ar-
    thropathy, 192
  joint effusion in, 192
  osteoporosis in, 192
Peritalar dislocation, *242*
Peroneal spasticity, 69
Perthes' disease, similarity to sickle cell
  anemia, 359
Phalanges, 77
Phlebolith, calcified thrombae, 147, *147,
  148*
Physiological anesthesia, after fracture,
  271
Pinhole columnator, in bone scanning,
  442
Plane of support, 57, *59*
Plantar fasciitis, bone scan diagnosis, 452
Plantar spur, in ankylosing spondylitis,
  219
Plantarflexed first ray, 101
Plantarflexed metatarsal, intractable
  plantar keratosis and, 116
Plasmacytoma, of bone in multiple mye-
  loma, 416
Plummer's disease, in hyperthyroidism,
  322
Polydactylism, 125, *126, 127*
Positional deformity, versus structural,
  103–104
Posttraumatic edema (*see* Edema, trau-
  matic)
Potts fracture, 261
Primary bone, reorganization of, 272
Primary cellular callus
  frature repair and, 271–272
  ossification of, 272
Primary fracture healing, 272–273
Progressive systemic sclerosis, as similar
  to atrophic arthropathy, 190
Pronation, 77
  of calcaneus, 39
  of navicular, 38

of talus, 38
  rheumatoid arthritis and, 206
Protrusio actabuli deformity
  in osteomalacia, 342
  in Paget's disease, 379
Proximal articular set angle, *56, 57*
  as structural deformity, 103–104
  deviated joint and, 109
  subluxed joint and, 110
Pseudoarthrosis
  bone scan diagnosis, 451
  non-union of fracture and, 274
Pseudocysts, in osteoarthritis, 223
Pseudogout, calcium pyrophosphate crystals and, 230, *230*
Pseudoperiostitis, 160–161
Pseudosinus tarsi, 58
Pseudofracture, in Paget's disease, 379
Pseudotumors, in hemophilia, 361
Psoriatic arthritis, 214–215, *214–218*
  as similar to atrophic arthropathy, 190
  deformities of
    main-en-lorgnette, 215, *216*
    pencil-in-cup, 192, 215, *215, 216*
  erosion in, 202, *203*, 215
  periostitis in, 215
  resorption of bone in, 204
  sausage-shaped swelling of digits, 214,
    215
  similarity to hyperparathyroidism, 323
  ungual tufts in, 215
Public Health Service, 2
Pulmonary hypertrophic osteoarthropathy, 159–160
  clubbing of toes and, 159, 160
  synovitis and, 159

Rad, defined, 3
Radiation (*see also* X-ray)
  effective shielding of non-essential tis-
    sue, 3
  effects on living tissue, 2–5
  free radicals and, 4
  long-term effects, 4–5
    genetic, 4
    somatic, 4–5
  low-level ionizing, 2
  maximum permissible dose, 11
  non-threshold dose-response relation-
    ship, 3, 4
  realtive cell sensitivity, 3, 3t
  scatter type, 5, 9
Radiation control, laws and, 10–12
  Federal Performance Standards Act, 11
  Federal Register's proposed rules, 11–
    12
  maximum permissible dose, 11
Radiation safety, 2–12
Radiographic contrast, control of
  kilovoltage and, 15
  milleamperage seconds and, 15
Radiolucency
  as sign of osteomyelitis, 179, *180, 181*
  defined, 6
Radionuclide
  decreased uptake of
    aseptic necrosis, 443
    congestive heart failure, 443
    in infarction, 443
  hot spot and, 443
  increased uptake of
    fracture, 443

infarction, 443
  neuropathy, 443
  osteomyelitis, 443
  stroke, 443
  sympathectomy, 443
  passive diffusion and, 443
  photondeficient area, 443
  photopenic area, 443
Radionuclide examination, in Köhler's
  disease, 170
Radionuclide imaging (*see* Bone scan and
  specific type)
Radiopacity, defined, 6
Raynaud's disease, as similar to atrophic
  arthropathy, 190
Reactive edema (*see* Edema, infectious)
Rearfoot, longitudinal axis of, 50, *51*
Rearfoot varus, 58
  compensated, 58, *60*
  pseudosinus tarsi and, 58
  uncompensated, 67, *68, 69*
Rectilinear scanner, minification and,
  442
Rectus forefoot, 55
Reflex neurovascular dystrophy, Sudeck's
  atrophy, 161
Relex sympathetic dystrophy syndrome
  (*see* Sudeck's atrophy)
Reiter's syndrome
  arthritis mutilans in, 216
  bone scan diagnosis, 452
  clinical features
    arthritis, 215
    balanitis circinata, 216
    conjunctivitis, 215
    keratoderma blenorrhagicum, 215
    mucosal ulcerations, 216
    non-specific urethritis, 215
  osteoporosis in, 216
  sacroiliitis in, 216
  similarity to hyperparathyroidism, 323
Relative metatarsal protrusion pattern
  determination of, *112*
  hallux-abducto-valgus deformity and,
    112
Rem, defined, 3
Renal disease, calcification of Baggenstoss
  and Keith and, 145
Renal osteodystrophy, 342–343, *349–352*
  insufficiency fractures and, 265
  osteomalacia in, 342–343
  osteosclerosis in, 343
  radiologic findings
    osteosclerosis, 343
    rugger-jersey spine, 343
    tumoral calcific mass, 343
Renal tubular acidosis, osteomalacia and,
  342
Reparation phase of fracture healing, 271
Reticuloendothelial and hematologic disease, 358–378
Reticulum cell sarcoma, 282–283, *292*
Retrocalcaneal spur, 62
Rheumatoid arthritis, 204–207, *205–213*
  as similar to atrophic arthropathy, 190
  claw toes development in, 206–207,
    208
  deformities of
    boutonniere, 205
    hallux-abducto valgus, 205, 206, *207,
      209*
    swan-neck, 205

disuse atrophy of, 205
early, 204–205, *205*
erosion in, 202, *203*, 205, *212*, *213*
insufficiency fractures and, 265
interstitial polymyositis in, 205
of the forefoot, *211*
osteoporosis and, 343
proliferative synovitis and, 204–205
pronation and, 206
steroid myopathy in, 205
Rickets (*see also* Osteomalacia), 342, *346–348*
in renal osteodystrophy, 342–343
radiologic findings
bowing deformity, 342
greenstick fracture, 342
paintbrush appearance of metaphysis, *346*
Rigid flatfoot
secondary to tarsal coalitions, 93
Roentgen, W. K., 1
Roentgen, defined, 3
Rugger-jersey spine, in renal osteodystrophy, 343, *351–352*

Saber shin, as sign of luetic osteomyelitis, 188
Salter-Harris classifications, *260*
Salter-Harris fracture, *260–261*
Sarcoid arthritis, *439*
Sarcoidosis, 432, *436–440*
acroosteosclerosis and, 432
arthritic involvement, *439*
enchondromatosis and, 432
fibrous dysplasia and, 432
gout and, 432
hypervitaminosis D in, 344
metastatic disease and, 432
of bone, *440*
tomogram, *438*
tuberculous dactylitis and, 432
tuberous sclerosis and, 432
Sacroiliitis, in Reiter's syndrome, 216
Sagittal plane analysis, in first ray deformity, 113
Scatter radiation, 5, 9
Scleroderma, 154, *155*
CRST syndrome and, *155*
resorption of bone in, 204
similarity to hyperparathyroidism, 323
Sclerosis, as sign of osteomyelitis, 179
Screen, x-ray and, 8
Scurvy, 344–345, *357*, *358*
ring epiphyses in, 345, *357*
white line of, 345
zone of provisional calcification, 345, *357*
Secondary fracture healing, 273
Secondary navicular (*see* Os tibiale externum)
Sensory neuropathic osteopathy, 190
Septic arthritis, technetium bone scan and, 443
Sequestrum
as sign of osteomyelitis, 179, *180*, 182
in diabetic osteopathy, 190
technetium bone scan and, 445
Sesamoid position, 102, *105*, 106
Sever's disease, 171, *175*
Shepard's crook deformity, in fibrous dysplasia, 380, *393*
Shin splint, bone scan abnormalities in,

452
Sickle cell anemia, 358–359, *361–366*
radiologic findings
bone infarction, 359
dactylitis, 359
hair-on-end pattern, 358, *361*
hand-foot syndrome, *363*
osteonecrosis, 359
similarity to Perthes' disease, 359
Siderophore, gallium-67 localization and, 445
Sinus tarsi, 57–58, *59*
Ski-jump projection (*see* Harris and Beath projection)
Snow-cap calcification, in multiple hereditary exostoses, *405*
Sodium thiosulphate, x-ray fixer and, 16
Soft tissue
atrophy of, 139, *156*
edema of, 132, *133–135*
emphysema of, 139, *141*
induced X-ray changes in, 132–159
ossification of, 156–157, *157*, *158*
Soft tissue calcification
calcinosis, 147–148, *149–152*
dystrophic, 140–146
metastatic, 152–156
secondary to metastatic calcium deposits, 324
Soft tissue effusion, joint space and, 202
Soft tissue injury, 231–236
anterior talofibular ligament and, 231
arthrography and, 231
calcaneofibular ligaments and, 231
drawer sign x-rays and, 231
inversion sprain of the ankle, 231, *232*, *236*
sprain, 231
strain, 231
stress inversion x-rays and, 231
Soft tissue mass, 132, *136–138*, *316*
cutaneous induration, *138*
ganglion, *136*
in Paget's disease, 380
Somatotropin, in acromegaly, 320
Spastic equinus, 80, *83*
Spiral fracture, 245
Sprain
defined, 231
inversion of the ankle, 231, *232*, 236
Starburst pattern, 280
Static edema (*see* Edema, traumatic)
Steatorrhea, osteomalacia and, 163
Steroid myopathy, in rheumatoid arthritis, 205
Strain
defined, 231
radiologic signs of, 231
Stress dorsiflexion view, 31, *31*, 32
Stress fracture, 264–270, *264–270*
bone scan diagnosis, 452
fatigue, 264
in fibrous dysplasia, 380
insufficiency, 264
osteonal remodeling and, 265
technecium bone scan and, 266
Stress inversion x-rays, 231, *232*
anterior talofibular ligament and, 231
calcaneofibular ligament and, 231
inversion sprain of ankle and, 231, *232*
of ankle, 30, *30*
soft tissue injuries and, 231

Stretch reflex, in gastrocnemius muscle, 80
Stroke, increased uptake of radionuclide and, 443
Structural deformity, versus positional, 103–104
Subchondral cyst, in hemophilia, 360
Subcutaneous calcinosis, 148, *149*
etiology of, 148
venous stasis and, 148, *149*
Subluxation, defined, 236
Subluxed joint, 40
defined, 108
increased proximal articular set angle, *110*
Subperiosteal calcification, as sign of luetic osteomyelitis, 188
as sign of osteomyelitis, 180, 181
Subtalar coalition, *71*, *73*
Subtalar joint, 26
Subungual exostosis, 119, *121*, *122*
Sudeck's atrophy, 344, *356*
as reflex neurovascular dystrophy, 161
juxta-articular demineralization and, 163
Sunburst reaction, 158, 159
Supernumerary bone, 40–45
os intermetatarsium, 45, *45*
os interphalangeum of the hallux, 43, *43*
os peroneum, 43, *43*
os subfibulare, *44*, 45Su
os subtibiale, 44, *44*
os supra naviculare, 40, *42*
os sustentaculi, 45, *45*
os tibiale externum, 40, *41*, 45
os trigonum, 40, *41*
os vesalianum, 44, *44*
Supination, of talus, 38
Surgical amputation, as similar to atrophic arthropathy, 190
Sustentaculum tali, 26, 39
Swan-neck deformity, in rheumatoid arthritis, 205
Swing phase, in normal gait, 80
Sympathectomy, increased uptake of radionuclide and, 443
Synchrondrosis, 93
Syndactylism, *126*, *127*
Syndesmosis, 93
Synostosis, bony, 93
Synovial sarcoma, *294*
Synovitis
bone scan diagnosis, 451, 452
hypertrophic pulmonary osteoarthropathy and, 417
inflammatory, 452
pulmonary hypertrophic osteoarthropathy and, 159
traumatic, 451
Syphilitic osteomyelitis, 187–188
Syphilitic tabes dorsalis, as basis for Charcot joint disease, 191
Systemic lupus erythematosus, 154, *154*, *155*

Talar declination angle, 57, *59*
Talipes, 77–99
calcaneo-abducto-valgus, 80, 84–86
equino-adducto-varus, 78, *78*
achilles tendon and, 79, *79*
talus neck and, 79

tibial tendons and, 79
etiological theories
  abnormal embryotic position, 78
  arrested anomalus embryotic development, 78
Talipes cavus, in atrophic arthropathy, 191
Talo-lesser tarsus angle (see Talonavicular angle)
Talocalcaneal angle, 51, 53
  calcaneovalgus and, 88
  collum tali axis and, 53
  metatarsus adductus and, 78
  neurological cavus and, 82
  vertical talus and, 91
Talocalcaneal coalition, 93–94
  halo sign and, 69
  Harris-Beath axial projections, 95
  types
    synchrondrosis, 93
    syndesmosis, 93
    synostosis, 93
Talocalcaneal notch, 39, 53
Talonavicular angle, 53, 54
Talonavicular beaking, 69
Talonavicular coalition, 96
Talonavicular fusion, 95
Talus, 17, 20, 38, 77
  fracture of, 251
  microtrauma of, 38
  pronation of, 38
  supination of, 38
Tarsal coalition, 69–70, 70–75
  calcaneonavicular, 74
  calcaneonavicular bar and, 70
  computerized axial tomography and, 454
  functional, 70, 71
  functional subtalar, 71
  signs
    peroneal spasticity, 69
    talonavicular beaking, 69
    standard views, 69–70
    talonavicular bar and, 75
Technetium bone scan, 442, 447–452
  concentration at epiphyseal plates and, 445
  dynamic, 443, 444
  in diagnosis of
    benign bone tumors, 445
    cellulitis, 443
    growing bone islands, 443
    hematogenous osteomyelitis, 443
    involucrum, 445
    malignant tumors, 445
    metastatic tumors, 445
    septic arthritis, 443
    sequestrum, 445
  static, 443
  stress fracture diagnosis and, 266
Technetium phosphate, bone scan and, 442
Thalassemia, 359–360, 367–371
  Erlenmeyer flask deformity in, 360
  hair-on-end pattern in, 360, 370
Thalassemia major (see Cooley's anemia)
Thallium, podiatric surgery and, 453

Thyroid acropachy, 322–323, 334
  digital clubbing and, 322
  disseminated periostitis in, 322–323, 334
  hyperthyroid disease and, 160
Tibial sesamoid
  erosion of crista, 107
  fracture of, 244
Toe-off in normal gait, 80
Tomogram
  neoplastic evaluation and, 285
  of metastases, 420
  of sarcoidosis, 438
Tophi, in gouty arthritis, 225, 229
Toxic nodular goiter (see Plummer's disease)
Toygar's triangle, 139, 139, 140
TPX System, 35
Transverse fracture, 243, 245
Transverse plane analysis, 91
  of first ray deformities, 102
Trauma, 231–277
Trench foot, as similar to atrophic arthropathy, 190
Tri-malleolar fracture, 261
Trident hand, in achondroplasia, 381
Tuberculosis dactylitis, 189, 432
Tuberculous osteomyelitis, 189, 189
Tuberous sclerosis
  osteopoikilosis and, 381
  sarcoidosis and, 432
Tumor (See Neoplastic evaluation and specific type)
Tumoral calcinosis, 148, 150

Ultrasonography, 35, 36, 36, 37
Ungual tuft, in psoriatic arthritis, 215
Uremic osteopathy (see Renal osteodystrophy)

Valgus, 77
Valgus deformity, 191
Varicosity, subcutaneous calcinosis and, 148
Varus, 77
Venous stasis, subcutaneous calcinosis and, 148, 149
Vertebra plana deformity, metastasis and, 415
Vertical talus, congenital, 91, 92
  pathological findings, 91
  radiographic findings, 91
Villonodular synovitis, 314
Vitamin C deficiency (see Scurvy)
Vitamin D deficiency, osteomalacia and, 163

Weightbearing lateral projection, 19, 19
  cuboid and, 19
  first and fifth metatarsals and, 19
  medial cuneiform and, 19
  navicular and, 19
Wimberger's sign of scurvy, 345, 357

X-ray (see also Radiation)
  angle and base of gait type, 50
  arithmetic speed and, 14
  average gradient, 14, 15

central ray, 6, 16
collimation of beam, 3, 7, 16–17
contrast and, 14–15
darkroom processing technique, 8
definition and, 15
density and, 15
distortion and, 15
evaluation of soft tissue, 132–159
exposure time and, 8
film
  emulsion layer, 13
  silver halides, 13
film base, 13
film position and, 9, 10
film speed and, 8
filtration of, 7, 15
focal spot and, 17
graininess of, 14
hard, 6
heel effect, 7
intensifying screen and, 8, 13–14
kilovoltage and, 7
lead apron and, 15–16
magnification technique, 32–33, 33
negative potential of, 1
object-film distance and, 9, 9, 17
primary beam, 6
projection and, 16
Rad and, 3
relative noise of, 14
Rem and, 3
resolution and, 14
roentgen and, 3
soft, 6
target-film distance and, 9–10, 10
  kilovoltage, 10
  Milliamperage times Time, 10
view and, 16
X-ray processing
  acid neutralizer and, 16
  developer, 16
  fixer, 16
X-ray projection
  angle and base of gait type, 32
  of ankle
    anterior drawer, 31, 31
    lateral, 28, 28
    lateral oblique, 28, 28, 29
    medial oblique, 28, 29
    mortise, 27, 27
    stress dorsiflexion, 31, 31, 32
    stress inversion, 30, 30
  of foot
    axial calcaneal, 24, 25
    axial sesamoidal, 24, 24, 25
    dorsoplantar, 17, 17, 18
    Harris and Beath, 26, 26
    lateral oblique, 22, 22, 23
    medial oblique, 21, 21, 22
    non-weightbearing medial, 20, 20
    weight-bearing lateral 19, 19
X-ray techniques, 13–37
  Polaroid radiographic system, 34–36
  xeroradiography, 34
Xenon-133, podiatric surgery and, 452–452
Xeroradiography, 34, 285